RHINOPLASTY
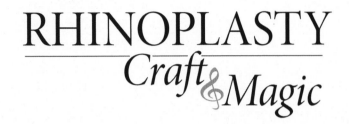
Craft & *Magic*

RHINOPLASTY
Craft & Magic

Mark B. Constantian, MD

Private Practice;
Active Staff, Department of Surgery/Plastic Surgery,
St. Joseph Hospital, Southern New Hampshire Medical Center,
Nashua, New Hampshire

MEDICAL ILLUSTRATOR
Amanda Yarberry Behr, MA, CMI

Quality Medical Publishing, Inc.
St. Louis, Missouri
2009

Printed in Italy

This book presents current scientific information and opinion pertinent to medical professionals. It does not provide advice concerning specific diagnosis and treatment of individual cases and is not intended for use by the layperson. Medical knowledge is constantly changing. As new information becomes available, changes in treatment, procedures, equipment, and the use of drugs become necessary. The editors/authors/ contributors and the publisher have, as far as it is possible, taken care to ensure that the information given in this text is accurate and up to date. However, readers are strongly advised to confirm that the information, especially with regard to drug usage, complies with the latest legislation and standards of practice. The authors and publisher will not be responsible for any errors or liable for actions taken as a result of information or opinions expressed in this book.

The publisher has made every effort to trace the copyright holders for borrowed material. If any have inadvertently been overlooked, we will be pleased to make the necessary arrangements at the first opportunity.

PUBLISHER: Karen Berger
EDITORIAL DIRECTOR: Michelle Berger
ASSISTANT EDITORS: Amy Debrecht, Taira Keele, Olivia Ayes, Becky Sweeney
PROJECT MANAGER: Keith Roberts
MANUSCRIPT EDITOR: Glennon Floyd
VICE PRESIDENT OF PRODUCTION AND MANUFACTURING: Carolyn Reich
PRODUCTION: Elaine Kitsis, Susan Trail, Sandy Hanley, Ngoc-Thuy Khuu
DESIGN AND ILLUSTRATION: Amanda Yarberry Behr
DIRECTOR OF GRAPHICS: Brett Stone

Quality Medical Publishing, Inc.
2248 Welsch Industrial Court
St. Louis, Missouri 63146
Telephone: 1-314-878-7808
Website: *http://www.qmp.com*

LIBRARY OF CONGRESS CATALOGING-IN-PUBLICATION DATA

Constantian, Mark B.
    Rhinoplasty : craft and magic / by Mark B. Constantian.
        p. ; cm.
    Includes bibliographical references and index.
    ISBN 978-1-57626-247-4 (hardcover)
    1. Rhinoplasty. I. Title.
    [DNLM: 1. Rhinoplasty--methods. 2. Nose--anatomy & histology. 3.
Postoperative Complications. WV 312 C758r 2009]
    RD119.5.N67C66 2009
    617.5'230592--dc22

                                        2009007093

QM/LG/LG
5 4 3 2 1

For my wife Charlotte

❧

And now I know a wish

comes true

…Because of you

FOREWORD

Thirty years ago Mark Constantian, a young plastic surgeon fresh out of residency, asked if he could come from the East coast to visit and watch me operate. Because there was interest in my unorthodox approach to rhinoplasty and I was eager to spread the word, I arranged a date for his visit. For most of my years in practice, my operating room was open to observers, but even though I had many who came to watch, very few followed up. Mark Constantian was an exception. I was unprepared for the intensity of his interest in rhinoplasty and his insatiable desire for detail. We invested numerous hours discussing cases that I had operated on and reviewing a growing file of photographs of patients who were scheduled for surgery. Those visits became an annual event that lasted until I retired in 2004. Since then the yearly visits and animated discussions have continued, but now they involve his cases.

Why another book on rhinoplasty? Because this particular book is the product of countless hours of thought, discussion, and analysis candidly presented by its author. It has distilled the most common pitfalls in diagnosis with a wealth of surgical material underscoring each anatomic variant or combination of variants. The young practitioner will benefit from the practical considerations laid out in detail— essentials such as how to approach the initial consultation or the value of dictating a preoperative plan with expected results and limitations. The more sophisticated surgeon will likely recognize that special problem patient he or she is about to operate on in one of the hundreds of cases that are detailed in these pages.

The most important prerequisite for producing meaningful new ideas is an obsessive passion for the subject—Mark Constantian certainly has that for rhinoplasty. But he has brought more to the table than just passion. In his early training, Mark was exposed to research and quantitative analysis. He has used that background to quantify his new ideas, providing a scientific basis for the conclusions drawn. There is valuable information on every page, but as a member of the emeritus group of surgeons who has devoted most of a professional life to delving into the many mysteries of this surgery, I was especially impressed by one chapter that should be mandatory reading for anyone performing nasal surgery—that is Chapter Four: "The Anatomy of Function and How Rhinoplasty Affects the Airway." This chapter is scholarly, factual, and extremely important. It is in sharp contrast to the thinking that prevailed 30 years ago, when most plastic surgeons avoided looking inside the nose, preferring to refer internal nasal airway problems to ENT colleagues, most of whom did not have the wealth of information that has been presented in this outstanding chapter.

This book is a gift to the profession by Dr. Constantian, beautifully presented and framed in the familiar excellence of QMP and its founder, Karen Berger. Every teacher, if fortunate, can, in retirement, relish the contributions made by a former student. I must say, I am justly proud of Mark Constantian for this superb addition to our understanding of the art and science of nasal surgery.

Jack H. Sheen

FOREWORD

Dr. Mark Constantian is not just my colleague, but a close friend, as is his wife, Charlotte, his partner in work and in life. These two volumes are a labor of love and, if not a love of labor, at least a tolerance for expending prodigious effort to complete a task. Ralph Waldo Emerson was correct when he stated that "Nothing great was ever achieved without enthusiasm." And there is no shortage of enthusiasm in these pages. Books of this size by a single person are increasingly rare in these times, and it is a refreshing departure from the usual multiauthor tomes.

In his debut discourse when inducted to the French Academy in 1753, the naturalist George Buffon stated, "The style is the man himself." So too with this book. Dr. Constantian is meticulously devoted to detail in everything he does, even when he accompanies himself on his guitar and when he records his playing with background band accompaniment. Who would not want their surgeon to be a perfectionist?

Dr. Constantian's professional life is proof that one need not be in a large metropolis to attract patients. Nashua, New Hampshire, where Dr. Constantian lives and works, has a population of about 90,000. I have been glad throughout the years to be able to refer some of my dissatisfied patients to Dr. Constantian, Nashua being about an hour's drive from Boston. On more than one occasion I have sent to him a new patient with a difficult nasal problem. In every instance, Dr. Constantian's rapport with the patient was excellent. He has often used the occasion of an unhappy patient to bridge the gap between us, even trying to lessen the patient's financial burden.

Dr. Constantian is more than a talented rhinoplastic surgeon; he is more than a student of rhinoplasty; he is a scholar of the various problems associated with nasal surgery. One will find in these pages honest appraisals of complications, some of them his own. Fortunately for the reader, he is an excellent teacher, more than willing to share his experience, the bad and the good, with anyone who is willing to study, not just read, this chef d'oeuvre. Throughout each chapter one feels the author's presence and benefits from his step-by-step pedagogy. He not only shows his techniques but discusses his reasons for choosing them. The reader soon becomes a participant.

Plastic surgery's ancient traces centered on the nose and its reconstruction. Through the centuries, the objective has always been a nose of normal appearance. In the latter part of the nineteenth century and the beginning of the twentieth, because of pioneers such as Roe and Joseph, improving the appearance of the nose became a desideratum.

Not all patients are happy after rhinoplasty. Dr. Constantian shares his views on how he deals with this unpleasantness for both patient and surgeon. His admonitions about patient selection should be heeded. He discusses patients to avoid, such as those with body dysmorphic disorder and others whose expectations are unrealistic.

He does not, however, mention surgeons to avoid, so let me tackle that question here. Briefly: The surgeon who does only an occasional rhinoplasty and the prospective patient should avoid each other. Does this mean that only experts such as Jack Sheen or Mark Constantian should undertake a rhinoplasty? No, but we must remember that every surgeon undertaking a procedure should be competent. The old saying "As plain as the nose on your face" should remind us that the result after rhinoplasty is visible to everyone. In this sense rhinoplasty is an unforgiving procedure.

For most of us, rhinoplasty was a mysterious procedure during our residencies. In my days of training (1961-1963) I never saw an open rhinoplasty. I had trouble visualizing what my mentor was doing in the nose with his chisel, rasp, and hammer. I could see the submucous resection, but that was about all. Today the average trainee probably understands less about and feels less competent performing rhinoplasty than any other cosmetic procedure.

Dr. Constantian and (the appropriately named) Quality Medical Publishing, in these beautifully presented and lavishly illustrated two volumes, have succeeded marvelously in providing a guide to improve the skills of anyone performing rhinoplasty—to the ultimate benefit of the patients to whose well-being every physician must be dedicated. Finally in this book we have a new tool—in addition to the historical methods of taking courses, watching videos, performing operations on cadavers, and visiting more experienced rhinoplastic surgeons to watch them work—that allows new rhinoplasty surgeons to become competent.

I feel I should point out that there is no "real" magic in rhinoplasty. As Dr. Constantian mentions in his preface, *magic* does not mean pulling a rabbit from a nostril. Instead, he calls our attention to how a properly executed anatomic change produces a balanced nose that may look smaller even when it has been augmented. He makes a point with which most rhinoplasty surgeons would agree: "Good rhinoplasty is also brain surgery, and can rehabilitate damaged self-confidence."

Blaise Pascal, the seventeenth century French mathematician and philosopher, speculated, "Cleopatra's nose, had it been shorter, the whole face of the world would have been changed." If Dr. Constantian had been living then and Cleopatra had had the good sense to have sought his services, there would have been no romance with Julius Caesar and no enervating war with Ptolemy. That *would* have been magic. But it is not too late. After having read this classic (and it is a classic) I wrote to the secretary-general of the United Nations to suggest thinking of rhinoplasty as a resource to prevent or end wars. Magic for peace—what better goal! In this regard we await with high expectations Dr. Constantian's next book.

Robert M. Goldwyn

PREFACE

I do not know what I may appear to the world;
but to myself I seem to have been
only like a boy playing on the seashore,
and diverting myself in now and then
finding a smoother pebble or a prettier shell than ordinary,
whilst the great ocean of truth lay all undiscovered before me.

SIR ISAAC NEWTON
Brewster's Memoirs of Newton

Why do so many smart surgeons struggle with rhinoplasty or stop performing it altogether? Is it the limited access? Is it the technical skill required, the complex anatomy, the narrow margin of error, or the lack of binocular vision? Or is it simply that the nose is an idiosyncratic little body part that will not follow the laws that Nature has established for every other type of surgery?

It was not always this way. During my plastic surgery residency in the mid 1970s, rhinoplasty was a simple operation. There were very few rules. Every preoperative nose was too big, and so the solution was always reduction. We were taught to recognize thick-skinned patients and not operate on them. If the airway was obstructed, we would remove part of the septum and reduce the turbinates. Patients who had imperfect outcomes were rejected for further surgery, because nothing could be done to help them. They had been poor rhinoplasty candidates.

Therefore many surgeons agreed with McDowell, writing in 1978:

> During the last 15 years, evidence has been increasing that the "pay dirt" lode in the great mine of rhinoplastic information is nearly exhausted. The nose is a small organ with a rather simple anatomical structure; in two-thirds of the century, the fine investigative surgeons at work seem to have exhausted most of the possibilities for desirable structural changes in this small and simple organ. The situation is not unlike that which has existed for 50 years with regard to operations for indirect inguinal hernia.

That very same year, the first edition of Dr. Sheen's *Aesthetic Rhinoplasty* was published. I met Dr. Sheen in July 1978, just after finishing my residency, and read a typescript of his book, then at the printer. I was captivated. The logic and order of the surgical steps made more sense than anything I had read on the subject, and I saw how his principles of support and structure applied not only to the unoperated nose, but could also be used to rehabilitate secondary and tertiary patients, whose deformities had been considered inoperable until then.

But Dr. Sheen's words were only part of the spark that ignited my interest in rhinoplasty: he performed magic in the operating room. Dr. Sheen was a rapid, efficient, technically gifted surgeon; but it was his clarity of goals, energy, and excitement—and even more than that, his *wonderment*—that made his surgery so remarkable and such a catalyst for my own work. Dr. Sheen's contributions to rhinoplasty expanded over the next 30 years. His techniques and innovative, often iconoclastic, observations became the modern framework within which we all discuss rhinoplasty: recognition of middle vault collapse, the inverted-V deformity, the patient's aesthetic, the importance of the "ethnic" nose, and the unbalanced top-heavy or bottom-heavy nose (disproportion); and his concepts of less resection—not more—for thicker-skinned patients, omitting osteotomy and the low-to-high osteotomy, the airway ramifications of the narrow nose, inadequate tip projection, camouflage for asymmetry, the two-surface concept for alar wedge resection, and the use of the alar lobule as a composite graft.

And these are the big contributions: dorsal and tip augmentation to treat supratip deformity; identification of the middle crus, the low radix, short nasal bones, and alar cartilage malposition; the techniques of spreader grafts, the shield tip graft, and crushed cartilage grafts; the use of the ear as a cartilage and composite graft donor site; and many new concepts for using rib grafts. His observations became our new paradigm, and his terminology became our rhinoplasty lexicon.

Armed with this new information, I entered practice in New Hampshire, eager to apply what I had learned and create astonishing rhinoplasty results—I fell flat on my face. Nothing I saw or did resembled the diagrams in my atlases or the magic that I had seen in Dr. Sheen's operating room. Nothing behaved the way it should.

When I reduced the dorsum, why did the middle third look narrower, and why did the nose shorten? Why had the columella become lower, the alar rims more arched, and the nasal base larger and blunter? I had not touched them. Why was rhinoplasty so different from all the other operations I had learned? This was not magic—it was black magic.

I determined to understand what was going on. I didn't believe in idiosyncrasy; I believed in biological laws—but I had to decipher what they were. I tried to relate the postoperative changes to what I had done and to the preoperative deformity. When there were outcome differences between apparently similar noses, there had to be a reason. And most important, what was the relationship between nasal appearance at the end of the operation and its appearance a year later? It made no sense to discuss aesthetic goals with my patients if I had no idea how to achieve them. How could the surgeon learn to control the postoperative result? I resolved to break The Rhinoplasty Code.

This book is a product of my 30-year adventure into nasal phenomenology, function, and technique. It summarizes what I know today. Because Dr. Sheen's texts have become such standard reference works, the reader familiar with them will recognize comforting similarities. My Patient Studies have used Dr. Sheen's format, describing the deformity and patient goals, the surgical plan, and the postoperative analysis. I have included many hundreds of intraoperative photographs that demonstrate those intraoperative changes that are important for the reader to learn and that show the grafts used in each patient. And I have included many examples of sequential postoperative changes so that the reader may observe how each type of nasal shape and intervention matures as time passes.

But there is much here that I hope the reader will find new and educational, and that will help direct treatment. Part I describes not only *static* anatomy but *dynamic* nasal anatomy—how things move during surgery and afterward—a phenomenon almost unique to rhinoplasty and one reason that it is so difficult to learn. Chapter 3 explains why rhinoplasty is a right-brain operation that trades heavily in balance and proportion, and shows the reader how to access right-brain function on command. Chapter 4 summarizes the results of 17 years of airway research and relates physiology to surgical practice so that surgeons can reliably ensure that each of their patients breathes better postoperatively. Chapter 5 analyzes the four critical anatomic variants that most often make the difference between successful and unsuccessful results.

Part II explores rhinoplasty as an operation: why rhinoplasty is difficult, rhinoplasty planning in the abstract, and applied concepts and aesthetics. It concludes with a widely applicable method for creating an operative plan.

Part III covers basic concepts and techniques in the primary surgery. I explain how a surgeon can teach himself or herself rhinoplasty in the same way that I did. In the operating room, I demonstrate the interactive nature of rhinoplasty step by step, so that the reader can learn to interpret intraoperative signals and artifacts as they occur, understand them, and react to them. Part III also details graft harvesting and technique for each graft used in primary rhinoplasty. Following this is a chapter that discusses the typical postoperative course and a chapter devoted to postoperative problems, including my own complications.

Rhinoplasty deformities may seem limitless, but they are not. By and large, they form patterns. Likewise, their surgical solutions form patterns. Part IV introduces an icon system that reduces the operative plan for each case to a schematic, located at the top corner of every page on which the case is described. Soon the reader will be able to link the schematics, relate the icons to the solutions and to the deformities that they correct, and therefore begin to see these deformities as recognizable groups with associated characteristics. This recognition is the beginning of familiarity with The Code. Part IV also contains analyses of the treatments of the common and less common primary rhinoplasty shapes.

Part V discusses secondary rhinoplasty—its unique techniques and donor sites—and treatment of regional or generalized deformities.

Not all unfavorable rhinoplasty results are technical. Perhaps even more unfortunate than unfavorable results are surgical successes in unhappy patients. These difficulties occur along a spectrum, and their pathophysiology is complex—related, I believe, to both the patient's self-esteem and prior interpersonal relationships. Part V therefore concludes with a discussion of body dysmorphic disorder and lessons that I have learned from my own unhappy patients.

As these volumes grew, so did the need for a certain amount of purposeful repetition. Though one clinical example might have sufficed in a few instances, I have tried to show several so that the interested surgeon might be able to match an upcoming case to elements of the clinical examples, and thus be more rapidly guided toward a successful solution. In doing so, I have tried to show ranges of outcomes; and where there were postoperative problems, I point them out. Showing only perfect results would not be teaching, but marketing, and that is not the purpose of this book.

There is still a void in rhinoplasty learning; therefore there must be a void in rhinoplasty teaching. Some rhinoplasty techniques have become devilishly complex and abstruse. I have deliberately tried to do the opposite in my own work and in my teaching. The reader may therefore wonder why there aren't many more technical variations. But rhinoplasty is not difficult because too few techniques have been described, but rather because many surgeons do not yet fully understand its right-brain nature, how to make a diagnosis that directs treatment, the importance of controlling skin sleeve movement, and that no rhinoplasty is a success unless it ensures an optimal airway. Nature's laws are consistent, regardless of the surgical approach. Thus the principles in this book apply whether the surgeon uses grafts or sutures, columellar or mucosal incisions. There is perhaps no other operation that so completely integrates balance and harmony with the surgeon's technical skill and spatial intelligence, and so thoroughly tests the surgeon's ability to uncover and produce the patient's aesthetic goals.

That is the *craft* of rhinoplasty. But there is also the *magic:* balanced noses look smaller than unbalanced noses, even when they have been augmented. Dorsal and tip grafts correct supratip deformity without skeletal reduction. Raising the dorsum decreases apparent nasal base size. There are many other apparently paradoxical effects unique to rhinoplasty.

Good rhinoplasty is also brain surgery. It can rehabilitate damaged self-confidence in ways that are best measured by changes in the patients' eyes. That is perhaps the greatest magic of all.

Most rhinoplasty surgeons have been confounded by the operation at one time or another. Even Dr. John Roe, to whom we are indebted for much of what we do in rhinoplasty today (including the endonasal approach) noted, after performing only four rhinoplasties:

> There is no class of operations that demands in every case a more careful preliminary study of all the conditions presented—not only in respect to the abnormal state of the tissues to be operated on, but also in respect to the possibility of obtaining the desired surgical result—than the operations required for the correction of nasal deformities.

It is to the surgeons who may benefit from a better understanding of the operation, and to all of our patients, that I offer the text that follows.

Tap into the magic.

Mark B. Constantian

BIBLIOGRAPHY

McDowell F. History of rhinoplasty. Aesth Plast Surg 1:321-348, 1978.
Newton I. Quoted in Sagan C. Cosmos. New York: Random House, 1980, p 71.
Roe JO. The deformity termed "pug nose" and its correction by a simple operation. Med Rec 31:621, 1887.

ACKNOWLEDGMENTS

Just like performing surgery, writing a book is a team project. Bigger books, especially those that take decades to come together, need bigger teams. During these years, I have been assisted by many staff in my office and in the hospitals where I perform surgery.

In my office: My operating room scrub and office nurse, Donna Morton, LPN; my patient coordinator and photo manager, Anita Serian; my aesthetician, Jennifer Cross; my typist, Melissa Rascoe; and Julie Murphy and my wife, Charlotte, who retrieved, logged, and scanned more than 5000 patient photographs and proofed and assembled the chapters.

Were I to list all the other contributions that Charlotte has made to *Craft and Magic*, the readers might wonder if I did anything myself except the surgery. She was there from the beginning, in the rhinomanometry, the teaching concept, the organization and planning, the cover design, the end pages, the icons, the textural flow, the revisions, and the morale. Without her, there might have been no book at all.

In the hospitals: Circulating nurses Susan Demers, RN; Carol Lajoie, RN; Patricia Hansen, RN; Kimberly Vissa, RN; and Christine Senel, RN. Scrub nurses Susan Harvey, RN; Patricia Manley, LPN; Catherine Porcello, CST; Dorothy Sowards, RN; and Janet Yorek, RN. Nurse anesthetists Jennifer Gagnon, CRNA; Laura Tashjian, CRNA; and Patricia Pare, CRNA. Intraoperative surgical sequences were patiently photographed by my wife, Charlotte, or by Christine Senel, RN.

At Quality Medical Publishing: Olivia Ayes, assistant editor; Amanda Behr, illustrator; Michelle Berger, DVDs and preproduction coordination; Sandy Hanley, production assistant; Elaine Kitsis and Susan Trail, composition artists; Carolyn Reich, vice president of production; Keith Roberts, project manager; Ngoc-Thuy Khuu, graphics technician; Brett Stone, director of graphics; Becky Sweeney, editing preparation; Suzanne Wakefield, director of editing; and Karen Berger, president of Quality Medical Publishing, who oversaw it all.

And in my life: Those wonderful people who educated me, encouraged me, believed in my work, and provided examples for me to follow: Velda S. Berberian, Mary and Neil Halkyard, Rt. Revs. William H. and C. Gresham Marmion; Eugene H. Courtiss, MD; Robert M. Goldwyn, MD; Courtland L. Harlow, MD; John R. McGill, MD; and Jack H. Sheen, MD, and Anitra Sheen.

To each one I express my deepest appreciation.

CONTENTS

PART III   CONCEPT AND TECHNIQUE IN PRIMARY RHINOPLASTY

14 Problems in the Postoperative Course 751

VOLUME II

PART IV PRIMARY RHINOPLASTY

15 Common Problems in Anatomy and Proportion 827

16 Exceptions to the Usual 951

DVD Contents

VOLUME I

 Primary Rhinoplasty With Lateral Crural Relocation

 Rib Harvesting and Perichondrial/Cartilage Strip

Rib Graft Harvesting, Perichondrial/Cartilage Strip, and Laminate

VOLUME II

 Secondary Rhinoplasty With Composite Grafts and Maxillary Augmentation

 Secondary Rhinoplasty With Ear Cartilage

A Note on Terminology

Because of the shape and location of the nose, traditional terms signifying position may not be intuitively obvious when discussing nasal anatomy. For example, is *superior* at the radix or along the dorsal edge? Is *inferior* along the columella or the nasal floor?

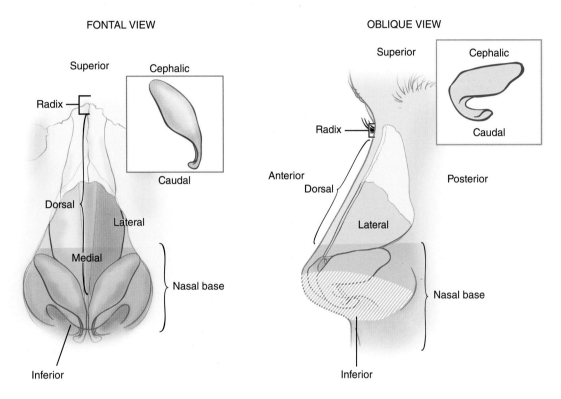

FONTAL VIEW

OBLIQUE VIEW

Therefore to avoid confusion we have adopted the following conventions when referring to various anatomic locations:

Radix/root: The discernible point or origin of the dorsal line

Nasal base: Composed of tip, columella, alar rims, lobules, and the anterior nasal floor

Anterior: Along the dorsal edge, around and including the tip lobule

Posterior: Toward the facial plane externally; toward the perpendicular ethmoidal plate internally

Dorsal: Along the highest point of the nasal bridge

Superior: Toward the nasal radix

Inferior: Underside of tip lobule, columella, alar rims, and lobules

Lateral: Sidewalls from the dorsal edge to the point at which the nose merges with the cheek

Caudal, Cephalic: Locations within a specific structure (for example, caudal septum).

PART IV

Primary Rhinoplasty

Perhaps the sentiments contained in the following pages are not yet sufficiently fashionable to procure them general favor; a long habit of not thinking a thing wrong, gives it a superficial appearance of being right, and raises at first a formidable outcry in defense of custom. But the tumult soon subsides. Time makes more converts than reason.

In the following pages, I offer nothing more than simple facts, plain arguments, and common sense; and have no other preliminaries to settle with the reader, than that he will divest himself of prejudice and pre-possession, and suffer his reason and his feelings to determine for themselves; that he will put on, or rather that he will not put off, the true character of a man, and generously enlarge his views beyond the present day.

THOMAS PAINE
Common Sense

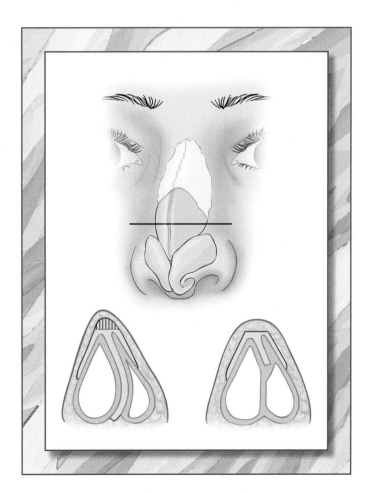

PART IV

Primary Rhinoplasty

CHAPTER 15

Common Problems in Anatomy and Proportion

And teach me how
to name the bigger light,
and how the less,
that burn by day and night.

WILLIAM SHAKESPEARE
The Tempest, Act I, Scene 2

"Of course they answer to their names?"
the Gnat remarked carelessly.
"I never knew them to do it," [said Alice.]
"What's the use of their having names,"
said the Gnat, "if they won't answer to them?"

LEWIS CARROLL
Through the Looking Glass

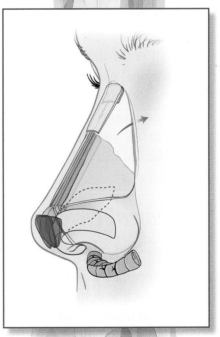

Introducing the Icons

Even though each human being has his or her own wonderful uniqueness, and each nose is in some way different, noses do not come in infinite varieties, which makes it much easier for a surgeon. Are the lateral crura orthotopic or malpositioned? Is the tip adequately or inadequately projecting? Is the dorsum low or high relative to the nasal base? What anatomy indicates preoperative airway obstruction? In different patients, common traits yield a common solution. The deformities can therefore be broadly classified into groups, which means that the reconstructive plans become similar, differing quantitatively but not qualitatively.

In Part IV, therefore, we use a series of icons—one of which is located in the upper right corner of every page on which a case is being discussed. The relevant icon will show, in broad terms, the reconstructive plan for that patient.

I do this for two reasons. First, it is important for a rhinoplasty surgeon to be able to quickly recognize patterns and relationships, decisions that can often be made by inspecting a nose without even touching it. Pattern recognition allows groupings of strategies and ideas, so that a surgeon does not become overwhelmed by apparently limitless combinations and permutations of reduction and augmentation techniques. It is helpful to know where to start for each case, to be able to begin to analyze the deformity within that patient group or pattern and therefore construct a surgical plan quickly and securely.

Second, surgeons may wish to refer to portions of this text to find help for particular cases, and in that regard, the icons become a sort of visual index that should make the search easier.

Dorsal Deformities
THE STANDARD RHINOPLASTY

In naming this section "The Standard Rhinoplasty," I am not being entirely facetious. Although each of these patients had a "bump" and wanted a smaller nose (characteristics that most primary rhinoplasty patients share), each has subsidiary anatomic quirks that must be taken into account. As is often true in rhinoplasty, a deformity may not be as obvious as it seems.

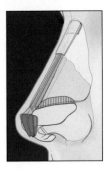

At this point you may wonder whether there is any rhinoplasty that I consider simple and straightforward or instead whether I secretly delight in composing convoluted solutions for even the simplest surgical problems. Why can't a nose job just be a nose job?

I have great sympathy for surgeons who feel that way. Remember, however, that traditional rhinoplasty has its own taxonomy of postoperative problems, from new airway obstructions to supratip deformities, loss of contour, and postoperative results that look pinched, artificial, and "surgical." Each of these unfavorable outcomes can be traced to an inadequate understanding of nasal structure, critical anatomic variants, interdependence of anatomic parts, soft tissue limitations, and how rhinoplasty affects the airway. It is perhaps easier to justify complex solutions when treating significant deformities; but because biologic laws behave predictably once they are understood, the same surgical rules must apply even when the deformities may not be as severe. These cases illustrate that principle.

PATIENT STUDY ONE*

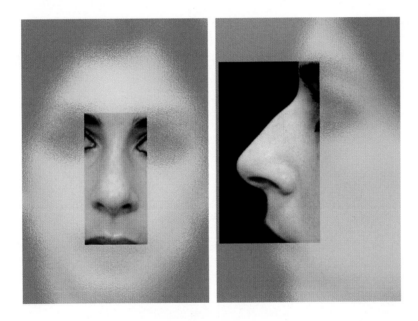

This woman's radix was slightly low, increasing apparent nasal base size; her nasolabial angle was 95 degrees; and her tip was inadequately projecting (note the lobule hanging from the septal angle). Although this tip requires grafts for increased projection, it is important to be conservative so that a larger postoperative nasal base does not exaggerate the preoperative imbalance (that is, the preoperative nose is already bottom heavy). The patient's goal was a straight dorsum without retroussé.

*This patient's intraoperative sequence is detailed in Chapter 11.

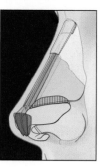

SUMMARY OF THE SURGICAL PLAN

1. Limited skeletonization over the bony and upper cartilaginous vaults
2. Dorsal reduction
3. Transfixing incision with trim of membranous and caudal septa (secondary adjustment after dorsal reduction)
4. Retrograde 2 mm trim of cephalic margins, lateral crura
5. Septoplasty
6. Spreader grafts
7. Thin radix graft
8. Tip grafts, crushed only
9. No osteotomy

Postoperative Analysis

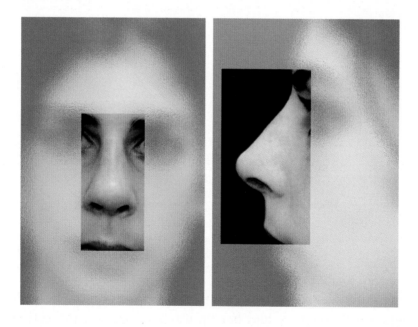

At 7 days, the dorsum is already straight and tip projection is adequate. Note that tip grafts support the tip, producing their effect; the soft tissues do not contract around the tip grafts to reveal them.

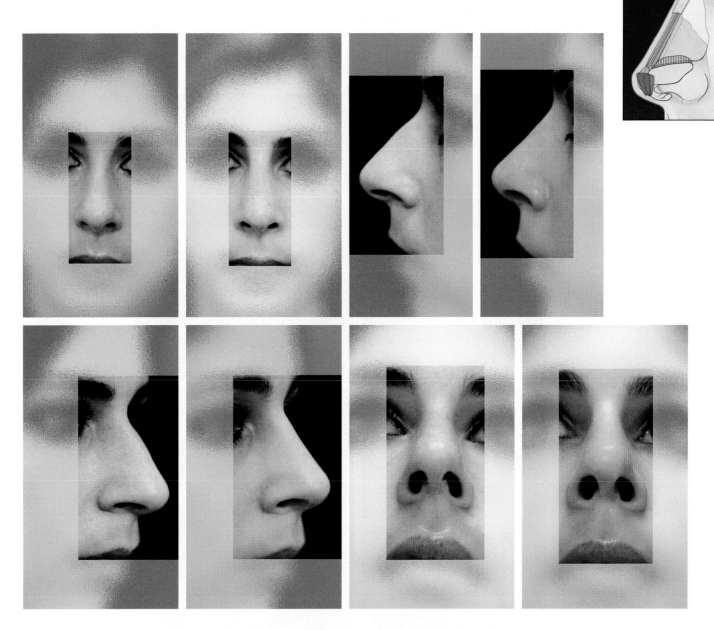

Without osteotomies, the relationship of the bony vault to nasal base width is appropriate, but the excessive middle vault narrowness has been corrected with thin spreader grafts, protecting the airway. On the lateral view, the tip is now adequately projecting and the nose appears less dominant in its lower third than it did preoperatively. The opposite obliques show an improved relationship between the elevated root and the augmented tip; contours are smooth and natural.

Note also that the lateral crura were malpositioned, but were not resected and replaced. The strong cartilages and thin soft tissues combined to threaten postoperative distortion if more complex techniques had been used. The patient did not object to her tip, and therefore its contour was managed by a very conservative resection and by rotating the nasal base slightly, which decreased the deformity visually but minimized the chance of a postoperative irregularity.

PATIENT STUDY TWO

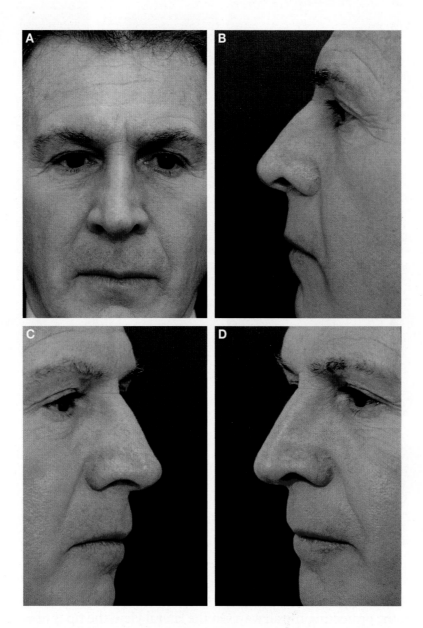

Likewise, this patient's nose has some quirks. Although he had adequate tip projection, airway obstruction was profound (notice the middle vault collapse on the left and the flared nostrils, contracted to support his airway). The alar walls are asymmetrical, the left being concave and the right convex. Tip projection is adequate on the left side *(C)* but inadequate on the right *(D)*, because of a difference in lateral crural rotation.

Notice how much information is available from the surface, without exposing the anatomy during surgery.

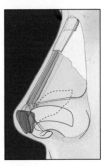

SUMMARY OF THE SURGICAL PLAN

1. Limited skeletonization over the bony and upper cartilaginous vaults

2. Dorsal reduction

3. Transfixing incision with modest trim of the caudal and membranous septum, anterior two thirds only

4. Resection and replacement of concave left lateral crus, inverting the cartilage so that the convexity faces laterally

5. Septoplasty

6. Asymmetrical spreader grafts: right graft thinner and convex to left, left graft thicker

7. Thin radix graft

8. Crushed cartilage tip grafts

9. No osteotomy

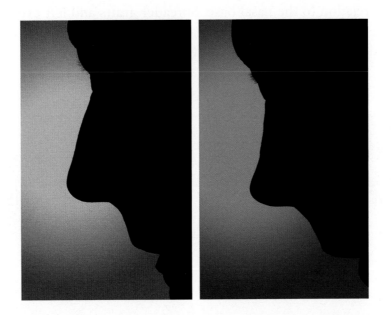

Soft tissue thickness makes significant reduction neither desirable nor possible in this patient. Even a slight dorsal reduction with tip grafts has allowed a dramatic change in the relationship of the dorsum to the nasal base.

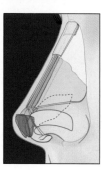

Postoperative Analysis

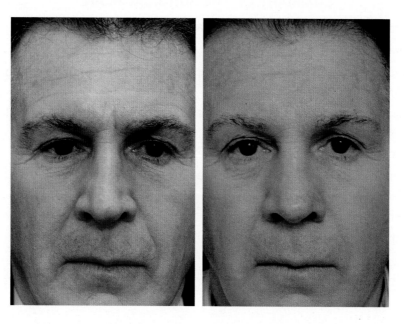

One year postoperatively and without osteotomy, the bony vault remains appropriately wide in relation to the nasal base. Spreader grafts and left external valvular support have improved the airway (note that the patient no longer flares his nostrils); the middle and lower thirds are now symmetrical.

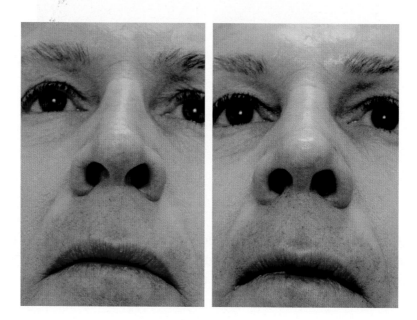

Tip symmetry has improved, the dorsum is now straight, and the tip projects above the supratip. The base remains unscarred, and the columella is narrow.

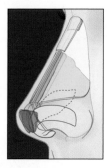

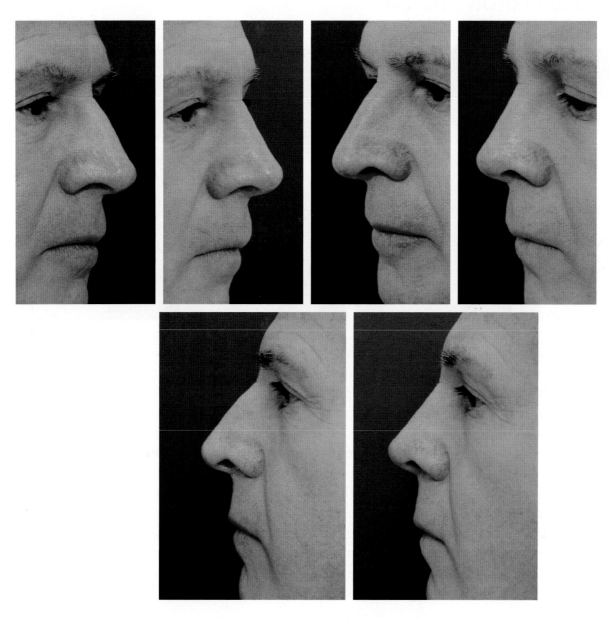

The obliques now match more closely, after left middle vault support and correction of inadequate projection in the right tip. Note also that the left alar wall hollow has disappeared, and retraction in the midpoint of the left rim has improved. The dorsum remains strong and straight, appropriate for an adult male, and without the loss of shape that would have accompanied soft tissue contraction.

LOW RADIX/LOW DORSUM

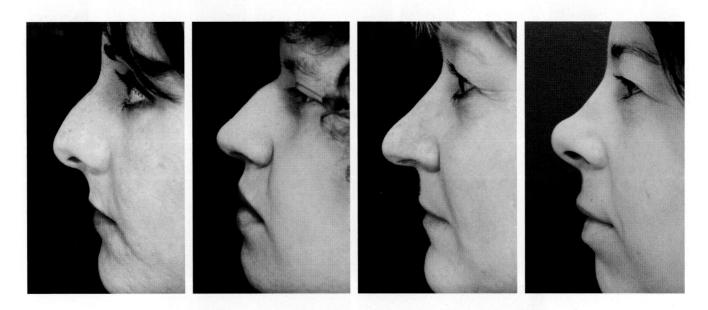

There is a sameness about the low radix/low dorsum variant (one of the four critical anatomic variants [see Chapter 5]), and the first clue is a preoperative imbalance. The base seems too large for the upper nose. Associated with a low radix and low dorsum may be orthotopic lateral crura; malpositioned lateral crura; and inadequate, adequate, or excessive tip projection. Remembering that malposition (or cephalic rotation of the lateral crura) often accompanies external valvular incompetence, and that a low dorsum often accompanies internal valvular incompetence, the surgical plan must therefore include three aesthetic goals:

1. Create adequate tip projection.
2. Improve alar wall contour by repositioning lateral crura, if necessary.
3. Improve nasal balance and proportion in one of two ways:
    a. If the dorsum is convex, reduce the high area and augment the low area.
    b. If the dorsum is straight, elevate the entire bridge to balance the base.

Each alternative minimizes an overall reduction in dorsal height, which would otherwise only exaggerate the preoperative imbalance.

LOW RADIX

PATIENT STUDY ONE

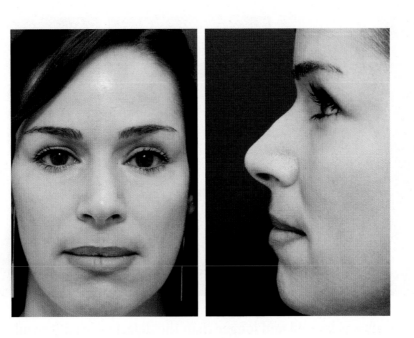

Adequate tip projection accompanied the low radix in this patient. However, the tip was blunt and there was a high septal deviation toward the left. The caudal septum protruded from the left side of the columella.

SUMMARY OF THE SURGICAL PLAN

1. Resect and replace caudal septum as a free graft
2. Limited skeletonization
3. Slight dorsal reduction
4. Septoplasty
5. Spreader grafts
6. Radix graft
7. Crushed cartilage tip grafts
8. No osteotomies
9. No alar wedge resections (preoperative tip lobule is already broad)

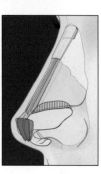

A thicker spreader graft was planned on the right to compensate for the high septal deviation toward the left.

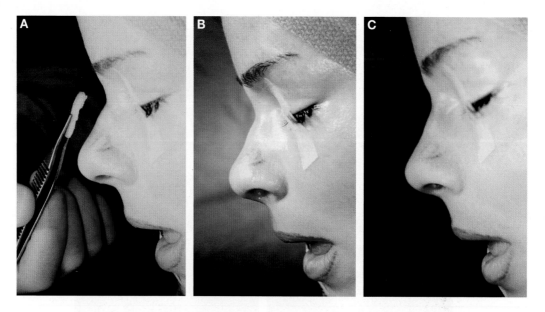

The radix graft was layered and longer than the defect, so that it would produce a smooth line when inserted *(A)*. The diminution in nasal base size after graft placement is immediate (compare *B* and *C*).

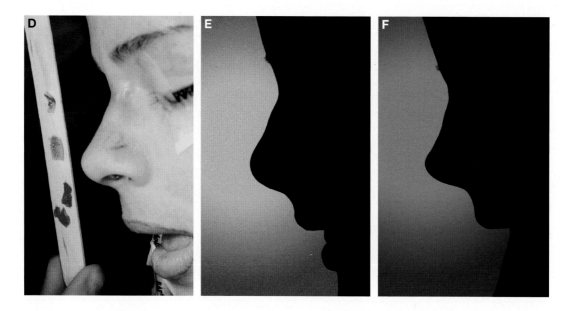

Multiple crushed tip grafts will support and refine the tip with less chance of visibility beneath thin skin *(D)*. Silhouettes dramatize the change in contour and proportion that occurred.

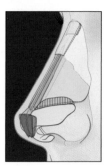

Postoperative Analysis

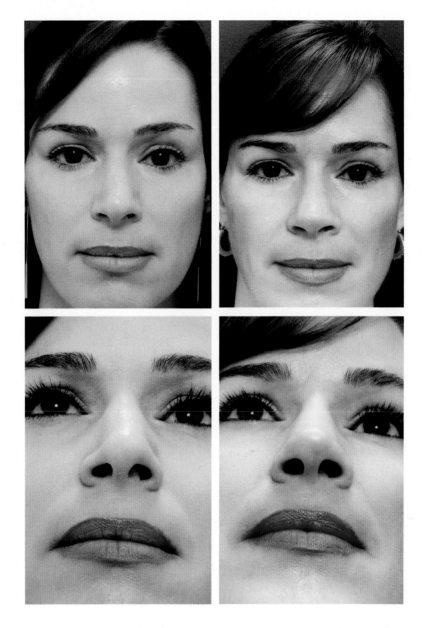

Fifteen months postoperatively, the nose is more symmetrical. From below, the dislocated caudal septum remains corrected. Tip grafts have narrowed the lobule. The base remains wide, but appropriately wide for tip lobular width.

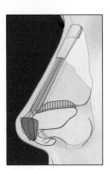

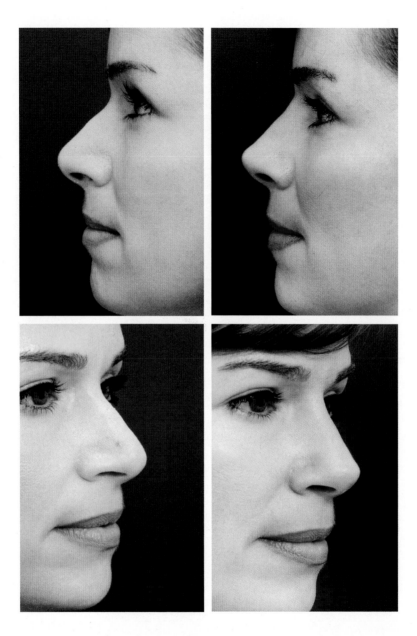

Lateral views show a straight dorsum with improved balance and apparent diminution in nasal base size, despite tip grafting. The oblique view reveals improved tip contour. Notice that increased tip lobular size has produced an apparent decrease in nostril length, even though alar wedge resections were not performed. Geometric mean postoperative airflow increased 2.6 times over preoperative values.

PATIENT STUDY TWO

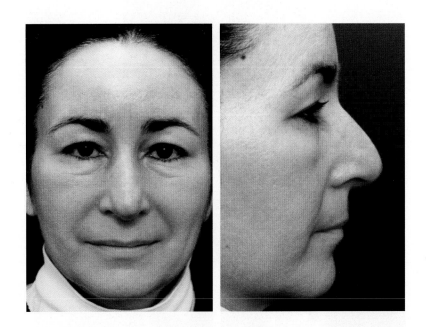

This patient had a deformity similar to that of the previous patient, with three differences: the imbalance is worse (the nasal base is larger), and the lateral crura are cephalically rotated—accompanied by inadequate tip projection, as often happens.

SUMMARY OF THE SURGICAL PLAN

1. Resection and replacement of alar cartilage lateral crura

2. Limited skeletonization

3. Dorsal reduction

4. Transfixing incision, slight shortening of caudal and membranous septa

5. Septoplasty

6. Asymmetrical spreader grafts, thicker on right

7. Radix graft

8. Multiple tip grafts

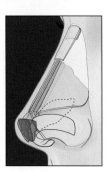

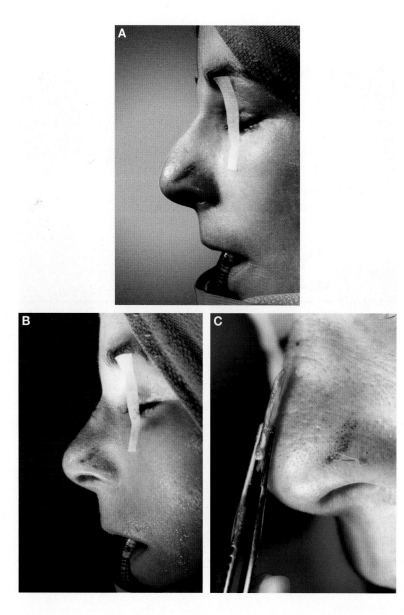

After dorsal reduction and relocation of the lateral crura *(B)*, the dorsum is straighter but the tip is still blunt and inadequately projecting. The dorsal resection is only 2 mm thick, but the span of the entire cartilaginous roof is visible on its undersurface *(C)*.

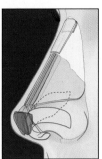

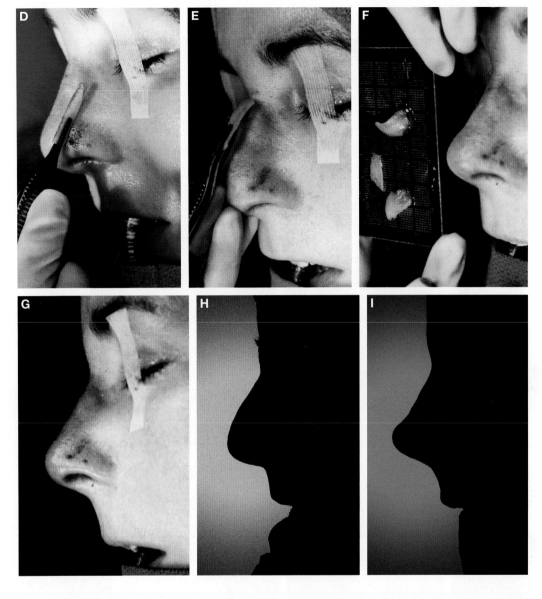

Septoplasty yields adequate material for spreader grafts *(D)*, a thin radix graft *(E)*, and tip grafts (solid and crushed) *(F)*. Notice how the radix graft reduces apparent nasal base size *(G)*. The silhouettes dramatize the changes in nasal balance and dorsum/tip relationships that have occurred.

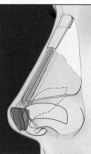

Postoperative Analysis

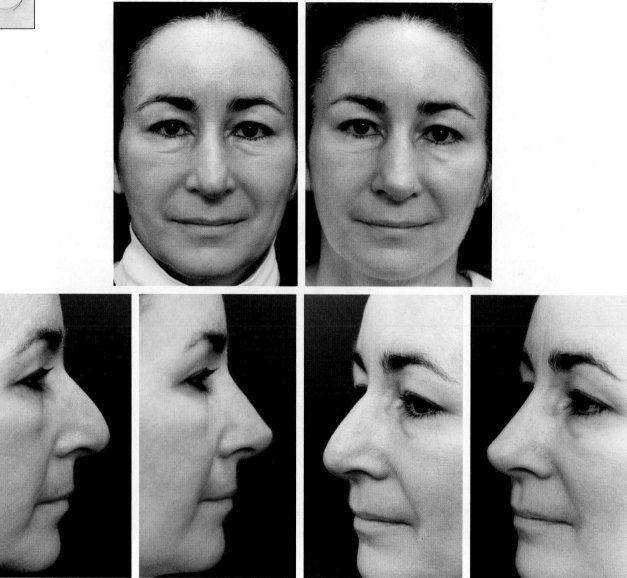

One year after surgery, despite medium-thickness soft tissues, the nose has better balance and more normal surface markings. The sidewalls are smooth and confluent, tip grafts are not visible, and tip anatomy is symmetrical. The positions of the lateral crura have been visibly altered, converting the tip to a more favorable contour. On the oblique and lateral views, the dorsum is straight, the tip is slightly above the dorsal line at the septal angle, and the alar hollows are ablated. Notice also that improved lateral crural support has braced the alar rims, blunting the central notch.

PATIENT STUDIES THREE, FOUR, FIVE, AND SIX

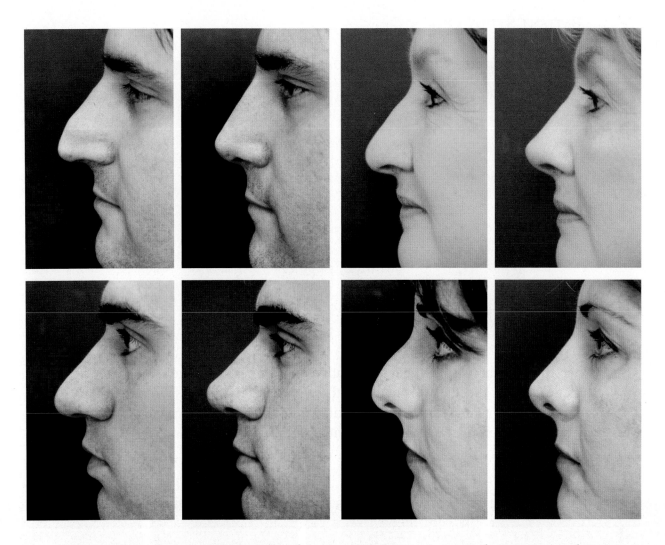

Low radixes occur in 30% to 50% of preoperative noses; its typical pattern must become instantly familiar to a surgeon. In the preoperative views, notice that the combination of low radix and inadequate tip projection act together to increase dorsal height and apparent nasal base size. Postoperatively, note the change in nasal proportion created by leveling the dorsum and raising the radix. The decision to elevate the radix, therefore, affects the amount of dorsal resection required (altering apparent nasal base size), and is particularly helpful for patients with thick skin and those whose noses are bottom heavy.

The traditional strategy of correcting a dorsal hump by removing everything above a line passing from the radix to the tip assumes three things: (1) the radix is optimally positioned; (2) the tip is adequately projecting; and (3) the skin can contract to the desired level dictated by the line. In many patients, at least one of these assumptions is wrong. The patterns, however, are consistent. Many other examples of the low radix follow in subsequent sections—note the similarities to these patients.

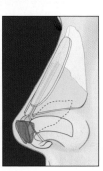

LOW DORSUM

PATIENT STUDY ONE

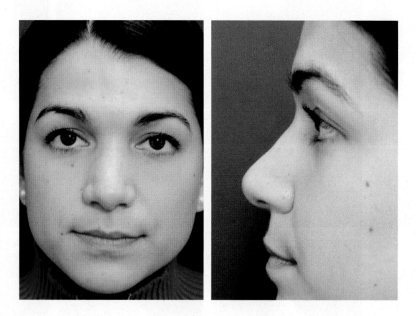

When the dorsum is straight but low relative to nasal base size, the same logic and strategy used for the low radix apply. In these patients, it is always tempting to accept dorsal height and reduce the tip cartilages significantly, so that the soft tissues will contract to produce a smaller base with better shape and balance.

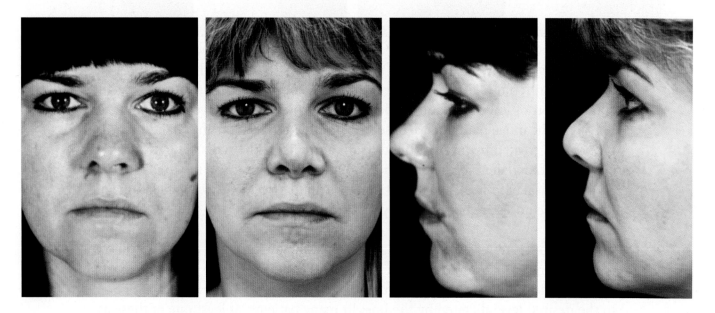

However, this is not what happens. Consider the operative sequence in this patient, whose nasal balance was similar.

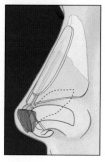

The patient's goal was to reduce the size of her nasal tip, but to not alter anything else. What occurred instead was the consequence of nasal structural interrelationships. (1) The surgeon reduced the width and projection of the tip cartilages. (2) Decreased tip projection produced an apparent dorsal convexity. The surgeon then reduced the dorsum. (3) Deciding that the dorsum had been overresected, the surgeon performed a septoplasty for graft material, reducing the dorsal strut to less than 5 mm, and apparently fracturing the dorsal strut. (4) Losing dorsal support, the surgeon placed a silicone implant. (5) Noticing that the nostrils were now flared (because of a change in dorsal height), the surgeon performed alar wedge resections.

The patient expected a tip reduction. She awoke with a saddle nose corrected by a silicone implant, a new airway obstruction, smaller nostrils, and incipient supratip deformity. Notice the changes that have occurred. On the frontal view, the nose is narrower (from the silicone implant and osteotomies). The upper lip has dropped posteriorly and lengthened. The midface seems to have flattened. On the lateral view, despite a dorsal implant, the dorsum/tip relationships are the reverse of what they were: the tip now hangs from the septal angle and implant, instead of projecting beyond it.

Even without this sequence of unfortunate events, the case illustrates the futility of reducing a large tip sufficiently to match a lower, smaller dorsum. The degree of alar cartilage resection necessary to produce the proper shape often exceeds the ability of the tip lobular tissues to adapt; tip support is lost, and concentric lobular contraction proceeds to supratip deformity.

In our case, the dorsum is even lower relative to nasal base size than it was in this historic parallel. However, patients do not see dorsal imbalance: they see the nasal base deformity and complain that their tips are too large. The surgical strategy is a combination of reshaping the tip and blending the dorsum to it as necessary.

SUMMARY OF THE SURGICAL PLAN

1. Limited skeletonization
2. Dorsal rasping for graft adherence
3. Resection and replacement of alar cartilage lateral crura
4. Septoplasty
5. Two-layer dorsal graft
6. Tip grafts with ethmoid buttress
7. Bilateral osteotomies

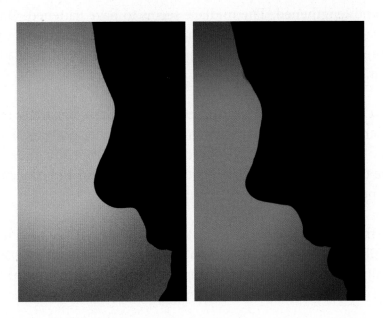

Silhouettes dramatize the resulting changes.

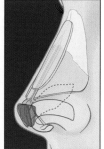

Postoperative Analysis

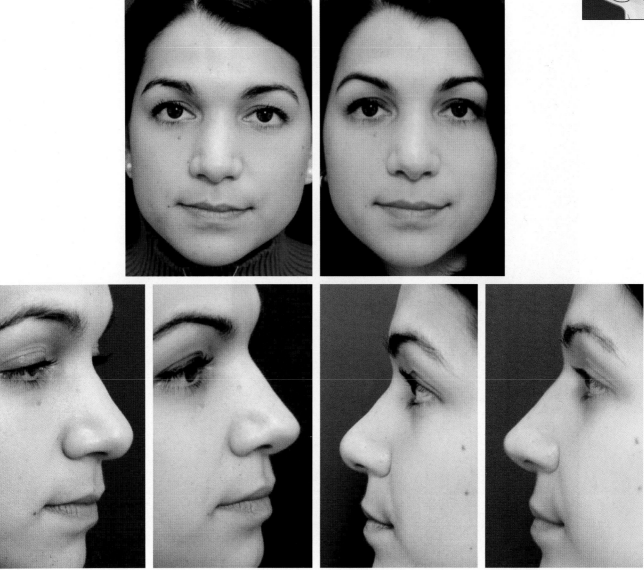

Postoperatively, the dorsum is narrower and longer, the supratip is flat, the tip is better defined, and tip lobular mass has shifted from cephalad to caudad.

A combination of tip reduction and dorsal augmentation has produced upper and lower hemi-noses that now fit, without producing a surgical appearance or loss of definition.

PATIENT STUDIES TWO AND THREE

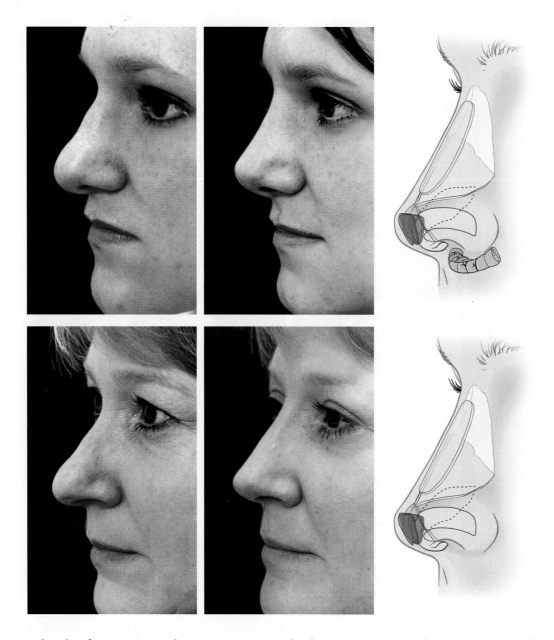

Like the first patient, these two patients had preoperative imbalances; the difference in their treatment is the management of their alar cartilages. In each case, the malpositioned lateral crura were relocated and the tips were grafted. The tips lost the peculiar flatness and apparent downward rotation that is characteristic of inadequate tip projection, and dorsal augmentation decreased the nasofacial angle and therefore diminished apparent nasal base size.

HIGH RADIX

A high radix is the exact inversion of the low radix, and therefore relevant considerations of dorsal and tip relationships also invert:

1. Dorsal reduction improves, rather than worsens, overall nasal balance.
2. Soft tissues at the radix, including the procerus muscle, may blunt or diminish adaption to the underlying skeleton in that area.
3. Particularly in men, the massiveness of the bony vault and overlying soft tissues often limit possible width reduction.

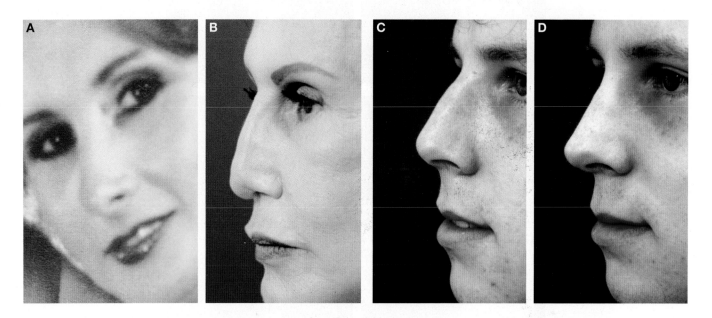

It is important to understand the imbalance. In the first patient (*A* and *B*), notice what happened to the nasal balance of this high-fashion model who followed her photographer's advice to have her "whole nose reduced, just a little." The subsequent cascade of operations, culminating in layered silicone dorsal implants and repeated base reductions, has completely altered her nasofacial angle.

Conversely, in the gentleman (*C* and *D*), reducing the bony and upper cartilaginous vaults combined with tip grafts has done just the opposite, releasing and lengthening the nasal base and increasing the nasofacial angle.

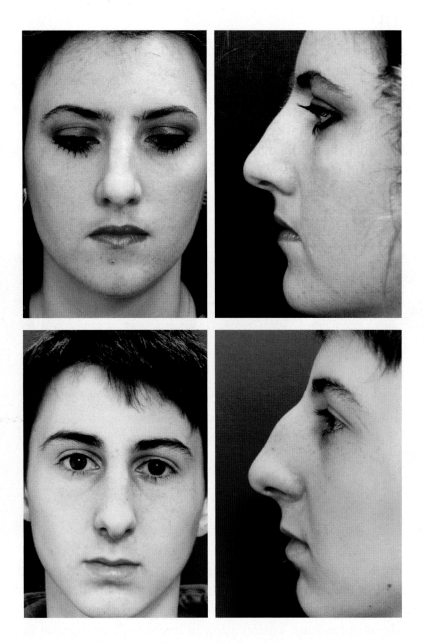

Here is the same preoperative deformity in two other patients. We consider them together.

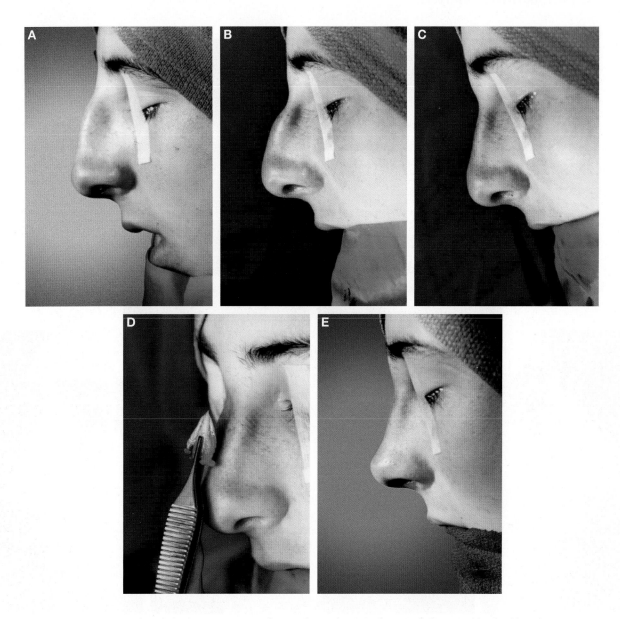

In this operative sequence, notice how the relationships of the nasal profile alter as the bony vault and then the cartilaginous dorsum are reduced (*B* and *C,* respectively). The 3 mm reduction of the cartilaginous vault has clearly opened the roof *(D),* thus requiring spreader grafts to reestablish equilibrium and internal valvular competence. After osteotomies and tip grafts, the amount of projection seems excessive, and the change in the nasofacial angle and dorsum/base prominence is significant *(E).*

Postoperative Analysis

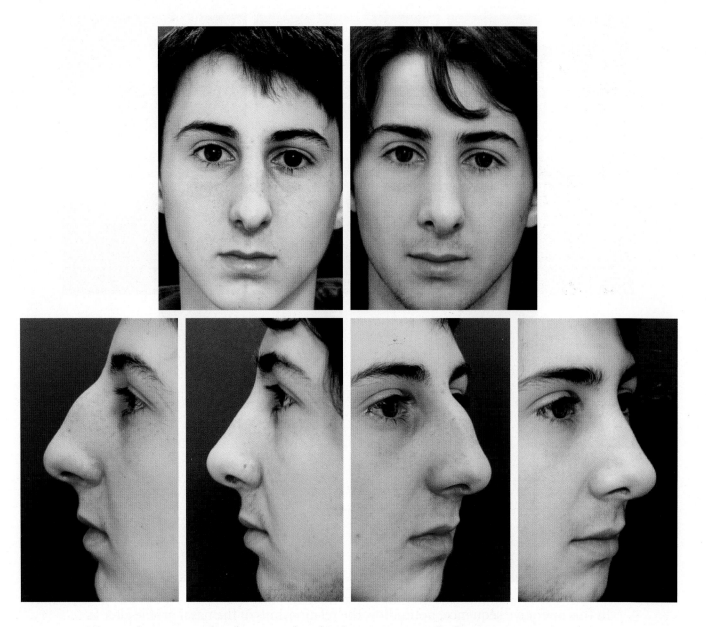

Notice, however, what happened as healing progressed: the apparent overcorrection disappeared. This characteristic postoperative change in such noses can be explained by the volume of skin covering the preoperative high bony arch: even in young patients, and more than 2 years postoperatively, the amount of soft tissue tightening that can occur is finite. Notice also the limited bony vault narrowing, despite a significant dorsal reduction. This is not to say that these noses should be overreduced, but the skeleton must be set to accommodate expected postoperative change. This type of technical fine-tuning is only possible to learn through serial intraoperative and postoperative photography. You will not remember 1 year later exactly how each nose appeared at the conclusion of the procedure.

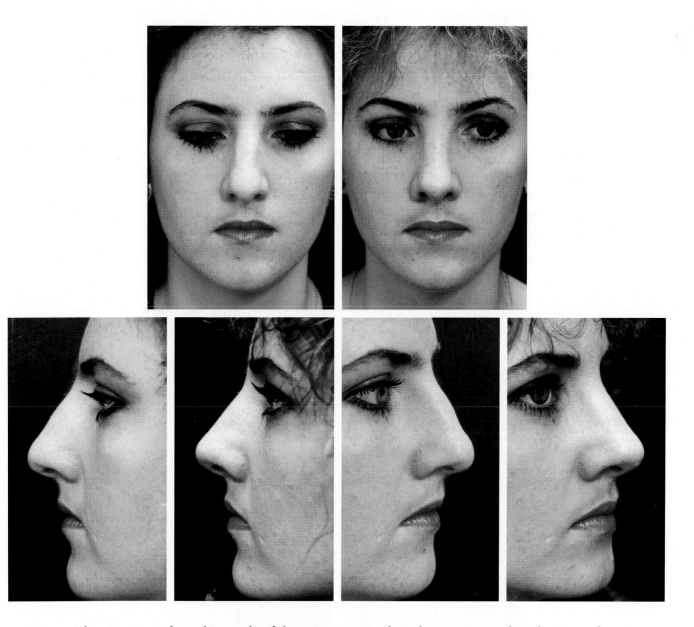

The common thread in each of these patients is dorsal resection with reduction of the radix, spreader grafts to reestablish middle vault continuity and valvular competence (asymmetrically thick, if necessary, to accommodate a high septal deviation), and multiple tip grafts for contour and support. In each patient, the nasofacial angle and the confluence among the upper, middle, and lower nasal vaults has improved. However, notice the limited postoperative narrowing, even late in the postoperative period. Frontal bossing is absent, leaving a relatively flat contour above the radix. Part of the difficulty of achieving a deeper nasofrontal notch is the lack of relief in the caudal frontal bone that might otherwise create more contrast; most patients with high radixes have this frontal bone configuration.

UNDULATING BRIDGE

There are some dorsal contours that cannot seem to make up their minds: some parts are too high, and some are too low. The most common configuration is a low radix, high mid dorsum, and low supratip, usually with adequate tip projection, cephalically rotated lateral crura, and thin skin. This combination makes the deformity tricky, because complex maneuvers on the lateral crura, whose postoperative flaws might be hidden by thicker soft tissues, will be visible under thin cover. Similarly, attempts to fill in the low spots at the radix and supratip, although logical and conceptually simple (and often successful for patients with thick skin), become disturbingly obvious in these configurations. Assuming that a good septal specimen can be obtained, I prefer to reduce the high point and re-create the entire dorsum with a single, straight graft, crushed and contoured to fit the deformity, and to add a second layer beneath its caudal end as needed to level the supratip.

PATIENT STUDY ONE

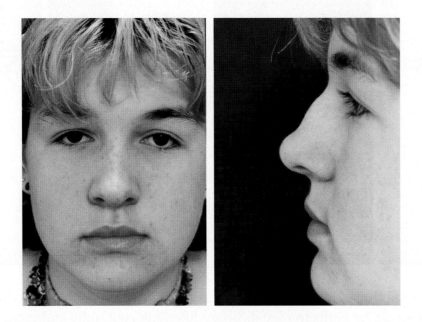

There are many women with this nasal shape who never seek rhinoplasty; the ones who do, therefore, are probably fastidious. The plan should be one that is going to work. Note the narrow middle vault, the site of this patient's airway obstruction. Notice also that her dorsal convexity is high, the supratip depression is deep, and the nasal base is large. Imagine how much larger the base would appear if the dorsal hump were leveled.

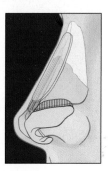

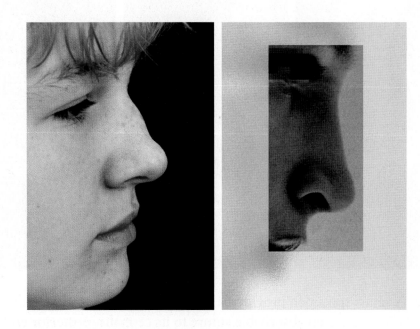

The patient illustrated her postoperative goal using a photograph of this woman, whose nose was shorter with a straighter dorsum, but whose tip and supratip were remarkably similar.

SUMMARY OF THE SURGICAL PLAN

1. Moderate skeletonization over the middle vault, narrow over the bony vault

2. Slight dorsal reduction

3. Retrograde cephalic trim of alar cartilage lateral crura

4. Transfixing incision with a 3 mm trim of the anterior caudal septum and a 2 mm trim from the membranous septum

5. Septoplasty

6. Spreader grafts

7. Layered dorsal grafts

8. No tip grafts

9. No osteotomies

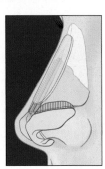

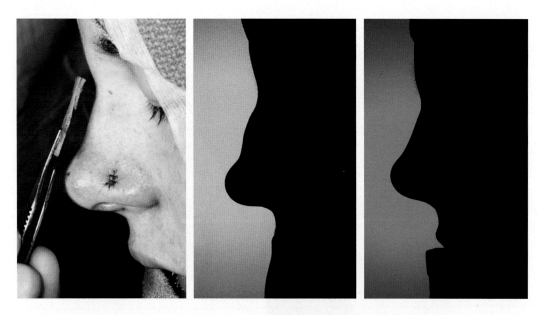

This patient's septal specimen provided a straight dorsal graft, and a second, thinner piece was fixed with an absorbable suture to its cephalic, posterior end. Dorsal reduction and lateral crural modification allowed slight tip rotation, shortening the nose.

Postoperative Analysis

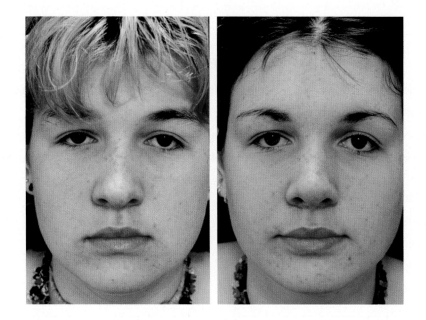

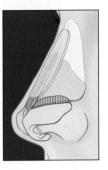

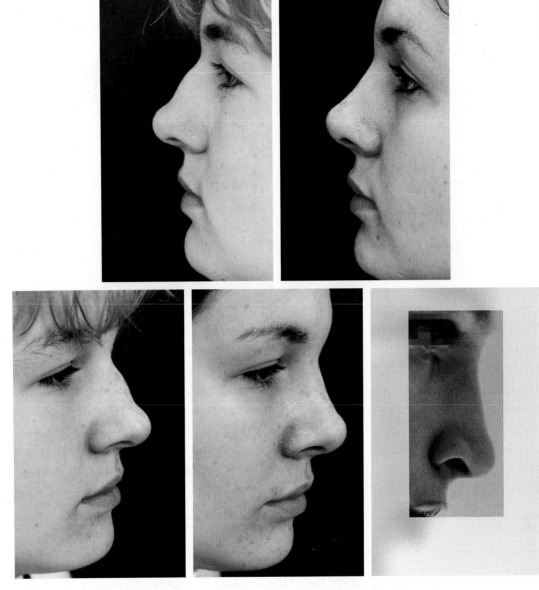

Postoperatively, the middle vault is slightly wider, but tip projection and contour have changed only minimally. The radix is slightly higher, but the dorsum and supratip are level, ending in a slight supratip depression that mimics the patient's preoperative goal. Postoperative airflow increased 1.9 times over preoperative values.

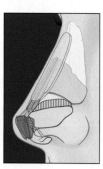

PATIENT STUDY TWO

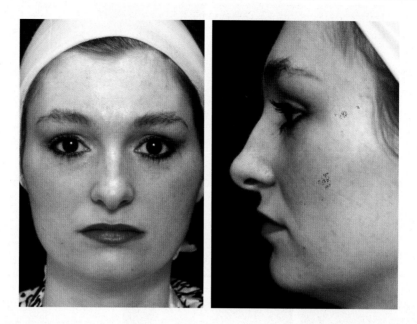

This young woman represents a more extreme variant: her skin is thinner, her alar cartilages are more convex and prominent, her middle vault is tighter, and her nose is longer, but her bridge still undulates. In addition to the dorsal graft needed to smooth bridge contour, the alar cartilages will be treated by a modest trim of the lateral crura and a vertical interruption of the domes, using crushed cartilage to reshape the tip and minimize the visibility of the lateral genua edges. An alternative would be lateral crural resection and replacement or transposition, but that is a riskier strategy when the cartilages are strong and the skin is thin, because postoperative deformation is much more likely.

SUMMARY OF THE SURGICAL PLAN

1. Wide skeletonization of the upper cartilaginous vault, limited over the bony vault
2. Reduction of the bony and cartilaginous dorsum
3. Transfixing incision with 3 mm trim of caudal septum and overlying mucosa
4. Delivery of alar cartilages through infracartilaginous incisions; 2 mm cephalic trim and 3 mm vertical wedge removed at each lateral genu
5. Septoplasty
6. Spreader grafts
7. Dorsal graft
8. Crushed cartilage tip grafts

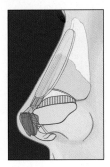

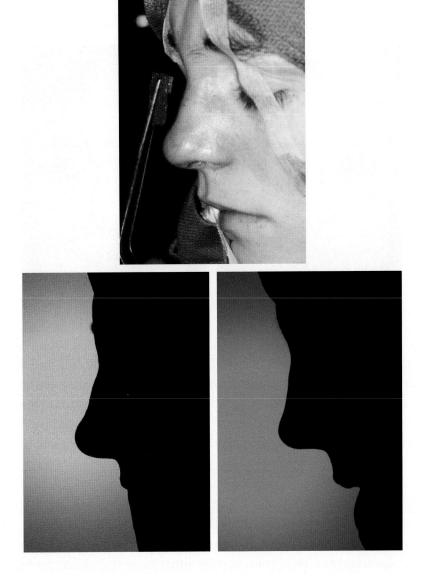

The primary septum yielded sufficient cartilage for a dorsal graft. Reduction of the dorsum, upper lateral cartilages, and caudal septum shorten the nose. It is important to resist the temptation to reduce the alar cartilages excessively, recognizing that soft tissue contraction will increase the effect that the surgeon sees on the table. Because tip grafts, not columellar struts, re-create projection, and because no permanent sutures have been placed, the tip is balanced on the alar cartilage arches.

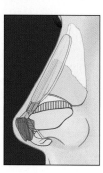

Postoperative Analysis

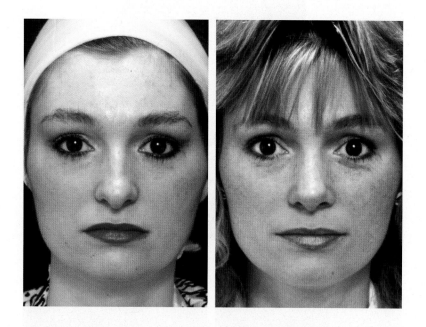

Postoperatively, there is confluence among the upper, middle, and lower nasal thirds after 3½ years. The upper third maintains its preoperative width but seems slightly wider because the dorsum has been reduced, the middle third has been opened by spreader grafts, and the lower third has been narrowed by reduction of the alar cartilage arch. The entire nose is slightly shorter, but the nasal base remains unscarred.

NOTE: Although interrupting the arch narrowed the alar cartilage arch, there is only a modest change in tip lobular width. It is important to remember that tip lobular width is not only cartilage width but also skin width. For the tip to narrow significantly, both cartilage and skin components must have the ability to tighten. Skin contraction is always finite, even when the soft tissue cover is thin.

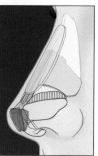

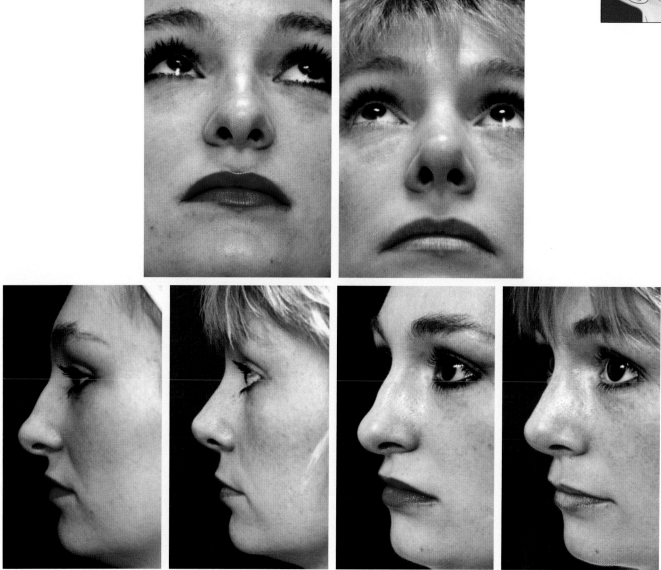

The dorsum is straight, the tip is adequately projecting, and the sidewalls are confluent but supported. The columella remains narrow. Crushed cartilage tip grafts are not visible, even under this patient's thin skin.

STRAIGHT DORSUM

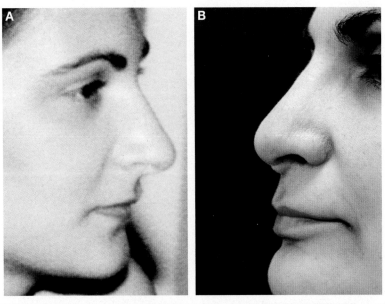

Original preoperative   Preoperative

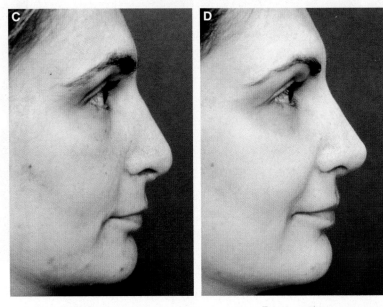

Preoperative   Preoperative

This patient's aquiline, straight dorsum was reduced, and her columella was resected, thickening her delicate skin, and costing contour and function. The smooth preoperative columellar contour was replaced by the knobby discontinuity visible in *B* and *C*.

Maxillary augmentation, nasal shortening, tip and columellar grafts, and revision of the columellar scar provided improvement *(D),* but the beauty of the original contours cannot be restored.

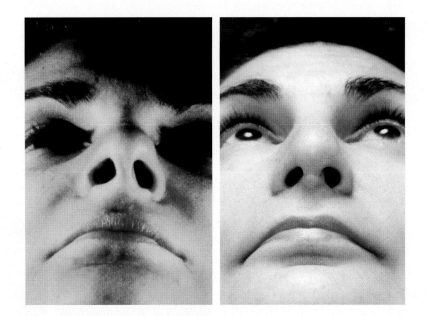

Comparing inferior views before and after columellar resection, the surgical changes are not flattering. *Although carefully performed open rhinoplasties can yield very good or even excellent scars, columellar resections never do.* The columella, already thickened by its central strut, develops discontinuities and deformities that are impossible to correct, because tissue is missing.

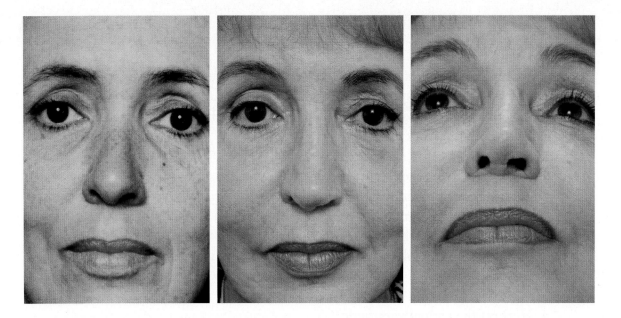

Even more interesting are the changes that have taken place on the frontal and inferior views. In an effort to reduce a large nasal base, made apparently larger by the dorsal resection, one of her surgeons resected a portion of the columella, along with the alar bases.

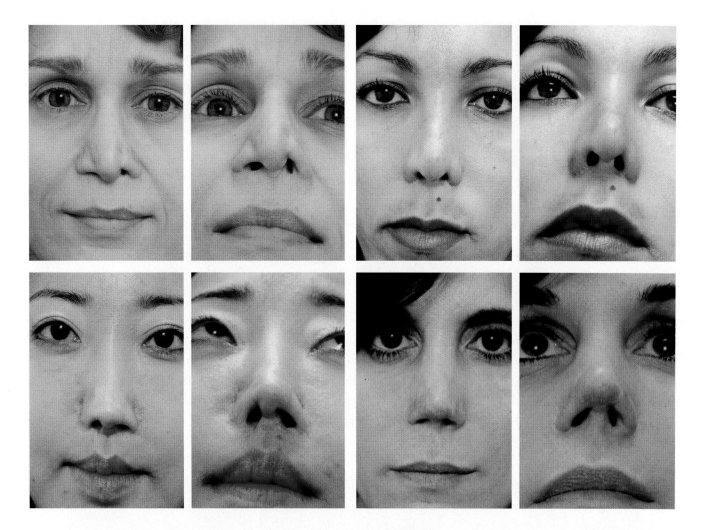

Here are other unhappy examples. In each case, the surgeon was trying to reduce a straight dorsum with a disproportionate nasal base. Nasal base reduction by direct excision should be filed with other well-intentioned techniques that succeed only on paper. It does not work.

An alternative, less destructive strategy is to use the principles outlined previously:
1. Ignore the false assumptions of reduction rhinoplasty, recognizing instead that soft tissue contractility is limited, not infinite, and that the nasal regions are interrelated, rather than independent.
2. Employ the principles of balance and proportion whenever reduction alone is not sufficient.
3. Maximize function.
4. Respect the patient's aesthetic.

In particular, recognize that a straight dorsum tests a surgeon's ability to do less of everything, which requires mastery of techniques that allow small, incremental changes and a light touch.

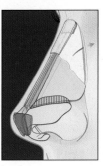

PATIENT STUDY ONE

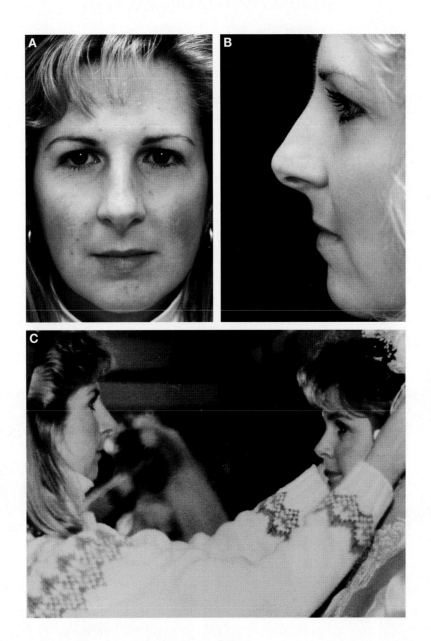

There is nothing strikingly wrong with this patient's nose. At most, it only has a little too much of everything: dorsal height, width, and length.

But the patient had a very definite idea of what she wanted: a nose resembling her sister's *(C, right)*. Achieving that goal within the patient's tissue limits meant small reductions in overall nasal size but more tip contour—increasing tip angularity without increasing projection.

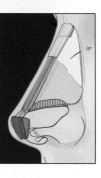

SUMMARY OF THE SURGICAL PLAN

1. Limited skeletonization
2. Rasping of bony vault
3. Trim of cartilaginous dorsum
4. Retrograde reduction of alar cartilage lateral crura (2 mm)
5. Transfixing incision with resection of caudal septum and mucosa
6. Septoplasty
7. Spreader grafts
8. Radix graft
9. Multiple crushed tip grafts
10. Bilateral osteotomies

Postoperative Analysis

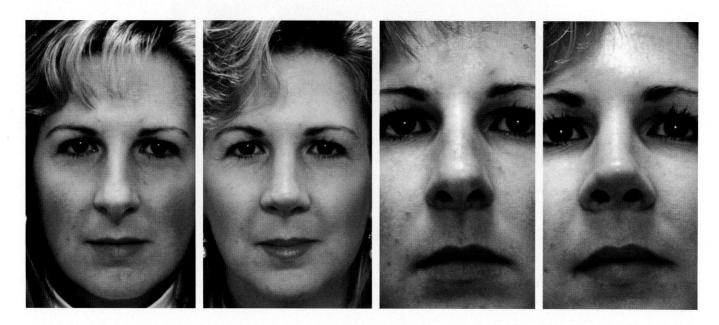

Two years later, the nose is narrower, and the middle vault remains stable and supported, despite dorsal resection. The nasal base is unscarred and the tip lobule is slightly narrower, but the external valves remain supported.

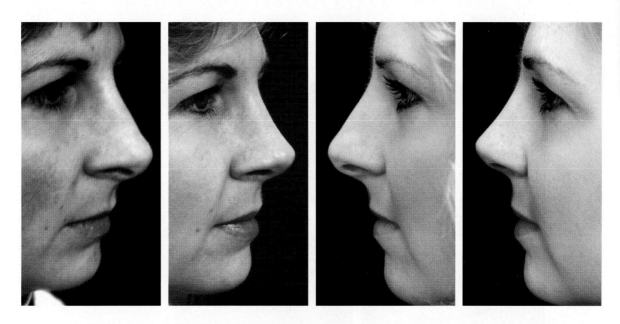

The dorsum is slightly lower but straight, and the tip remains projecting but narrower and more defined. Her result more closely resembles the familial appearance that the patient wished to share.

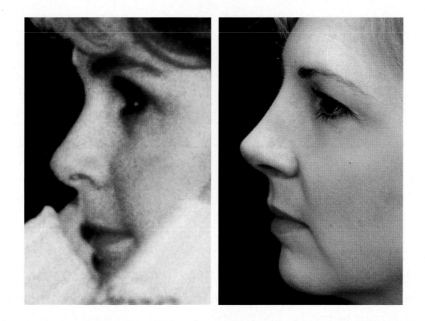

This is an operation measured in millimeters. It is surprising how such small resections and augmentations can alter contour. The dorsum is now slightly lower and the tip is more projecting, the radix graft has altered the balance between dorsal length and nasal base size, and the combination of lateral crural reduction, tip grafting, and elevation of the caudal and membranous septa has added delicacy to the nasal base.

Patient Study Two

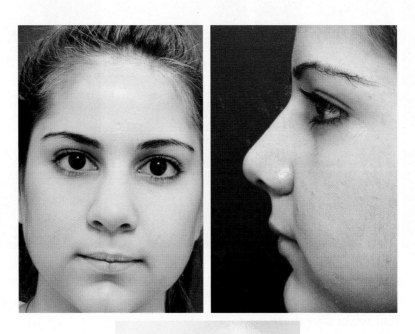

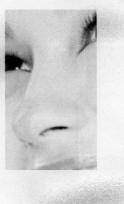

The straight nose seems simple, because none of its regional deformities are very remarkable. However, that is exactly what makes this type of nose so treacherous. The diagnosis must be precise, and individual maneuvers must be carried out sufficiently but not in excess, because the space between "too little" and "too much" is tight. Here, the patient's goals were a lower dorsum and a narrower, more projecting tip. Notice the radix position (slightly low) and the tip contour (blunt). The patient's lateral crura are malpositioned. Her nostrils are small relative to her tip lobular size.

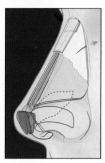

SUMMARY OF THE SURGICAL PLAN

1. Resection and replacement of alar cartilage lateral crura
2. Resection of medial crural footplates through short overlying incisions
3. Slight dorsal reduction, not opening cartilaginous roof
4. No transfixing incision
5. Septoplasty
6. Single-layer radix graft
7. Multiple tip grafts with buttress
8. Bilateral osteotomies

Postoperative Analysis

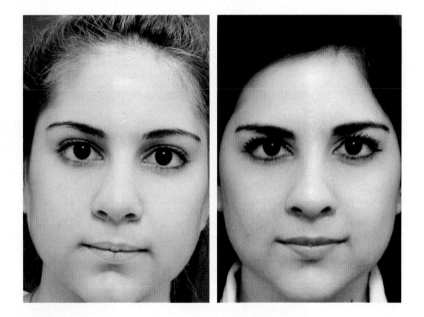

The patient is shown 5 years postoperatively. Dorsal reduction and osteotomies have narrowed the upper nose, and spreader grafts were unnecessary because the cartilaginous roof was not opened.

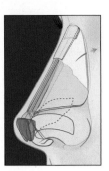

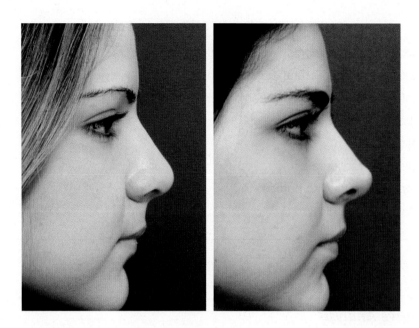

The dorsum is still straight, but its relationship to the tip has changed, in concert with the patient's wishes.

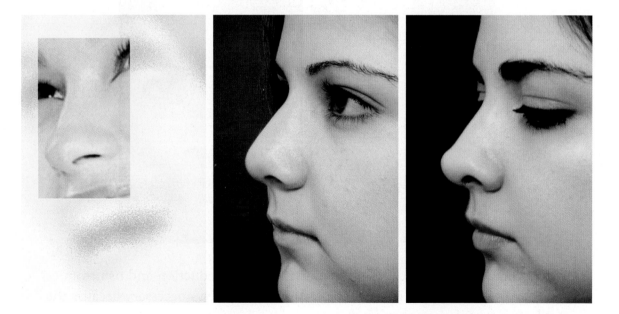

The 5-year, postoperative oblique view shows the change in nasal balance that has occurred with radix and tip grafting, particularly from the left side, where the preoperative inadequate tip projection is more obvious. Without augmentation, more refinement could not have been obtained beneath this soft tissue cover, and without elevating the radix, the postoperative nose would have been unbalanced.

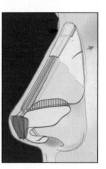

PATIENT STUDY THREE

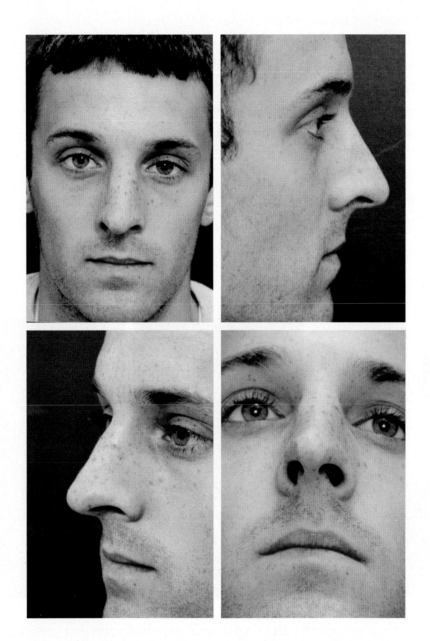

This young man had sustained previous trauma that caused the left nasal bone to protrude through the skin. It was subsequently removed by his first treating physician. There was a high septal deviation toward the right, and the caudal septum protruded from the right side of the columella. Although the dorsum is straight on the lateral view, the right oblique draws the low radix/inadequate tip projection combination into relief.

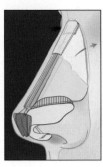

SUMMARY OF THE SURGICAL PLAN

1. Relocate the caudal septum
2. Minimal skeletonization
3. Slight dorsal trim
4. Septoplasty
5. Asymmetrical spreader grafts, thicker on left
6. Lateral wall graft over left bony vault depression
7. Thin radix graft
8. Two crushed tip grafts
9. Bilateral osteotomies

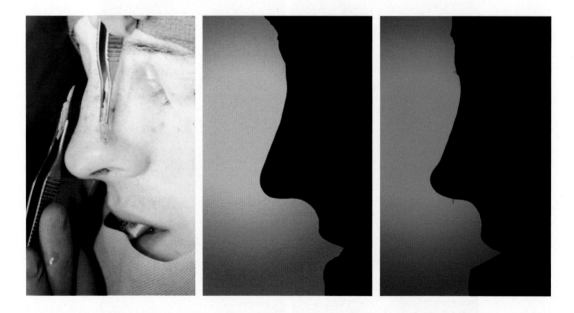

Despite previous trauma, the septal specimen supplied sufficient cartilage. Notice that there is asymmetry in spreader graft thickness to compensate for the high septal deviation, with the left much thicker than the right. A thin radix graft has altered the nasofacial angle, and tip grafts have brought the tip above the septal angle.

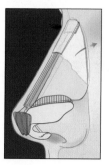

Postoperative Analysis

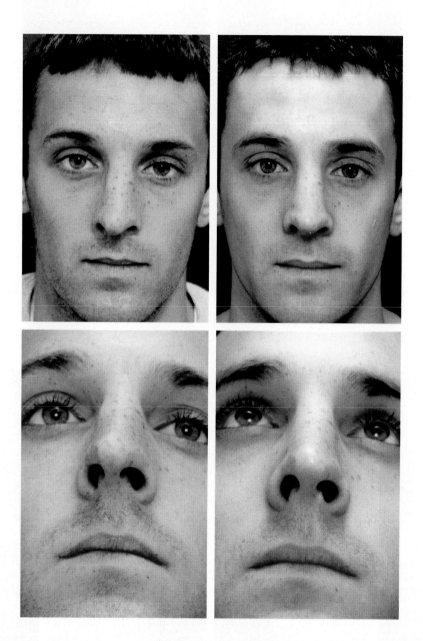

Postoperatively, the nose is symmetrical, the sidewalls are smooth, and the lateral wall graft has filled the depression left by the excised nasal bone. The resected caudal septum supports the columella as a free graft and remains midline.

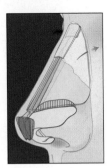

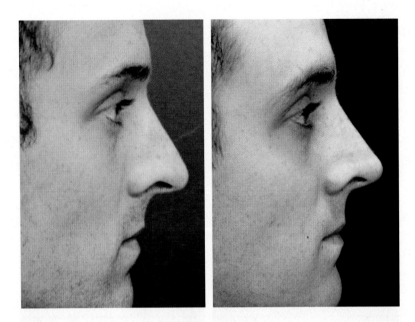

Without a columellar strut, tip projection has been increased, and lobular contour appears normal.

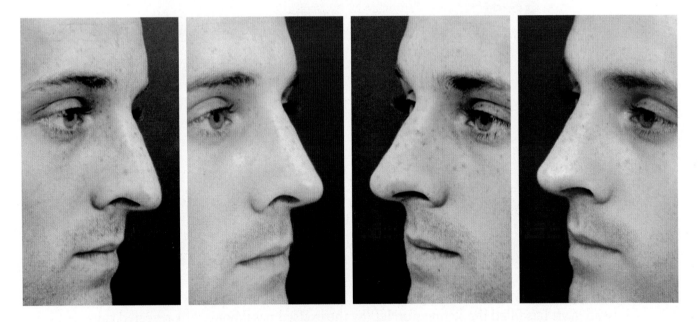

The oblique views now match for this previously asymmetrical nose. The nasofacial angle has improved. Notice that all surface markings remain identifiable (the bony vault edges and the lateral crural contours).

Middle Vault Problems
NARROW MIDDLE VAULT/NARROW NOSE

A narrow nose or narrow middle vault indicates a nose already in jeopardy. A suboptimal airway almost certainly exists, and dorsal resection will incapacitate the internal valves and can reduce nasal airflow up to 50%, according to our rhinomanometric measurements. It is worth making this diagnosis preoperatively.

PATIENT STUDY ONE

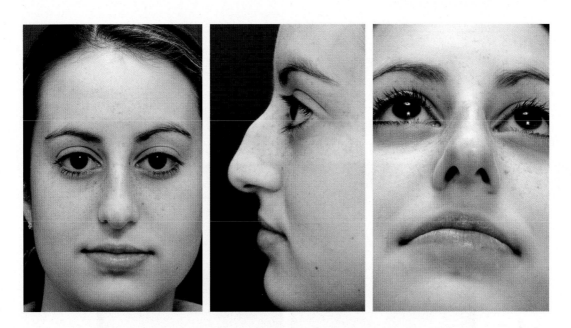

Although patients' eyes are drawn to the height of their dorsa and the width of their tips, the surgeon should look elsewhere. Consider how disproportionately narrow the middle third is and its implication for the patient's airway. Without a basis for comparison, such patients may not be aware of their preoperative obstructions, but symptoms can often be elicited. Observation frequently shows a patient who mouth-breathes through the initial interview, and sidewall support with a cotton-tipped applicator during inspiration brings immediate improvement. The surgeon must not forget the consequences of dorsal reduction without also stabilizing the middle vault.

In this patient the dorsum is high, the radix is low, the tip is inadequately projecting, and the cephalically rotated lateral crura have abandoned the external valves and left them flat and unsupported.

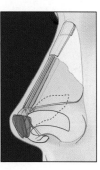

SUMMARY OF THE SURGICAL PLAN

1. Resection and relocation of alar cartilage lateral crura
2. Limited skeletonization
3. Dorsal reduction
4. Transfixing incision; shortening of the caudal and membranous septum
5. Septoplasty
6. Spreader grafts
7. Radix grafts
8. Multiple tip grafts

Postoperative Analysis

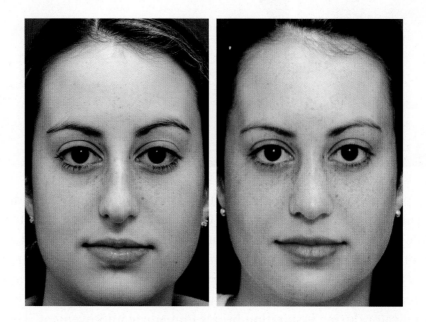

Three years after surgery, the nose is symmetrical and the sidewalls are smooth. The nose progressively widens from top to bottom, without the preoperative hourglass shape that constricted the airway. Postoperative airflow increased 12.9 times over preoperative measurements.

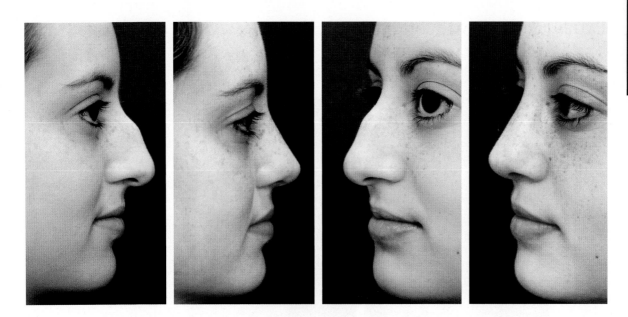

Despite tip grafting, the higher radix has favorably altered nasal base size, and the overall appearance has created an integrated nose, with each third fitting the adjacent one and the whole.

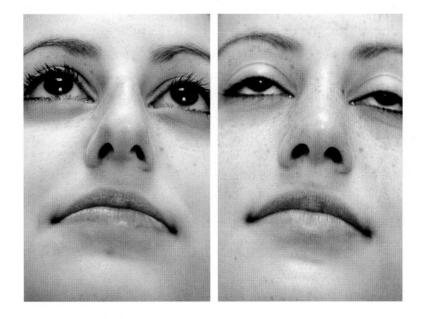

The combination of a lower dorsum and a repositioned lateral crura has produced oval, stable nostril openings.

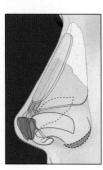

PATIENT STUDY TWO _____

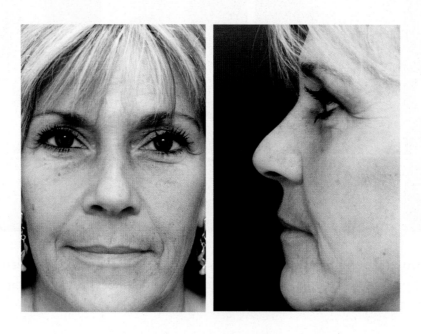

A narrow nose can coexist with a low or high dorsum. When it accompanies a low dorsum, short nasal bones are usually present, as in this patient.

The shorter the nasal bones are, the relatively longer the upper lateral cartilages are. Like a sail without a batten, the long expanse of upper lateral cartilage is frequently unstable, unsupported by a high, broad dorsum or long, sturdy nasal bones. When the lateral crura are cephalically rotated, even the external valves function poorly. This patient flares her nostrils to support her airways.

Notice that the cephalic end of the middle vault hollow indicates that the bony arch extends only 20% of the distance from the radix to the tip.

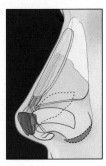

SUMMARY OF THE SURGICAL PLAN

1. Resect and replace alar cartilage lateral crura

2. Minimal skeletonization

3. Rasp bony vault for graft adherence

4. Septoplasty

5. Bilateral spreader grafts, single layer dorsal graft, thicker at root

6. Tip grafts

7. Bilateral alar wedge resections, removing 3 mm of external skin and 2 mm of vestibular skin

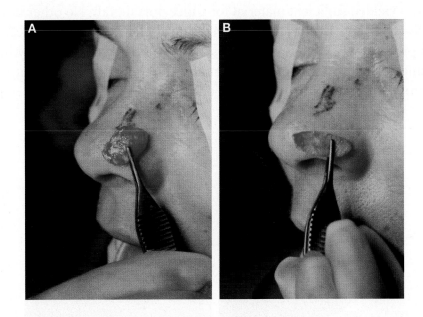

Each lateral crus was dissected free from its external and vestibular skin and resected at the lateral genu *(A)*, crushed, trimmed, and replaced along the alar rim in an orthotopic position *(B)*. A septal cartilage graft is another alternative, but using the patient's lateral crura spares more donor material.

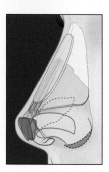

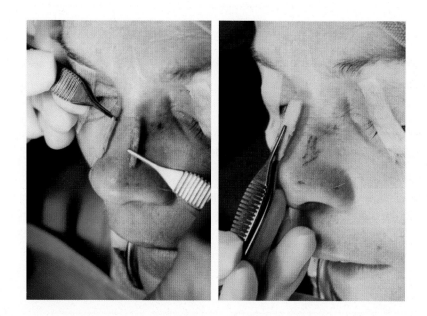

The septum yielded sufficient material for a nice dorsal graft. No other nasal skeleton was resected. Spreader grafts and a thin dorsal graft were fashioned. If the septum had provided less material, the dorsal graft alone would probably have provided sufficient internal valvular support and functional improvement, but both spreader and dorsal grafts provide width and stability.

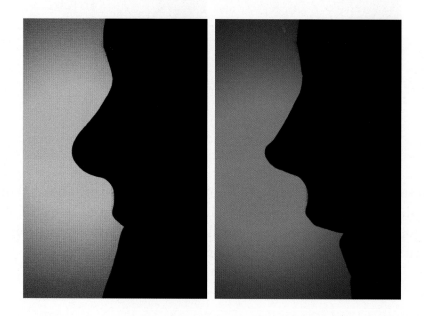

Silhouettes dramatize the effect of tip reduction and skeletal rearrangement. Notice that no contraction is required for the surface effect to appear.

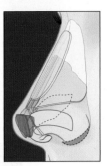

Postoperative Analysis

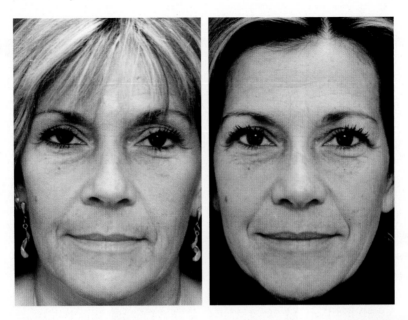

One-year postoperative views show smooth, continuous dorsal lines. The middle vault is slightly wider.

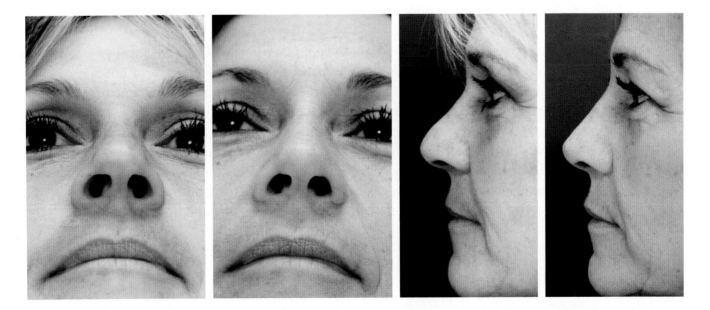

The dorsum is now straight, ending in a defined point of maximum projection. The inadequate tip projection often associated with alar cartilage malposition has been corrected by tip grafts, using neither a columellar strut nor sutures. The thin dorsal graft has raised the radix slightly and diminished apparent nasal base size. The base is slightly narrower, the patient no longer flares her nostrils, and the nostril sills are smooth. Postoperative airflow increased 4.6 times over preoperative values.

WIDE NOSE

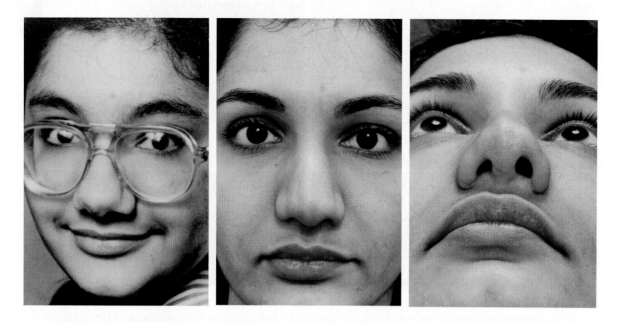

Like thick skin, wide noses dramatize the error of False Assumption Number One: nasal soft tissues do *not* have an infinite ability to contract to the shape of any underlying skeleton. Skeletal reduction, even accompanied by alar base resections, only creates soft tissue distortion, not a smaller nose.

Because human beings often seem to want the opposite of what they have, most patients with wide noses and/or thick skin describe or bring photographs of noses that are narrow and angular. If these patients are not to be disappointed, surgeons must channel these goals into results that can actually be achieved: even if the postoperative tip is not narrower, would a more angular tip be acceptable? Even if the postoperative dorsum is not narrower, would a straight dorsum be acceptable? If surgeon and patient can agree on essentials and find practical common ground, it is safe to proceed. Some patients, however, cannot abandon an ideal but surgically impossible objective, in which case these consultations can be long and unsuccessful.

PATIENT STUDY ONE

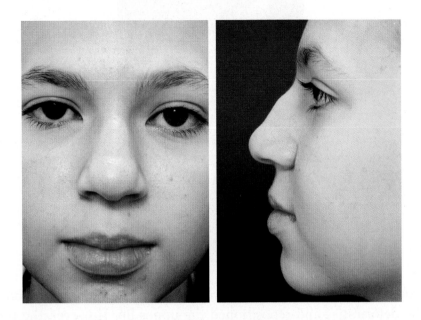

As this delightful young woman noted, "My nose spoils my image." Although the bony vault seems wide, it is still appropriate for the nasal base width; although the base seems wide, the tip lobule consumes most of its transverse dimension. This patient's frontal contours demonstrate nicely how many rhinoplasty decisions must be based on the relationship of one nasal part to another, even more than on the relationships of nasal parts to other ideal measurements or to the face as a whole. In practical terms, making a nose that fits the face translates to making the best possible nasal contours. The surgeon can really do no more than that.

SUMMARY OF THE SURGICAL PLAN

1. Maxillary augmentation, greater in the perialar areas

2. Minimal skeletonization and no transfixing incision

3. Dorsal reduction

4. Resection and replacement of the alar cartilage lateral crura

5. Septoplasty

6. Bilateral spreader grafts, with convexities toward the right for a high septal deviation to the left

7. Harvest ear cartilage

8. Radix graft

9. Tip grafts of ear cartilage (insufficient septal cartilage)

10. Columellar grafts of ear cartilage

11. No osteotomy

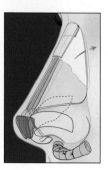

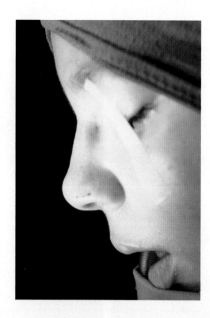

Dorsal reduction, lateral crural relocation, and maxillary augmentation have removed the deformities and repositioned the upper lip. However, the tip lobular skin remains soft and unsupported, and if left alone, the skin would retract to a supratip deformity.

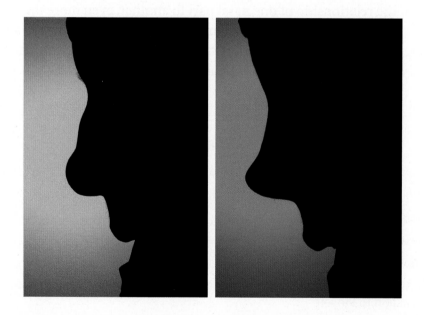

Spreader, dorsal, tip, and columellar grafts support the skin sleeve in a new shape. Dorsal reduction, maxillary augmentation, and columellar grafts have shortened the nose. The nose seems smaller.

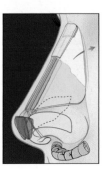

Postoperative Analysis

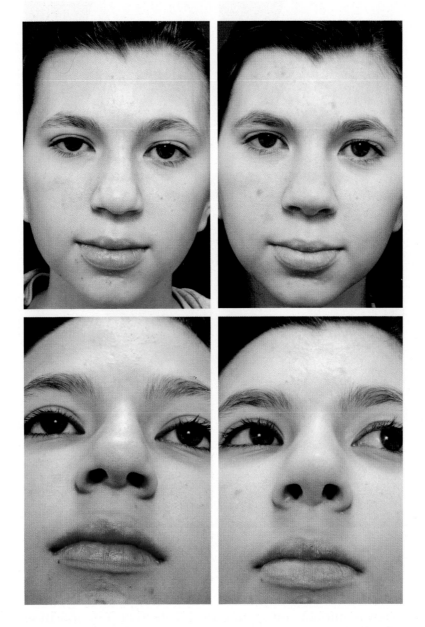

Without osteotomies, but with lateral crural repositioning and dorsal grafting, the nose seems narrower and shorter. The cephalically rotated lateral crura are now orthotopic. Lateral crural repositioning and tip grafting have altered the nostril axis. Geometric mean postoperative airflow has increased 2.6 times over preoperative values.

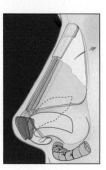

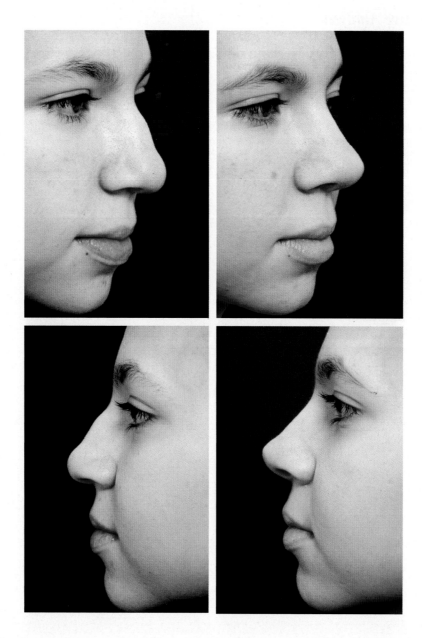

The oblique view is smooth and symmetrical. Lateral crural repositioning has ablated the alar wall hollows. Despite greater tip projection, the dorsal graft has maintained nasal balance, maxillary augmentation has moved the upper lip forward slightly (which is even more apparent on the frontal view), and columellar grafts have provided additional caudal displacement without widening the columella. These grafts extend the length of the columella only, and are not struts.

PATIENT STUDY TWO

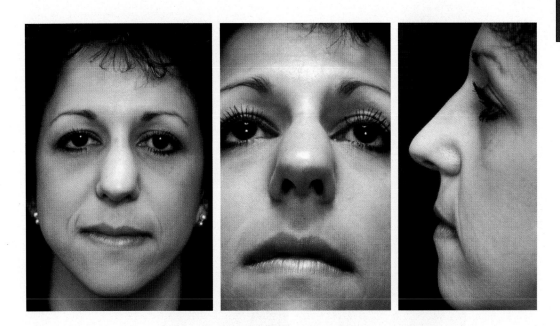

The deformity seen here is less common, and it cannot be treated by dorsal resection, because the dorsum is already at the proper height. Instead, the surgeon must think in three dimensions and narrow the shoulders of the bony and upper cartilaginous vaults without narrowing the dorsum, and then reestablish lateral wall position with spreader grafts.

SUMMARY OF THE SURGICAL PLAN

1. Limited skeletonization
2. Rasping bony vault shoulders, lowering bony sidewalls to allow 2 mm medial movement with osteotomies
3. Trim upper lateral cartilages to allow similar movement
4. Septoplasty
5. Spreader grafts
6. Crushed cartilage tip grafts
7. Bilateral osteotomies

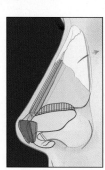

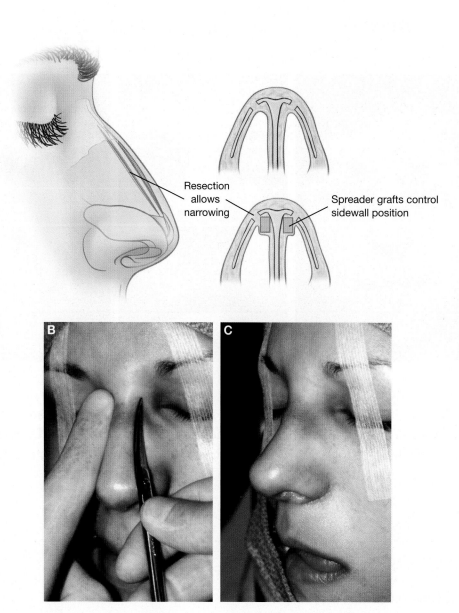

A

Resection allows narrowing

Spreader grafts control sidewall position

B

C

This is the single circumstance in which I will separate the upper lateral cartilages from the dorsal septal edge, to facilitate technical reduction of the upper lateral cartilages without touching the dorsal septal edge *(A)*. My finger and the scissors denote the space created between the sidewalls and the dorsum in *B*. The oblique view shows the expected middle vault collapse *(C)*. Notice the relatively short bony vault. Septoplasty cleared the airway and provided material for spreader and tip grafts.

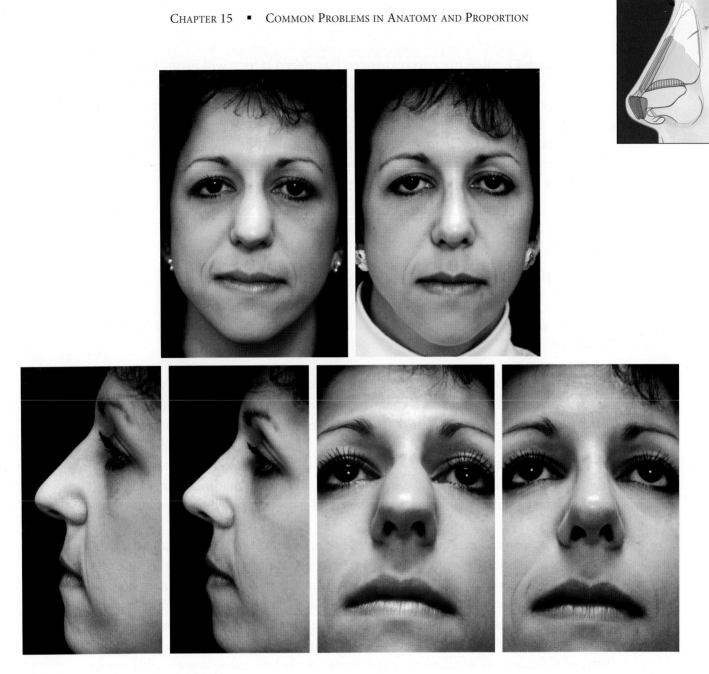

Postoperatively, the bony and upper cartilaginous vaults are narrower, but spreader grafts have established the position of the middle third and internal valves, preserving function. Without them, the intraoperative inverted-V deformity would have become permanent. Crushed tip grafts have lifted the point of maximum tip projection slightly, but the profile line is essentially unaltered, as the patient wished.

Wide noses with thick skin are rarely discussed among surgeons, because they are so difficult to treat using conventional methods. Absolute skeletal reduction in all areas would yield supratip deformity, because the tissues cannot change their dimensions. The surface effect of complex skeletal maneuvers is blunted or lost.

However, some limited improvements can be offered if they will meet the patient's stated and unstated goals. Tip grafts improve contour. Dorsal reduction and/or re-arrangement can improve shape and balance. These changes can be subtle or un-acceptable to some prospective patients. I always show a series of postoperative re-sults, including patients whose noses changed only modestly, and try to gauge a new patient's reaction. If he or she cannot accept the limited improvement that I can offer, it is better for me not to operate.

Tip Problems
INADEQUATE TIP PROJECTION

Inadequate tip projection ranks high among concepts that rhinoplasty surgeons must fully grasp, and for which they must have a dependable and reliable corrective technique.

Even though inadequate tip projection is one of four common anatomic variants that must be diagnosed preoperatively to avoid an adverse result (see Chapter 5), many rhinoplasty surgeons have their own unique definitions of what tip projection is, how to define whether tip projection is adequate, inadequate, or excessive, and there-fore how to correct each of these subtypes. It is also easy to confuse excessive tip projection with a large nasal base, a distinction that I have made earlier (see Chap-ters 1, 2, and 7). If the diagnosis is inaccurate, the correction will be unsuccessful.

Adequate tip projection must be adequate relative to something—in this case the nasal dorsum. Unless the alar cartilages are strong enough to support the tip inde-pendent of dorsal height, the patient cannot have a straight profile. *Any tip that projects to or beyond the level of the anterior septal angle is adequately projecting, and any tip that does not project to the level of the anterior septal angle is inadequately projecting.* The tip lobular/septal angle relationship is independent of nasal base size (instead reflecting skin volume and distribution), and therefore is applicable to any nose.

Tip projection denotes cartilage strength, not skin volume—a concept that may seem obvious but that becomes diffused or lost if the surgeon adds parameters such as the distance from the upper lip to the tip-defining point, the proportion of the nasal base in front of the anterior facial plane, or the ratio of base dimension to dorsal length, all of which are really skin volume and distribution estimates.

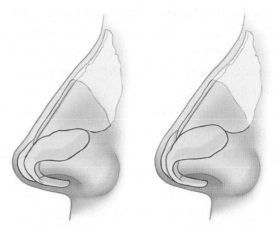

But there is an even easier way of defining inadequate tip projection: by learning to recognize what it looks like. The key to much of rhinoplasty is learning to see what is beneath the skin surface—what combination of anatomic shapes has created a particular surface configuration. In this case, the relevant anatomy is middle crural length. Adequate tip projection indicates a middle crus that is long enough to project the tip to the level of the septal angle or beyond *(left)*. When the middle crus is too short, the tip lobule seems to hang from the septal angle, which is inadequate tip projection *(right)*.

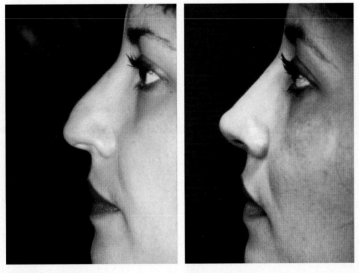

Preoperative   Postoperative

Even without a schematic to guide you, the anatomic shape that creates this patient's tip strength is obvious. The medial, middle, and lateral crura can only have one dimension based on their surface impact. A surgical dissection is not necessary.

As you examine each of the preoperative photographs throughout this text, imagine the underlying shape that must exist—the responsible anatomy.

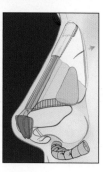

Inadequate tip projection is common, approximately 40% in primary patients and 80% in secondary patients. *Perhaps more than any other single nasal anatomic feature, inadequate tip projection impacts nasal aesthetics and surgical strategy.* The surgeon new to rhinoplasty should therefore remember seven points about inadequately projecting tips:

1. Adequate tip projection is essential for a straight postoperative profile.
2. Inadequate tip projection profoundly affects the entire profile line, causing some patients to view their noses as hooked, when the actual problem is tip lobular shape, not nasal length. Shortening the nose does not correct inadequate tip projection.
3. Inadequate tip projection reflects a short middle crus.
4. Adequate tip projection must be adequate relative to something—in this case the septal angle.
5. Tip projection reflects cartilage strength, not skin volume; the treatment for inadequate tip projection therefore depends on skeletal change, not skin thinning or supratip suturing.
6. Inadequate tip projection cannot be rendered adequate by reducing the tip.
7. The surgeon cannot correct inadequate tip projection by a larger dorsal resection. The solution is to set the dorsum at the proper level, and to bring the tip forward by lengthening the middle crural segment.

PATIENT STUDY ONE

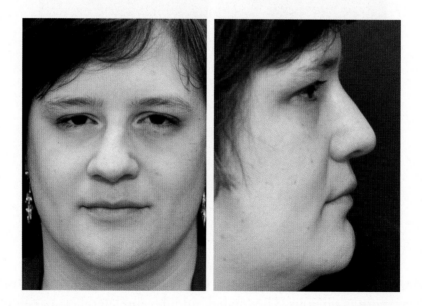

This patient's inadequate tip projection is accompanied by a slightly low radix and significant asymmetry in the middle vault. Previous trauma had injured the septum, causing airway obstruction and upper lip recession. Notice that, on the frontal view, the high septal deviation begins just below the medial canthi, at the caudal end of the bony arch, thus indicating short nasal bones.

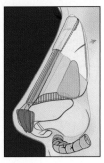

SUMMARY OF THE SURGICAL PLAN

1. Maxillary augmentation
2. Resection and replacement of the caudal septum
3. Dorsal reduction
4. Retrograde reduction of alar cartilage lateral crura
5. Septoplasty
6. Thick left spreader graft
7. Onlay to upper cartilaginous vault
8. Thin radix graft
9. Multiple tip grafts
10. Right osteotomy

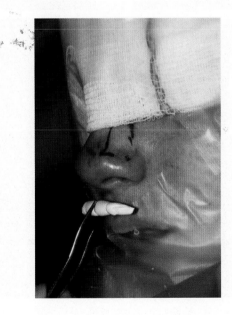

A sheet of 1 mm Gore-Tex was rolled into an implant, trimmed, and fixed circumferentially with 6-0 nylon sutures. The implant was inserted through an incision in the right nasal floor into a subperiosteal pocket dissected high over the maxillary arch and tight against the piriform aperture. In this nonmobile position with thick soft tissue cover, the implant is comfortable and effective, and it has a very low complication rate (unlike alloplastic nasal augmentation, which I do not perform).

Septoplasty cleared the airway and provided excellent building material. However, previous trauma had increased calcification in the septal segments. Accordingly, cartilage was saved for the dorsal and tip grafts. Calcified cartilage or bone can be used for spreader grafts, and the ethmoid makes an excellent lateral wall graft.

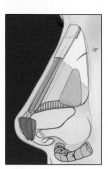

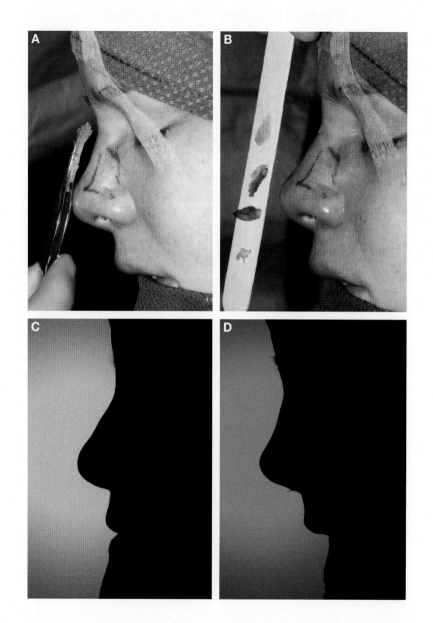

Notice the position of the vertical plane of the lip after maxillary augmentation. A radix graft has been fashioned, its edges have been beveled, and the graft has been crushed and contoured to the defect (thickest at the root) *(A)*. The only pieces left for tip grafting are small scraps, none of which form a traditional shield graft *(B)*. However, because the tip lobular pocket is intact, the dissection can be high and limited so that maximum effect can be obtained from the limited material.

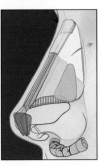

Postoperative Analysis

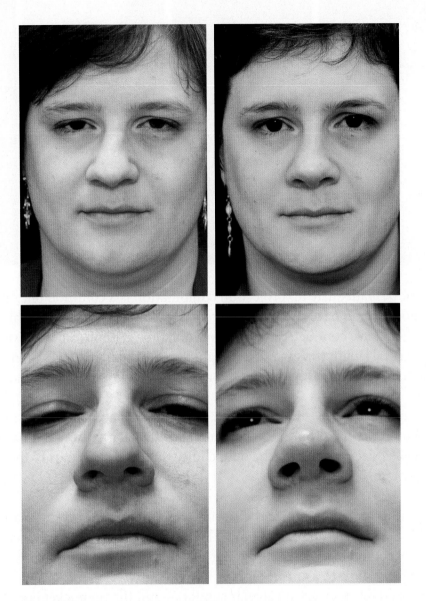

At 1 year postoperatively, frontal contours are smooth and more symmetrical. There is a slight residual depression in the left cartilaginous vault. Although absolute symmetry would have been better, asymmetries such as these are better left undercorrected than overcorrected: patients accept a familiar asymmetry that has been improved more than a nose that is straighter but much wider.

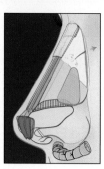

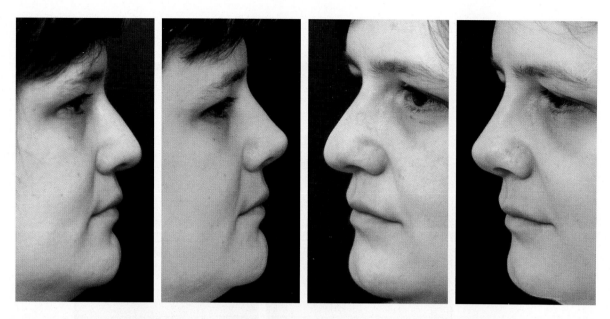

The low radix/inadequate tip projection combination is a common one. Dorsal reduction alone would have enlarged apparent nasal base size, and such thick tissues are unlikely to have contracted over a lower dorsum. Without an effective increase in middle crural length (tip grafts), a straight dorsum could not have been achieved. The nose seems shorter even though the nasolabial angle was not altered.

Two little augmentations—radix and spreader grafts—have completely altered the relationship of the nasal tip to the dorsum, and the balance between nasal length and nasal base size. That so much could come from so little is part of the magic of rhinoplasty.

Throughout this chapter, notice the similarities among the surgical plans for patients with inadequate tip projection. If the dorsum is high, it is reduced, but not with an expectation of seeing a straight profile until tip projection increases. As little as possible is done to alar cartilages—only enough to remove the deformity and maintain or establish external valvular support—and the tip pocket is not violated by other maneuvers, ensuring secure graft placement.

Notice also that increasing tip projection always obliges the patient to accept a slightly larger tip lobule, regardless of how the surgeon decides to increase projection. Increases in projection mean equivalent increases in tip lobular size, whether the projection is created by a columellar strut, by tip grafts, or by forcing the alar cartilage arches into new positions with sutures. Nature has only one set of rules, and skin sleeve distribution imposes limits on surgeons. My preference for tip grafts rests on its anatomic logic: grafts augment the deficient cartilaginous area, a quality not shared by borrowing cartilage from another deficient area with sutures or by forcing the tip skin forward with pressure from the nasal spine.

Because inadequate tip projection is so common and so critical to recognize (see Chapter 5), there are many examples of it throughout this text. All examples of inadequate tip projection share common traits. Once recognized and integrated into your right brain, the pattern and its underlying anatomy are impossible to miss, which is fortunate, because failure to correct this anatomic variant is one of the most common causes of an unfavorable rhinoplasty result.

The good news is that the anatomic defect—a short middle crus—is consistent and always responds to augmentation of the deficient cartilaginous segment.

BOX TIP, BALL TIP, AND ALAR CARTILAGE MALPOSITION

Boxy and ball nasal tips are widely recognized as aesthetically complex surgical problems, and they have inspired imaginative solutions to correct the deformities they impart.

The overwhelming majority of boxy and ball tips, however, have an importance outside the lobule that has been understated in the surgical literature and that eluded me for many years: both tip types represent variants of alar cartilage malposition (cephalic rotation). In fact, both boxy and ball tips occur uncommonly in patients with orthotopic alar cartilages, but instead appear most often as foreshortened variants of alar cartilage malposition. Therefore the major importance of either the boxy or the ball tip is not its cosmetic configuration within the lobule, but rather its functional ramifications outside the lobule at the external nasal valve.

Definition of Terms

The terms *ball, broad, bulbous,* and *boxy* have been used differently and sometimes interchangeably in the literature. According to most prior usage, ball and bulbous tips should be equivalent. However, neither *broad* nor *bulbous* defines the convexity (the ball) nor the angulation (the box) of the lateral crura.

The characteristics that distinguish ball and boxy tips from their flatter counterparts are best recognized from inferior views.

Distinguishing Criteria

Distinguishing Criteria for Boxy and Ball Tips

Type	Angle of Divergence	Lateral Genu	Lateral Crural Shape
Flat	60 degrees	Well defined	Flat
Boxy	90 degrees	Well defined	Usually convex
Ball	60 degrees	Poorly defined	Usually convex

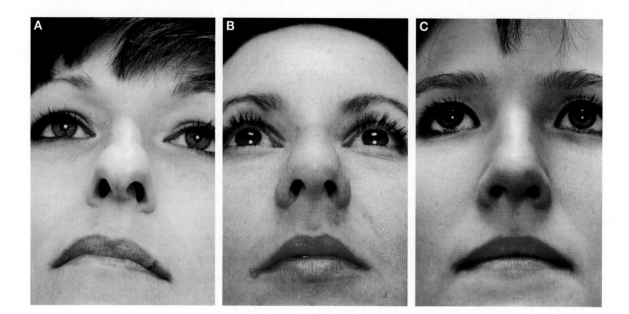

The boxy tip *(A)* imparts a square perimeter to the nasal base, in which there is a wide divergence between the medial crura (often approaching 90 degrees) and a relatively sharp angulation at the lateral genua, creating the corners of the box. Associated lateral crura usually have varying degrees of convexity. The ball tip *(B)* has a narrower, more ideal angle of divergence (closer to 60 degrees) and lateral crural convexities that often seem to efface the lateral genua entirely. Tips that are not clearly boxy or ball shaped are therefore relatively flat *(C)*, and so have clearly demarcated lateral genua and discrete middle crural segments that create angles of divergence close to 60 degrees. These characteristics apply whether the alar cartilages are adequately or inadequately projecting.

Association of Lateral Crural Orientation and Tip Contour in 200 Consecutive Rhinoplasty Patients

Lateral Crural Orientation	100 Consecutive Primary Patients		100 Consecutive Secondary Patients	
	Number	Incidence in Subgroup (%)	Number	Incidence in Subgroup (%)
Orthotopic	32		13	
Flat	27	84	2	15
Ball tip	5	16	10	77
Boxy tip	0	0	1	8
Malpositioned (cephalically rotated)	68		87	
Flat	18	26	24	28
Ball tip	31	46	36	41
Boxy tip	19	28	27	31

This table indicates the relationship between lateral crural orientation and tip contour in 100 primary and 100 secondary consecutive rhinoplasty patients.* Notice several important points:

1. Among the primary rhinoplasty patients, only 32% had orthotopic lateral crura, again dramatizing the prevalence of cephalic rotation (malposition).
2. Within that orthotopic group, the comparative relative frequency of occurrence of the ball tip was only 16%.
3. There were no boxy tips among the primary patients, and the remaining 84% of patients had flat lateral crura.
4. Alar cartilage malposition occurred in 68% of primary patients and 87% of secondary patients.
5. Among these primary and secondary malposition patients, each tip variant occurred at the same relative frequency: The ball tip was the most common in both groups, the boxy tip was second most common, and flat lateral crura were least common.

*Fisher z-tests were performed with a significant difference between independent proportions for each proportion. A 2×6 chi-square for the entire table was 25.8; $df = 5$, $p < 0.0001$. A 2×2 chi-square for lateral crural orientation by primary and secondary patients was 10.35, reduced to 9.3 using the Yates correction; $df = 1$, $p < 0.01$.

Association of Lateral Crural Orientation, Tip Contour, and Projection in 100 Consecutive Primary Rhinoplasty Patients

Lateral Crural Orientation	Incidence in Entire Patient Group (%)	Incidence in Subgroup* (%)
Orthotopic	32	
Adequately projecting		
Flat	10	31
Boxy or ball	2	6
Inadequately projecting		
Flat	17	53
Boxy or ball	3	9
Malpositioned (cephalically rotated)	68	
Adequately projecting		
Flat	7	10
Boxy or ball	7	10
Inadequately projecting		
Flat	20	29
Boxy or ball	34	50

*Upper and lower halves of the columns do not total 100% because of rounding.

This table reflects the association of lateral crural orientation, tip contour, and tip projection among the 100 primary patients only.* Note the following:

1. Inadequate tip projection was significantly more common among patients with malposition than among those with orthotopic lateral crura.
2. Similarly, boxy or ball tips were much more common among primary patients with malposition than among patients with orthotopic lateral crura, regardless of tip projection.
3. The most common configuration in patients with orthotopic lateral crura was flat, inadequately projecting alar cartilage (53%).
4. In contrast, the most common phenotype among patients with malposition was inadequately projecting ball or boxy tip (50%).
5. Adequate tip projection in patients with malposition was relatively uncommon (only 20%), regardless of tip or lateral crural configuration.

What does all this mean? First, the data reaffirm that malposition is common, not only in primary patients but especially in secondary patients, which is why malposition qualifies as one of the four anatomic variants that predispose to unfavorable results (see Chapter 5).

*A $2 \times 2 \times 2$ chi-square test (crural orientation by projection by contour) gave a value of 21.2; $df = 1$, $p < 0.001$.

The data also indicate that the overwhelming majority of ball and boxy tips are associated with lateral crura that are malpositioned and not orthotopic. Finally, both ball and boxy tip lateral crura (particularly the latter) are foreshortened, as if crural length has been used up in the arch that it forms in the axial plane, relocating the posterior insertion of the crus. *Therefore boxy and ball tip lateral crura are both malpositioned and relatively short, increasing the skeletal deficit and its effect on external valvular function.* In the cases that follow, notice the posterior alar hollow in the preoperative views and its improvement once the lateral crura have been relocated.

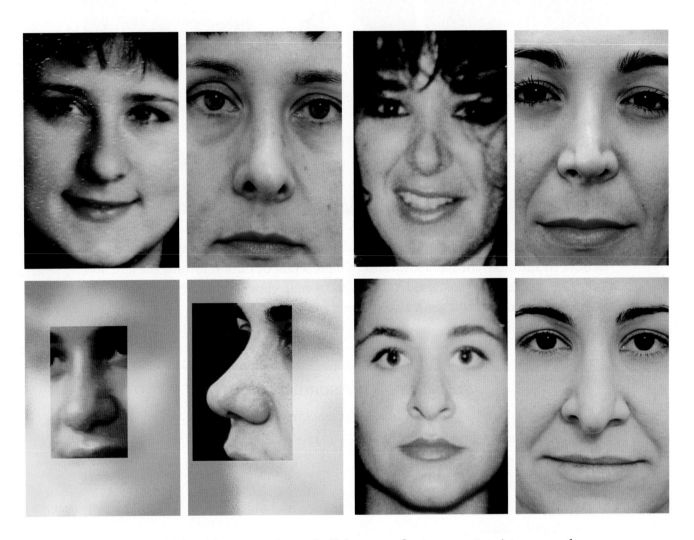

If unrecognized, malposition (in its ball, boxy, or flat incarnations) imparts characteristic secondary deformities. Patients frequently flare their nostrils to stabilize their external valves; in some patients, the soft tissue deficit becomes significant enough to require composite grafts, which not only replace the vestibular skin deficiency but also supply ample alar rim support. Among 100 secondary patients requiring composite grafts, the overwhelming proximate cause of the deformity was a preexisting alar cartilage malposition (80%).

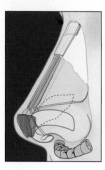
BOXY TIP

PATIENT STUDY ONE

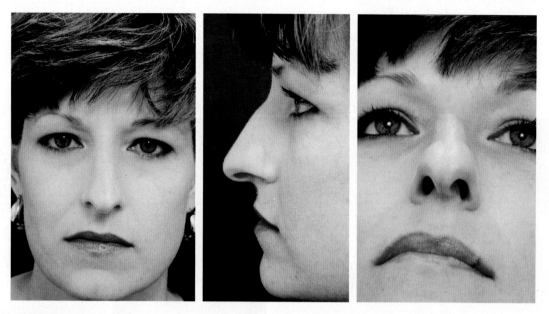

This patient illustrates the common association of a boxy tip with inadequate projection. In addition, she has a low radix, a high septal deviation toward the left, and upper lip retrusion (most evident on the frontal view)—a common secondary rhinoplasty characteristic seen also in some primary patients.

SUMMARY OF THE SURGICAL PLAN

1. Gore-Tex maxillary augmentation, right side thicker than left

2. Resect and replace lateral crura

3. Minimal skeletonization

4. Transfixing incision

5. Shorten anterior caudal and membranous septa

6. Dorsal reduction

7. Septoplasty

8. Asymmetrical spreader grafts, thicker on right than left

9. Radix graft

10. Tip graft with buttress

11. No osteotomies

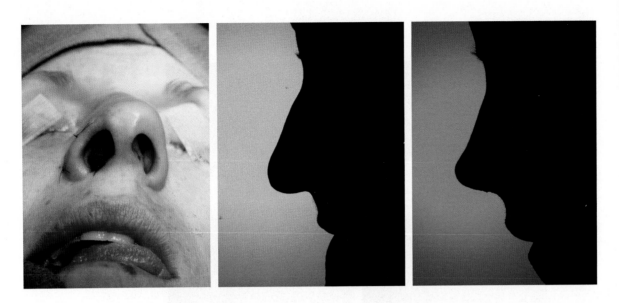

The right lateral crus has been resected and relocated, moving the natural convexity from the tip (where it causes a deformity) to the alar wall (where it converts flat to oval). Skeletal rearrangement has reduced the deformity but rebalanced the nose and increased tip projection. Notice the change in upper lip carriage created by maxillary augmentation.

Postoperative Analysis

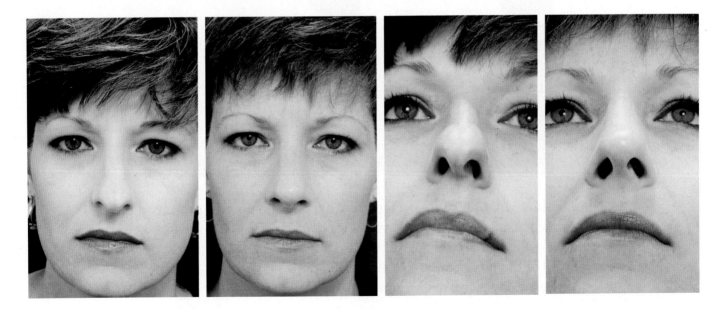

Two years postoperatively, the nose is slightly shorter, the sidewalls are confluent and symmetrical, the high septal deviation is camouflaged and straightened by spreader grafts, and the upper lip is more vertical. Resection and replacement of the lateral crura have altered the nostril contour favorably and reduced the bulk of the squared preoperative basal perimeter.

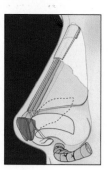

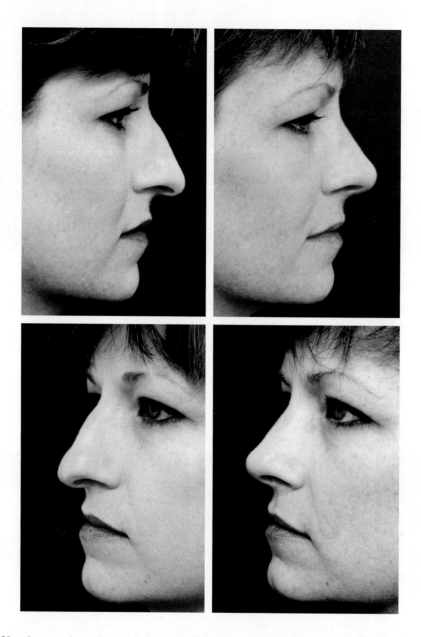

The profile shows that the radix is slightly higher and the tip now projects slightly beyond the septal angle. The oblique views particularly dramatize the unfavorable preoperative tip shape, reconfigured by lateral crural repositioning and tip grafting. Notice that the preoperative alar hollows have disappeared. Geometric mean postoperative airflow increased 3.6 times in this patient.

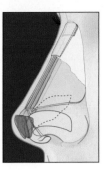

PATIENT STUDY TWO

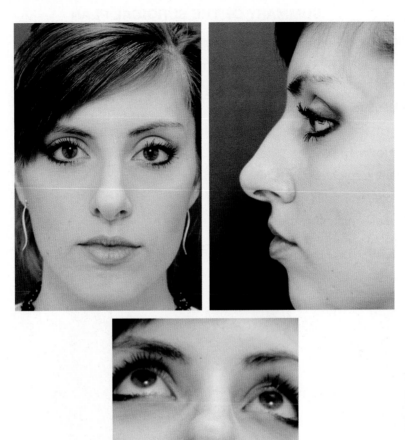

This patient demonstrates the less common combination of the boxy but adequately projecting tip (represented by only 7% of our series of 100 consecutive primary patients). Typical of so many patients with boxy and ball tips, her skin is thin and her cartilages are stiff and bossed. Her caudal septum protrudes into the left airway. There is a slight dorsal hump, and her low radix position increases apparent nasal base size. Notice that there is a broad angle between her middle crura and the foreshortening that her lateral crural bossing causes.

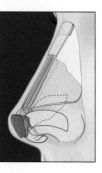

SUMMARY OF THE SURGICAL PLAN

1. Relocate caudal septum through hemitransfixing incision
2. Resect and replace lateral crura
3. Moderate skeletonization
4. Resect dorsum 2 mm
5. Trim membranous septum, shortening the nose
6. Septoplasty
7. Bilateral spreader grafts (thicker on left than right)
8. Single-layer radix graft
9. Multiple crushed cartilage tip grafts

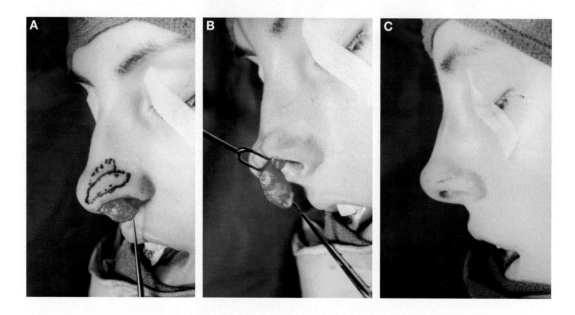

After relocating the caudal septum, the lateral crura were dissected free from their external and vestibular skin coverings to rotate them caudally as flaps. In *A,* note the original, cephalically rotated position (dotted line) and the intended new position (solid line). However, once fully dissected, the lateral crura proved too irregular and distorted for the flap procedure *(B);* thus each crus was resected, crushed, trimmed, and replaced along its alar rim. After all resections, nasal contours seem improved, but the soft tissues are unsupported; without reequilibration, contraction would yield a supratip deformity *(C).*

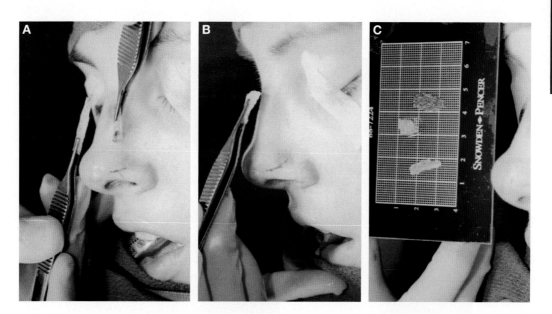

Substantial spreader grafts will support the narrow middle third and adjust the high septal deviation *(A)*. A thin radix graft will lift the root slightly *(B)*. Multiple tip grafts will reform the lobule *(C)*.

Postoperative Analysis

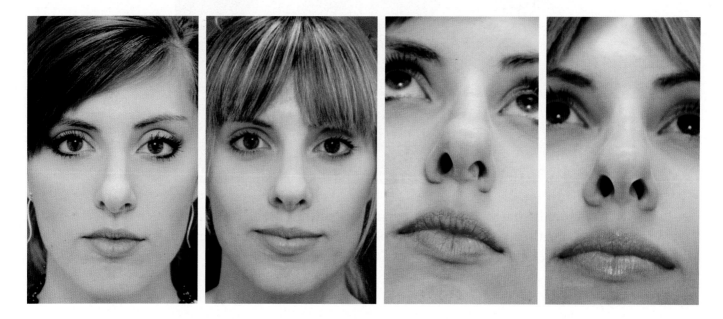

Fifteen months postoperatively, the nose is more symmetrical and the sidewalls are smoother. Notice, however, that the strong lateral crura retain a natural convexity, despite crushing. The columella remains narrow, and the caudal septum is now midline.

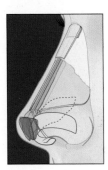

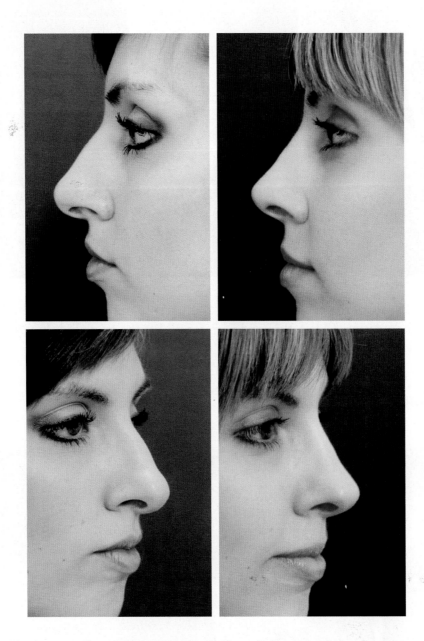

The dorsum is straight and better balanced, and the nasal base retains much of its native shape (in accordance with the patient's wishes) but seems less massive. The external valves are supported.

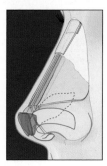

BALL TIP

PATIENT STUDY ONE _____

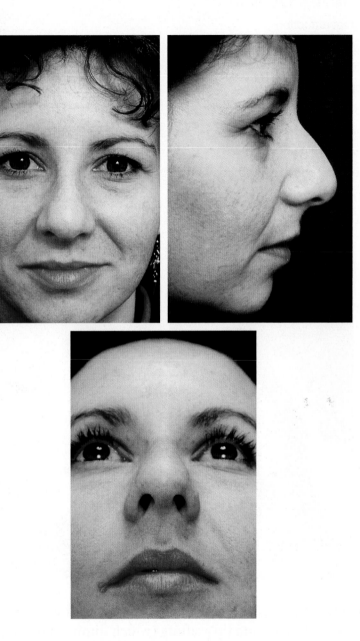

Among the boxy, ball, and flat malposition subtypes, the most common is the malpositioned ball tip with inadequate projection (31% in my series). Like the others, the deformity has cosmetic and functional components. Notice the normal angle of divergence of the medial crura (60 degrees), but the poorly defined lateral genu extend into the convex lateral crura. A low radix accentuates the large nasal base, and the small tip lobule (short middle crus) seems to hang from the septal angle.

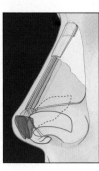

SUMMARY OF THE SURGICAL PLAN

1. Resect and replace lateral crura

2. Minimal skeletonization

3. Dorsal reduction

4. Transfixing incision with reduction of nasal spine and caudal septum, and excision of medial crural footplates

5. Septoplasty

6. Spreader grafts

7. Layered radix graft (one longer piece with two additional pieces posteriorly at the cephalic end)

8. Multiple lightly crushed tip grafts with a buttress

9. No osteotomies

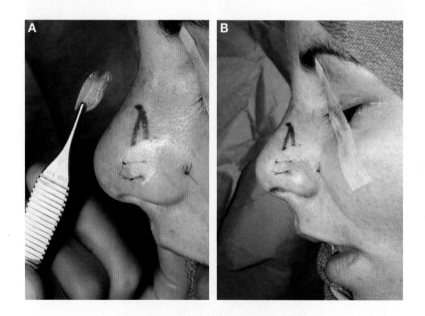

After resection and replacement of the lateral crura, the dorsum is trimmed in anticipation of both radix and tip grafting (which diminish the required dorsal resection). Notice that even this thin resection has opened the cartilaginous roof *(A)*. In configurations such as these, dorsal reduction alters the profile very little *(B)*. The caudal ends of the bony arch and the middle vault hollow were marked preoperatively.

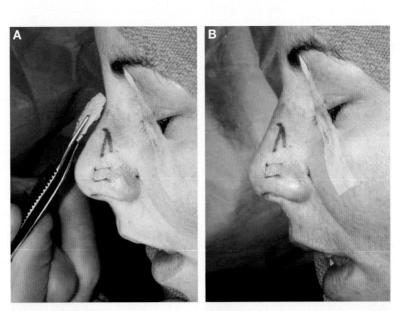

A layered radix graft was sized to the defect *(A)*. Compare the appearance after radix grafting *(B)* to the appearance after dorsal resection (*B* in the previous figure). Notice how radix elevation has straightened the dorsal line and decreased apparent nasal base size.

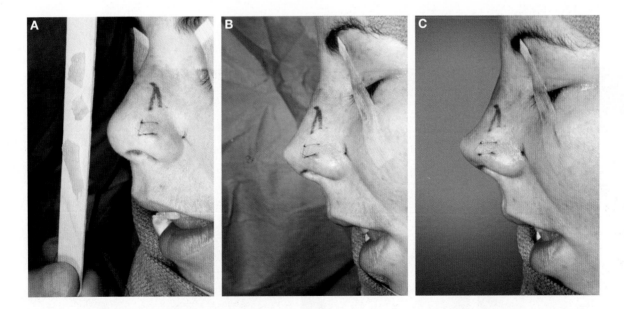

Tip grafts have been selected and lightly crushed, but they have been left untrimmed until their necessary length has been determined *(A)*. A small ethmoid buttress lies on the tongue blade center. After buttress placement, the point of maximum projection has been set, but the tip is artificially angular *(B)*. Crushed grafts inserted anterior to the ethmoid buttress soften the contour and further increase projection *(C)*.

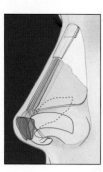

Postoperative Analysis

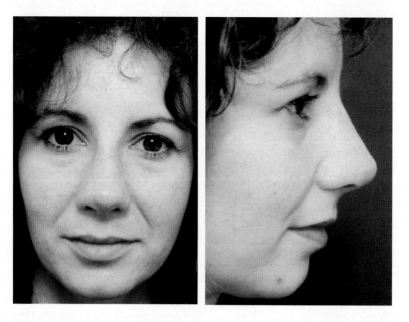

Even at 1 month after surgery, the nose has begun to take shape. The lobule has started to narrow, and the profile is straight. Notice the change from the blue card picture: serial intraoperative photographs strengthen a surgeon's judgment and teach *feel*.

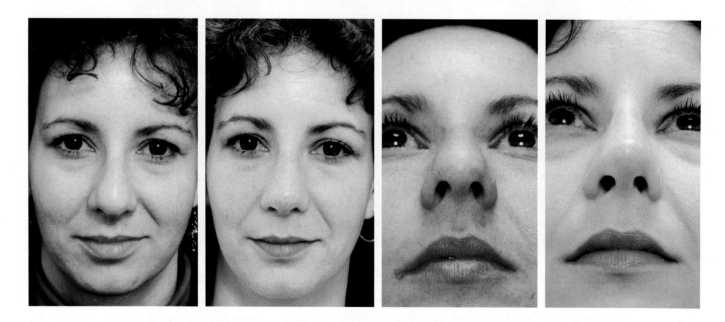

At 1 year, the tip has narrowed. Without osteotomy, the narrower upper nose now fits the wider nasal base. The external valves are supported.

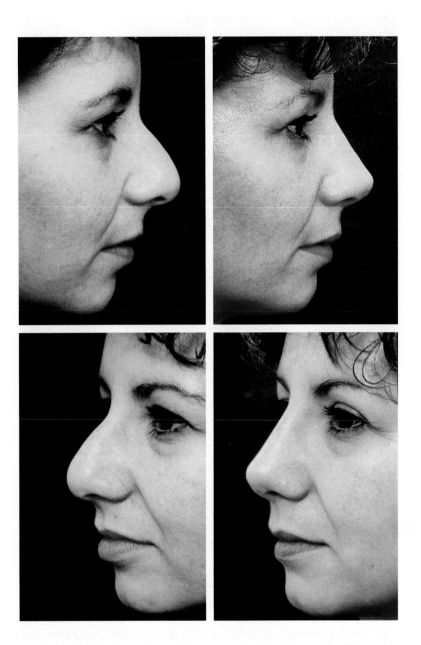

On the profile and oblique views, the nose remains balanced and less bottom heavy. Lateral crural repositioning has ablated the alar wall hollows. Geometric mean postoperative nasal airflow increased 2.5 times over preoperative values.

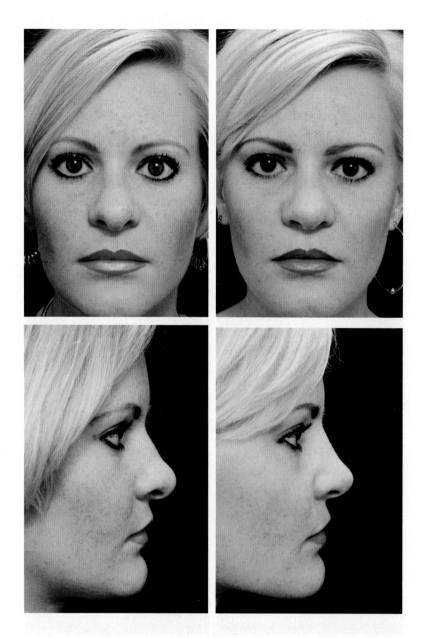

This patient, like the previous one, has thick soft tissues. Lateral crural resection and replacement creates conditions under which the tip lobule can narrow. However, a surgeon cannot force the narrowing—individual soft tissue characteristics prevail. Compare the postoperative results of the previous patient and of this patient, also at 1 year. This patient's tip was treated in the same way, but although the profile has improved, her tip lobule (now soft and unsupported) has not narrowed. Patients must accept this possibility beforehand so that they do not confuse the uncontrollable for the uncontrolled.

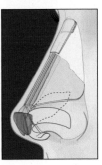

PATIENT STUDY TWO

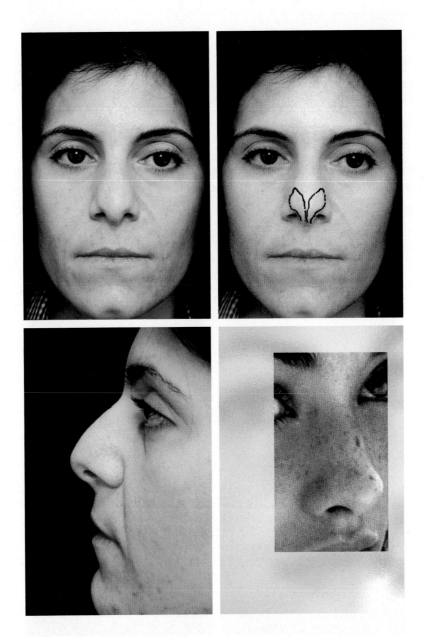

This patient's thinner skin highlights the malposition. The alar walls are unsupported and grooved, and the broad sweep of her cephalic lateral crura overpowers the short middle crural segments. The bony vault, however, is appropriately narrow relative to nasal base width. Characteristically, she wants what she does not have: retroussé and tip projection.

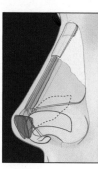

SUMMARY OF THE SURGICAL PLAN

1. Relocate lateral crura
2. Minimal skeletonization
3. Dorsal reduction
4. Transfixing incision with nasal spine, caudal septal, and medial crural foot-plate reductions
5. Septoplasty
6. Radix graft
7. Asymmetrical spreader grafts, thicker on the left than on the right (high septal deviation to right, masked by malposition)
8. Tip grafts with buttress
9. No osteotomies

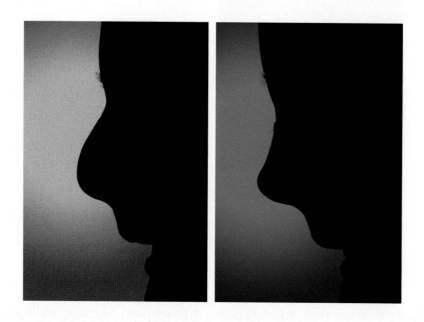

NOTE: Retroussé is produced by adequate projection beyond a straight dorsum, not by thinning or suturing the supratip skin (the upper nasal sutures represent an incidental scar revision).

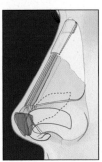

Postoperative Analysis

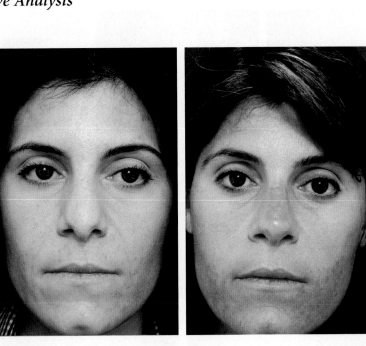

Twenty months postoperatively, the tip is narrower, more angular, and projecting. Middle crural length is adequate. Even without osteotomy, the narrow bony vault balances nasal base width.

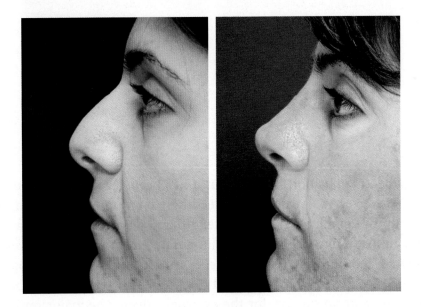

Despite unfavorable soft tissues, the combination of dorsal reduction, radix grafts, and tip grafts have achieved the patient's aesthetic goals. Spreader grafts and lateral crural repositioning stabilized the airway. Repositioned lateral crura support and reshape the alar rims. Postoperative nasal airflow increased 4 times over preoperative values.

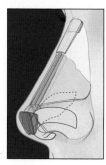

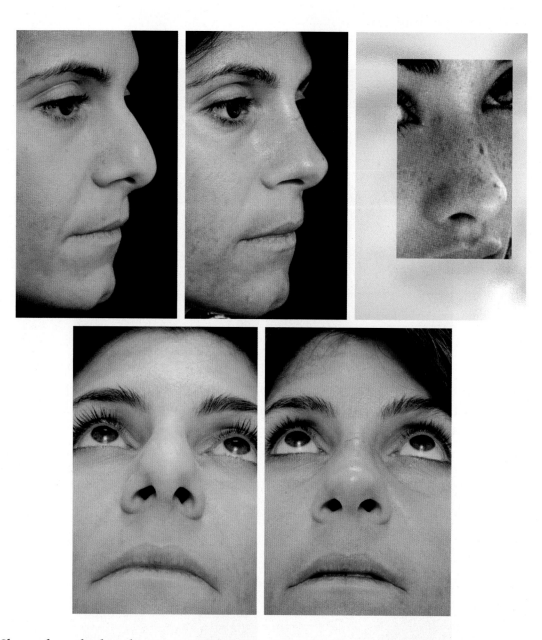

Sheen described malposition in 1979, but it has been regarded as an uncommon phenotype. However, malposition is exceedingly common, even among primary patients. Malposition affects alar crease length and alar margin shape and height, and occurs almost universally with cleft lip nasal deformities, as we shall see. The data presented here indicate that the lateral crura of most boxy and ball tips are malpositioned (cephalically rotated) and foreshortened in their axial planes, and provide poor structural support for the external valves. The major importance of ball and box tips is therefore not only the lobular deformity, but also the functional deficit associated with them.

KNUCKLED TIP OR NARROW TIP

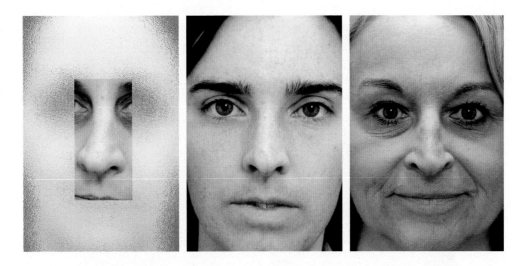

A subtype of primary deformity has as its most prominent characteristic a narrow tip with knuckles at the lateral genua, which patients characterize as "a witch's nose." Commonly associated with this tip configuration are thin skin, short nasal bones, and a disproportionately large nasal base. The dorsum may be straight or high. Tip projection may be adequate or inadequate. A short bony vault increases the proportion of cartilaginous sidewall support, so high septal deviations and valvular incompetence are usually obvious.

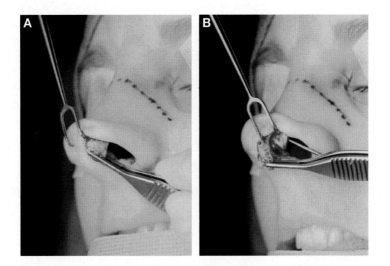

The knuckled alar domes are delivered *(A)*, and they are treated by vertical wedge resections through cartilage that spare lining *(B)*. There are surgeons who object to disrupting the alar cartilage arch because it alters tip projection, and this is a valid argument. But trouble only arises when the surgeon does nothing to compensate. If the tip is reconstructed with multiple crushed grafts, projection can be maintained, reduced, or augmented to satisfy the patient's wishes.

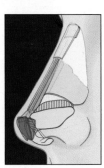

PATIENT STUDY ONE

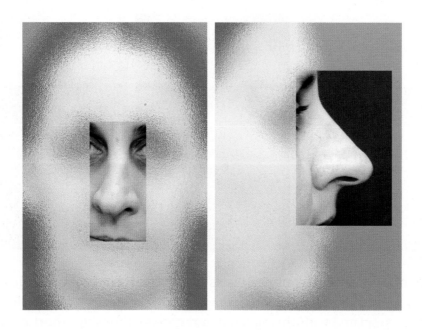

Typical of this subtype, short nasal bones support significant septal deviation poorly, leaving concave sidewalls. Although the domes are knuckled, the lateral crura are also concave, and valvular support is poor.

SUMMARY OF THE SURGICAL PLAN

1. Wide skeletonization over middle vault, narrow over bony vault
2. Retrograde reduction of alar cartilage lateral crura with 4 mm resection from domes
3. Submucosal 3 mm trim of caudal ends, upper lateral cartilages
4. Reduction of cartilaginous dorsum only
5. Complete transfixing incision, shortening caudal and membranous septa
6. Septoplasty
7. Asymmetrical spreader grafts, thicker on left than right
8. Upper dorsal graft
9. Multiple crushed tip grafts
10. Columellar grafts
11. No osteotomies

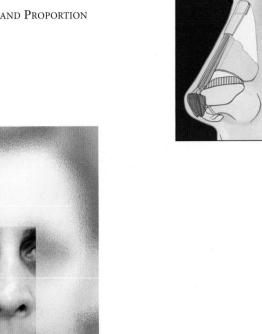

Postoperative Analysis

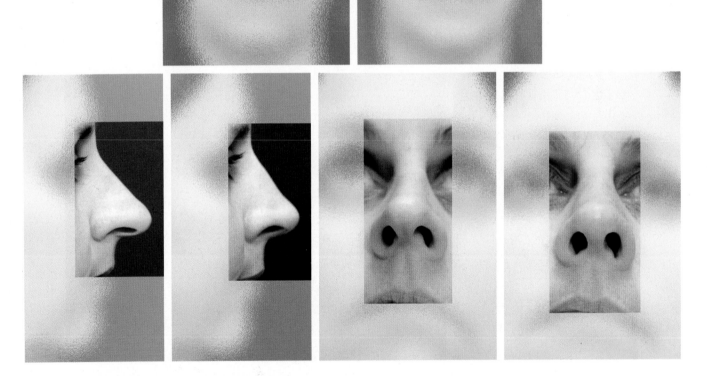

Eighteen months postoperatively, the long middle vault remains straighter, guided by the spreader grafts. Slight shortening has resected some of the caudal septal deflection. The tip is less projecting but normally contoured, without projecting edges, and cartilaginous dorsal resection and radix grafting have altered the nasofacial angle, diminishing apparent nasal base size. Geometric mean nasal airflow increased 12 times over preoperative measurements.

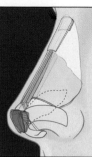

PATIENT STUDY TWO

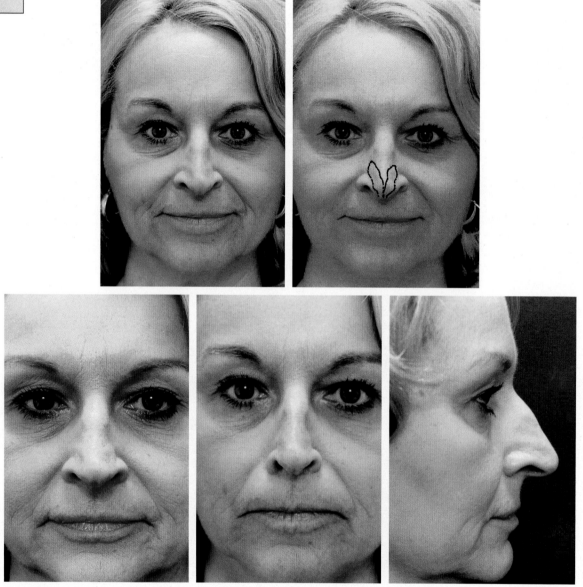

This patient shares similar characteristics with the previous one, with striking side-wall collapse in a nose doubly handicapped by short nasal bones and malposition. Unlike the previous patient, however, this woman has a high dorsum; but because the radix is similarly low, the same imbalance exists.

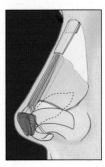

SUMMARY OF THE SURGICAL PLAN

1. Wide skeletonization
2. Resect alar cartilage lateral crura, medial to the deformed lateral genua; crush; and replace the long alar rims
3. Dorsal reduction
4. Transfixing incision, shortening caudal and membranous septa
5. Septoplasty
6. Asymmetrical spreader grafts, thicker on left than right
7. Layered radix graft
8. Multiple crushed tip grafts
9. No osteotomies

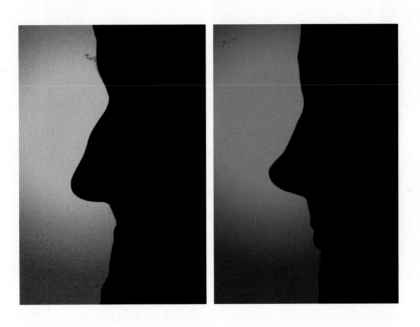

At the conclusion of the surgery, the upper nose is smaller but the radix is higher and the base is rotated, each of which helps to improve nasal balance.

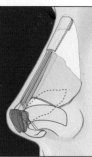

Postoperative Analysis

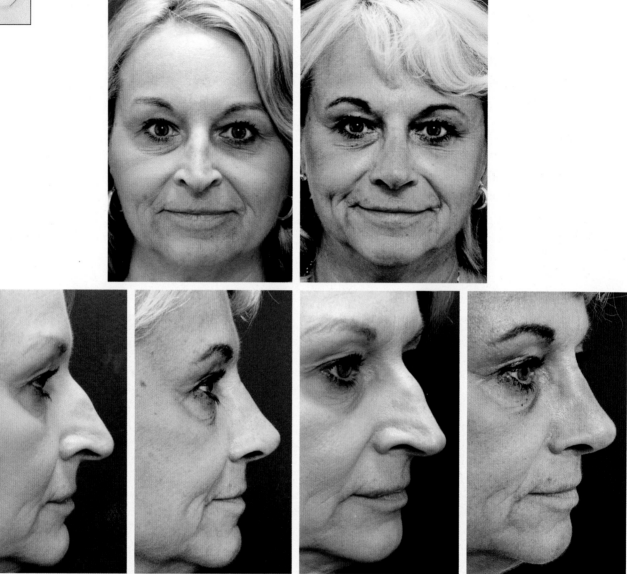

Two years postoperatively, the narrow, knuckled tip has disappeared, and spreader grafts have aligned the walls, softening the depressions at the caudal end of the bony arch. Geometric mean nasal airflow increased 12 times over preoperative measurements, a value that is artifactually high because of abnormally poor preoperative values.

Lateral crural repositioning has improved alar wall contour and ablated the hollow, so the patient no longer flares her nostrils to support her airways. Notice that no alar wedge resections were performed. The apparent reduction in nostril size stems from an improvement in alar flare and from the increased tip lobular size (the result of grafting).

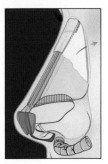

Problems of Length and Balance
SHORT NASAL BASE/SHORT NOSE

In patients with relative or absolute skin sleeve deficiency, skin expansion is not practical and stretch is limited. However, a surgeon can achieve what is possible by small expansions and reductions and by the sleight of hand that stems from improved balance and proportion.

SHORT NASAL BASE

PATIENT STUDY ONE

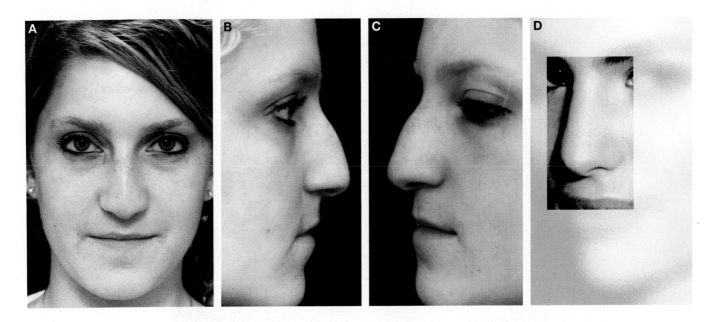

This is a slightly long nose with a tight nasal base and a vertical nasofacial angle.

Dorsal reduction and shortening alone will not provide the nasal balance that this patient prefers *(D)*. Her surgeon must move the nasal base forward visually. The following tools are potentially available:
1. Reduce dorsal height, if needed.
2. Increase tip projection.
3. Augment the columella (not as a strut but to increase medial crural strength).
4. Augment the maxillary arch, if needed.

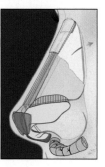

SUMMARY OF THE SURGICAL PLAN

1. Two-piece maxillary augmentation, widest in perialar areas
2. Limited skeletonization
3. Dorsal reduction
4. Retrograde lateral crural reduction, 2 mm
5. Transfixing incision, shortening the caudal and membranous septa, 3 mm
6. Septoplasty
7. Spreader grafts
8. Thin radix graft
9. Multiple tip grafts with buttress
10. Columellar grafts
11. Bilateral low-to-high osteotomies

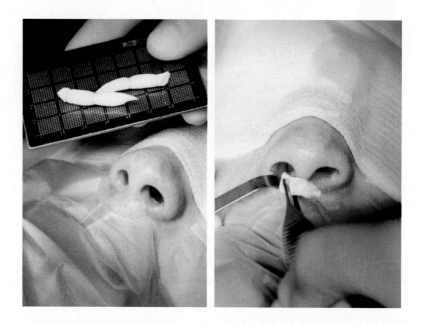

A piece of 1 mm Gore-Tex sheeting is rolled to form a tapered implant, split, and placed into a subperiosteal pocket, high over the maxillary arch and tight against the piriform apertures. The implant is placed as the first step, using a no-touch technique (see Chapter 17).

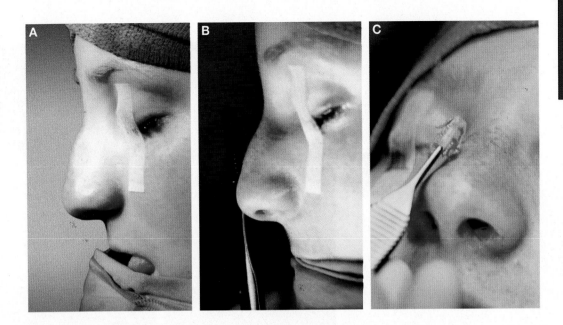

Reduction of the bony vault increases apparent cartilaginous dorsal height (compare *A* and *B*). Maxillary augmentation and dorsal resection have moved the nasal base anteriorly *(B)*. The cartilaginous resection is thin, but sufficient to open the roof *(C)*.

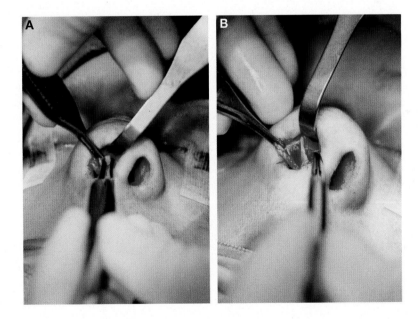

After placing the left spreader graft *(A)*, both internal valves have been reconstructed *(B)*.

929

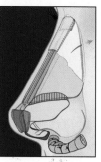

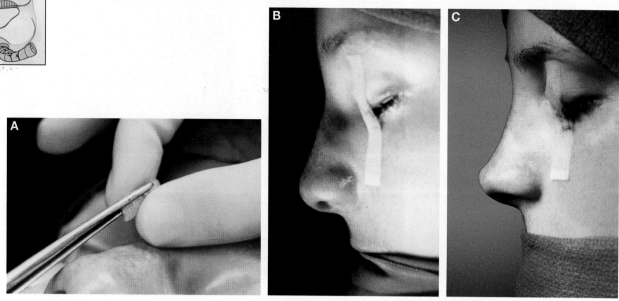

Septal cartilage is crushed to make a pliable graft *(A)*, which is placed at the radix under direct vision. The dorsal line is thereby straightened *(B)*. Tip grafts are added, completing the reconstruction *(C)*.

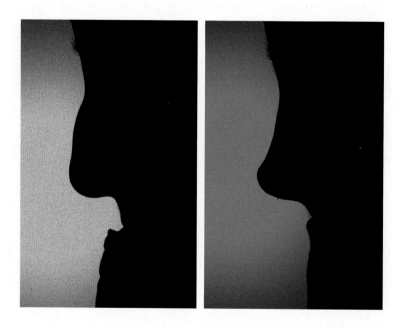

Silhouettes demonstrate the change in nasal base position and balance that has occurred.

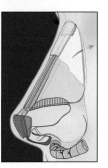

Postoperative Analysis

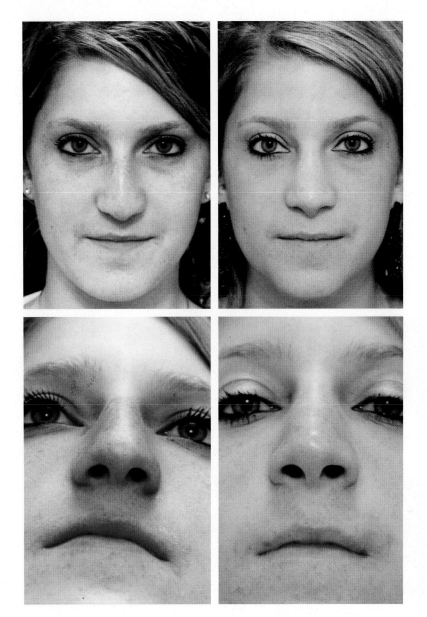

One year postoperatively, the improvement in nasal base projection is evident, even on the frontal view. The subnasale seems less compressed. Any change in postoperative nostril visibility alarms some patients, particularly if they do not anticipate it. The surgeon is wise to obtain explicit consent preoperatively. Notice the effect of maxillary augmentation.

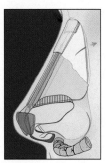

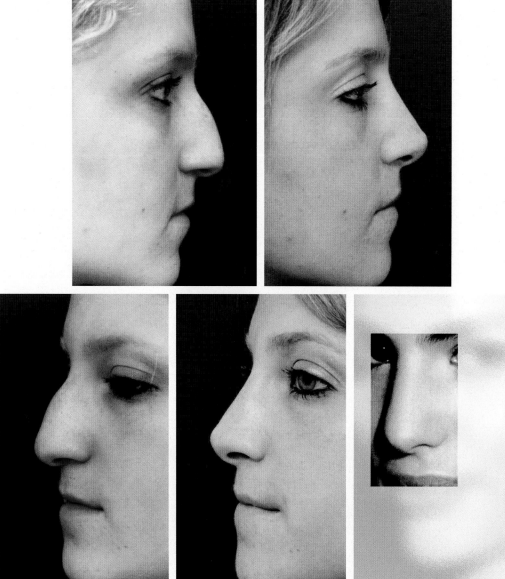

Tip and columellar grafts have moved the nasal base forward and increased projection. It may have been possible to perform this rhinoplasty without the radix graft, particularly considering the short nasal base. But the combination of a low radix and inadequate tip projection creates the appearance of the nose sliding down the patient's face; this and the patient's postoperative goal influenced my surgical plan.

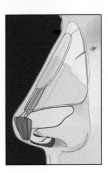

SHORT NOSE

Primary rhinoplasty patients with short noses seem to have too much skeleton for the amount of soft tissue, but the soft tissue is normally elastic. This anatomy must be distinguished from that in secondary cases, in which the skin deficit is the result of direct excision or contraction after skeletal reduction and in which the soft tissues are now often tight and inelastic.

The logic of the corrective plan is to reduce skeletal volume where possible in a way that will lengthen the nose or add soft tissue (particularly lining). In addition, augmenting the cephalic and caudal ends of the nose (radix, tip lobule, and columella) creates absolute and relative increases in nasal length by forming a nose that begins higher and ends lower.

PATIENT STUDY ONE

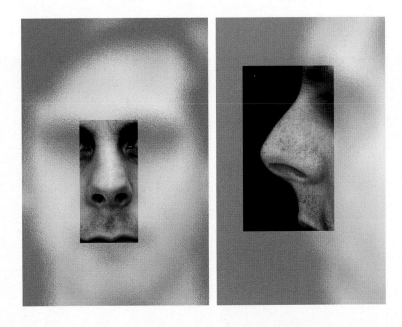

This patient is a tall man with a short nose. The dorsal skeleton pulls his inadequately projecting tip and alar rims cephalad, braced only by the caudal septum. The tendency of dorsal reduction to shorten the nose further must be overcome by dorsal augmentation at the cephalic end and by rotating the nasal base caudally. This is a shape in disequilibrium: a skin sleeve too small to accommodate its skeleton, creating a so-called *tension nose* characterized by a high dorsum, an obtuse nasolabial angle, and elongated nostrils (not all tension noses are short).

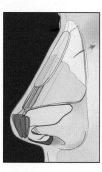

SUMMARY OF THE SURGICAL PLAN

1. Limited skeletonization
2. Minimal reduction of bony dorsum
3. 3 mm reduction of cartilaginous dorsum
4. Transfixing incision; resection of posterior caudal septum with overlying mucosa
5. No modification of tip cartilages
6. Septoplasty
7. Asymmetrical spreader grafts (thicker on right than left)
8. Upper dorsal graft
9. Tip grafts with ethmoid buttress, caudally positioned
10. Bilateral osteotomies
11. Augmentation mentoplasty

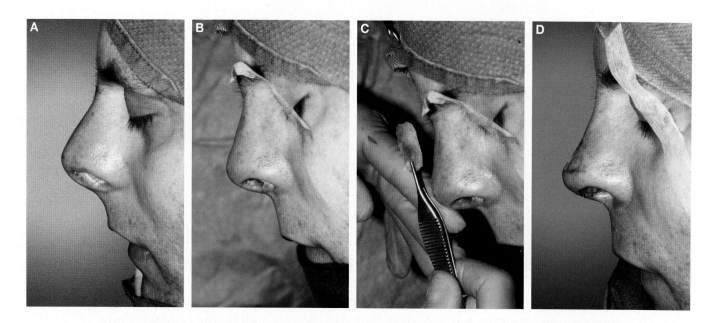

Dorsal reduction releases skin tension, and caudal septal resection allows the base to rotate inferiorly *(B)*. Septoplasty yielded a specimen that was thin and largely bony. The best piece was selected for the dorsum *(C)*. The dorsal graft and tip grafts draped the skin sleeve cephalad and caudad. Notice that the tip buttress was placed to set the desired angle of rotation, and other grafts added to it forced the tip and columellar skin inferiorly, adding absolute and relative nasal length *(D)*.

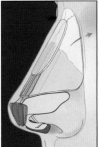

Postoperative Analysis

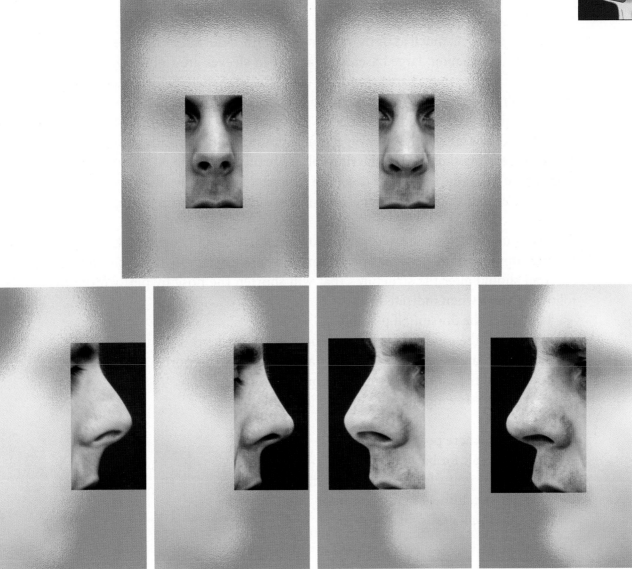

At 3½ years postoperatively the nose is more symmetrical, corrected by asymmetrical spreader grafts (thicker on the right than the left). Dorsal reduction and caudal rotation of the base have decreased nostril visibility. Tip projection is greater, and the tip lobule is appropriately larger, representing an increase in projection and middle crural length. Dorsal reduction has relieved anteroposterior nostril tension, converting tight slits to ovals.

Problems of Volume

LARGE BASE/LARGE SKIN SLEEVE

Large bases and large skin sleeves are two variations on a theme and so can be considered together. As much as or more than any of the deformities that we have considered in this chapter, large bases and large skin sleeves are right-brain surgical problems, because they share a common characteristic: there is too much skin for the preoperative skeleton. The surgeon has a problem, because skin sleeve contraction is limited (in contradistinction to False Assumption Number One, which states that the nasal soft tissue cover has an infinite ability to contract to the shape of any underlying skeleton). If the rhinoplasty reduces net skeletal volume, but the skin sleeve (already excessive) does not contract sufficiently, the nose will not shorten. Hence the aphorism that "Long noses become long again postoperatively."

The way out of this puzzle is a combination of reduction and augmentation, maintaining support where possible and adding it where needed. In specific terms, the surgeon should alter the structures that will shorten the nose by performing the following steps when indicated:

1. Reduce the dorsum, if possible.
2. Shorten the caudal ends of the upper lateral cartilages submucosally.
3. Reduce lateral crural width, maintaining valvular support.
4. Shorten the caudal and membranous septa.
5. Avoid narrowing the nose by osteotomy.

And augment where possible:

1. Radix graft for balance
2. Spreader grafts for middle vault width
3. Tip and columellar grafts for nasal base support
4. Lateral wall grafts for symmetry

PATIENT STUDY ONE

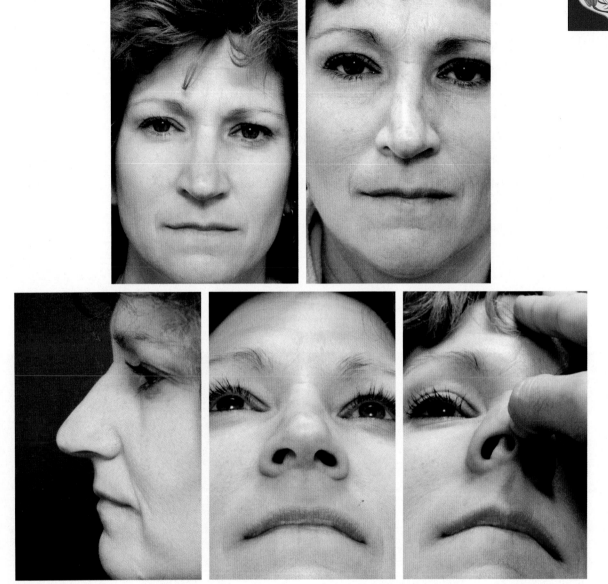

Paralleling the long nose in this woman is a severe functional problem, signaled by the flared nostrils as she tries to support her airways. Her middle vault is asymmetrically narrow after a high septal deviation to the right, and her caudal septum deflects into the right airway. Her base is long and large, unbalanced by her slightly low radix. Her soft tissues are moderately thick.

Aside from the functional correction, the aesthetic key in this nose depends on diminishing apparent nasal base size by improving nasal balance—the necessity of illusion.

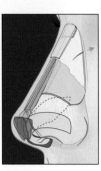

SUMMARY OF THE SURGICAL PLAN

1. Resect and replace lateral crura
2. Resect and replace dislocated caudal septum as free graft
3. Wide skeletonization
4. Shorten membranous and caudal septa through transfixing incision
5. Dorsal reduction, right greater than left
6. Septoplasty
7. Asymmetrical spreader grafts, thicker on the left than right
8. Thin radix graft
9. Multiple crushed cartilage tip grafts, no buttress
10. Columellar grafts
11. No osteotomy

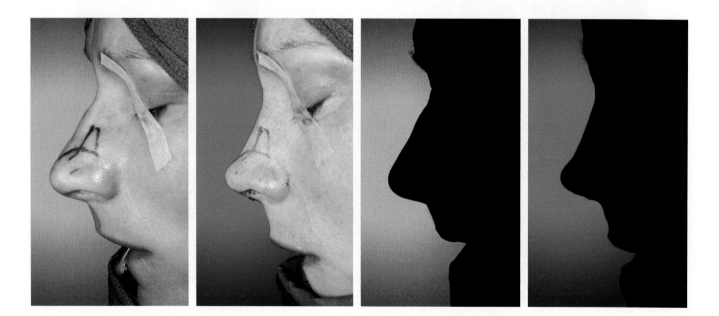

Let your technique-oriented left brain relax, and enjoy the right-brain changes: dorsal reduction and nasal shortening have reduced apparent nasal base size, and the radix graft altered the balance.

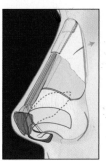

Postoperative Analysis

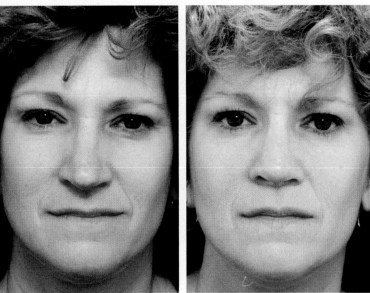

Preoperative   Postoperative

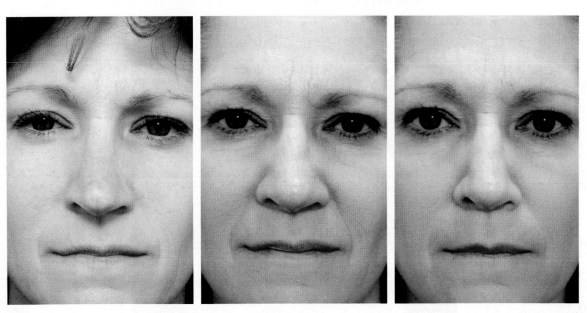

Preoperative   Postoperative   Postoperative with inspiration

Five years postoperatively, the nose is shorter and the patient no longer flares her nostrils to support her airways. The sidewalls are confluent, and even without osteotomy, the width relationship of the upper and lower nasal thirds is appropriate.

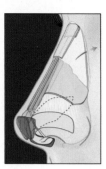

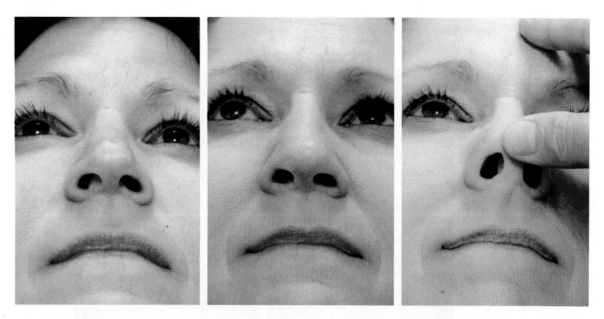

Lateral crural relocation has altered alar wall contour. The tip is symmetrical, the base is unscarred, and the resected and replaced caudal septum supports the columella without relapse of the curvature.

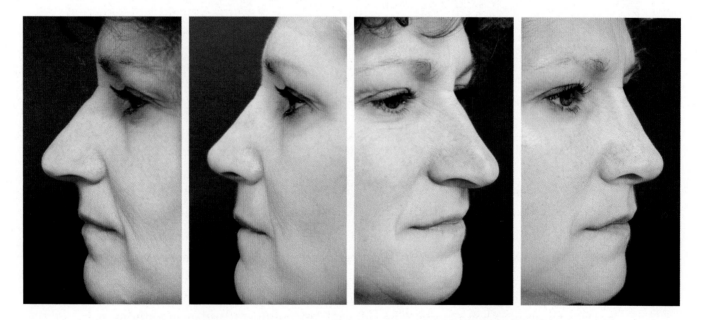

Repositioned lateral crura have ablated the alar wall hollows. Tip grafts have altered tip contour, columellar grafts support the nasal base, and slight nasal shortening and radix grafts have altered nasal balance. Although no skin contraction has occurred (not possible with this skin sleeve), the nose seems smaller. This is the magic of rhinoplasty. The dorsum is still straight, but the aesthetics improve with better balance.

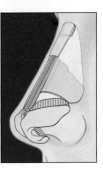

PATIENT STUDY TWO

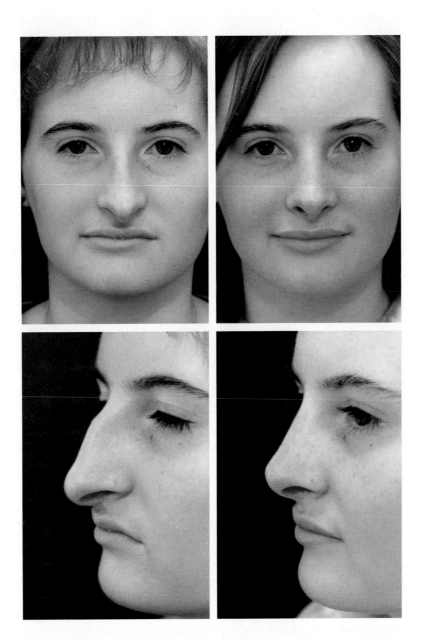

This patient is younger, with thinner skin that arguably will contract more. The upper nose is excessively narrow, the large and long base crowds the upper lip, and the skin sleeve is large. A significant reduction will cost the patient contour. The short nasal bones and narrow middle vault signal a poor airway.

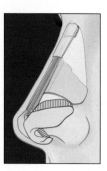

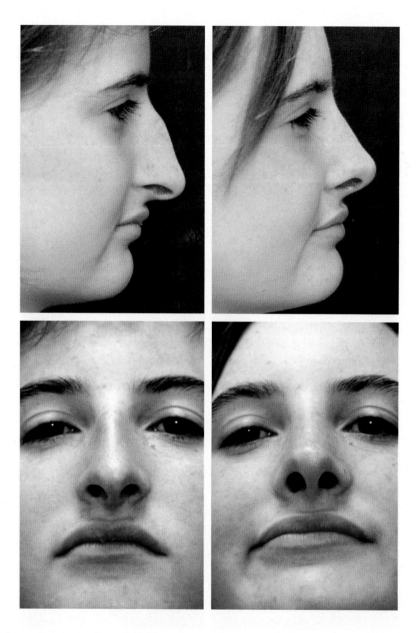

Wide skeletonization, dorsal reduction, submucosal upper lateral cartilage shortening, caudal septal resection, and thin radix and spreader grafts widen and support the new nose and maintain the airway. Postoperatively, dorsal height balances the large base (which seems smaller), and the middle vault is now appropriately wide, bringing the whole frontal view into better proportion. The nose seems to have moved visually cephalad on the patient's face.

PATIENT STUDY THREE

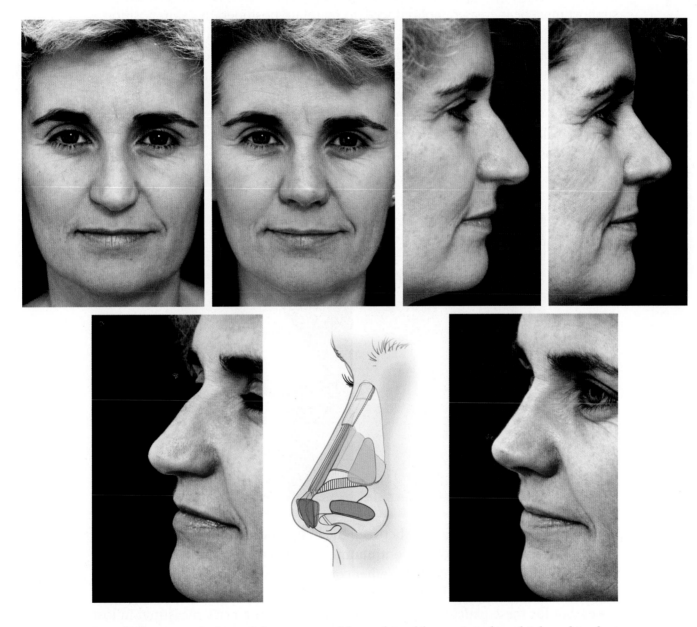

In a different variation of the same problem, this older patient has thicker skin, but with the same low radix/large nasal base. She has a narrow middle vault with a high septal deviation toward the left, and dimples marking the wavy lateral crura. The plan is the same: reduce the deformity, stabilize the airway, and support the skin sleeve, with dorsal reduction, nasal shortening, and radix, spreader, lateral, tip, and alar wall grafts. Twenty months after surgery, the symmetry, airway, and nasal shortening remain.

The long nose has many parallels with the ptotic breast. Both have excess skin relative to underlying support. Unless a surgeon plans to resect skin, the underlying support must be increased, not reduced, to maintain postoperative skin position.

But noncontractile skin may lengthen postoperatively, despite the surgeon's best efforts. Additional secondary shortening or augmentation may improve the result further. As is true in breast surgery, recurrent ptosis may be a problem. Direct skin excision can assist unusual cases (see Chapter 16). The key, however, remains equilibrium: balancing skeletal support to skin sleeve volume. The surgeon who controls the postoperative equilibrium controls the postoperative result.

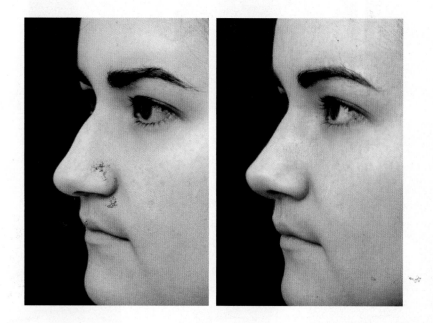

You may not see much difference between the long nose and the large base patient studies, which do occur along a continuum. The difficulty for most patients, and many surgeons, is not technical but rather conceptual. All of the preoperative noses in this section are large, and the patients know it. Their goals are uniformly smaller noses, but for these patients truly smaller noses come at a price measured in lost function, contour, and proportion.

The solution, therefore, is not a philosophical one; that is, it does not depend on whether a surgeon likes large noses or likes small noses. Successful treatment of a long nose/large nasal base requires a strategy that respects what Nature can and cannot do. If thick, large skin sleeves cannot contract, the postoperative plan cannot depend on contraction. During the consultation, these patients' surgical goals must be reframed from "smaller" to "better function, better shape, and better proportion." In doing so, most patients achieve what they believe is a smaller nose, because proportion reduces apparent size; but they may have achieved success by an unexpected route.

BIBLIOGRAPHY

Adamson PA, McGraw-Wall BL, Morrow TA, et al. Vertical dome division in open rhinoplasty. An update on indications, techniques, and results. Arch Otolaryngol Head Neck Surg 120:373-380, 1994.

Adamson PA, Morrow TA. The nasal hinge. Otolaryngol Head Neck Surg 111:219-231, 1994.

Adham MN. A new technique for nasal tip cartilage graft in primary rhinoplasty. Plast Reconstr Surg 97:649-655, 1996.

Aiach G, Levingnac J, Riu R. La Rhinoplastie Esthétique. Paris: Masson, 1989, pp 84-90.

Ali-Salaam P, Kashgarian M, Davila J, et al. Anatomy of the Caucasian alar groove. Plast Reconstr Surg 110:261-266, 2002.

Anderson JR. A reasoned approach to nasal base surgery. Arch Otolaryngol 110:349-358, 1984.

Arregui JS, Elejalde MV, Regalado J, et al. Dynamic rhinoplasty for the plunging nasal tip: functional unity of the inferior third of the nose. Plast Reconstr Surg 106:1624-1629, 2000.

Beekhuis GJ. Nasal tip projection. Eye Ear Nose Throat Mon 51:92-99, 1972.

Beekhuis GJ, Colton JJ. Nasal tip support. Arch Otolaryngol Head Neck Surg 112:726-728, 1986.

Behmand RA, Ghavami A, Guyuron B. Nasal tip sutures part I: the evolution. Plast Reconstr Surg 112:1125-1129, 2003.

Belinfante LS. Nasal tip modification using four distinct methods. J Oral Maxillofac Surg 51:506-516, 1993.

Berman WE. Changing the nasal tip: Part III. Ear Nose Throat J 75:71, 1996.

Berman WE. Changing the nasal tip: Part IV. Ear Nose Throat J 75:131, 1996.

Berman WE. Changing the nasal tip: Part V. Ear Nose Throat J 75:198, 1996.

Berman WE. Changing the nasal tip: Part VI. Ear Nose Throat J 75:280, 1996.

Bernstein L. A basic technique for surgery of the nasal lobule. Otolaryngol Clin North Am 8:599-613, 1975.

Burres S. Tip points: defining the tip. Aesthetic Plast Surg 23:113-118, 1999.

Cachay-Velásquez H. Surgical lengthening of the shot columella: division of the depressor septi muscles. Eur Arch Otorhinolaryngol 249:336-339, 1992.

Cárdenas JC, Carvajal J, Ruiz A. Securing nasal tip rotation through suspension suture technique. Plast Reconstr Surg 117:1750-1755, 2006.

Chait L, Ritz M. A new approach for the refinement of the very broad nasal tip. Br J Plast Surg 44:572-574, 1991.

Close LD, Schaefer SD, Schultz BA. The over-projecting nasal tip: precise reduction without rotation. Laryngoscope 97:931-936, 1987.

Collawn SS, Fix RJ, Moore JR, et al. Nasal cartilage grafts: more than a decade of experience. Plast Reconstr Surg 100:1547-1552, 1997.

Constantian MB. Closed rhinoplasty current techniques, theory, and applications. In Mathes SJ, Hentz VR, eds. Plastic Surgery, vol 2, 2nd ed. Philadelphia: Saunders, 2005, pp 517-572.

Constantian MB. Elaboration of an alternative, segmental, cartilage-sparing tip graft technique, experience in 405 cases. Plast Reconstr Surg 103:237-253, 1999.

Constantian MB. Experience with a three-point method for planning rhinoplasty. Ann Plast Surg 30:1-12, 1993.

Constantian MB. Four common anatomic variants that predispose to unfavorable rhinoplasty results: a study based on 150 consecutive secondary rhinoplasties. Plast Reconstr Surg 105:316-331, 2000.

Constantian MB. Functional effects of alar cartilage malposition. Ann Plast Surg 30:487-499, 1993.

Constantian MB. Grafting the projecting nasal tip. Ann Plast Surg 14:391-402, 1985.

Constantian MB. Indications and use of composite grafts in 100 consecutive secondary and tertiary rhinoplasty patients: introduction of the axial orientation. Plast Reconstr Surg 110:1116-1133, 2002.

Constantian MB. Narrow middle vault and unrecognized alar cartilage malposition: the face of secondary rhinoplasty today. Presented at the New England Society of Plastic and Reconstructive Surgeons, Inc. Lenox, MA, June 2004.

Constantian MB. Rhinoplasty in the graft-depleted patient. Oper Tech Plast Reconstr Surg 2:67-81, 1995.

Constantian MB. The boxy tip, the ball tip, and alar cartilage malposition: variations on a theme—a study in 200 consecutive primary and secondary rhinoplasty patients. Plast Reconstr Surg 116:268-281, 2005.

Constantian MB. The incompetent external nasal valve: pathophysiology and treatment in primary and secondary rhinoplasty. Plast Reconstr Surg 93:919-931, 1994.

Constantian MB. The middorsal notch: an intraoperative guide to overresection in secondary rhinoplasty. Plast Reconstr Surg 91:477-484, 1993.

Constantian MB. The septal angle: a cardinal point in rhinoplasty. Plast Reconstr Surg 85:187-195, 1990.

Constantian MB. The two essential elements for planning tip surgery in primary and secondary rhinoplasty: observations based on review of 100 consecutive patients. Plast Reconstr Surg 114:1571-1581, 2004.

Constantian MB, Clardy RB. The relative importance of septal and nasal valvular surgery in correcting airway obstruction in primary and secondary rhinoplasty. Plast Reconstr Surg 98:38-54, 1996.

Daniel RK. Rhinoplasty: a simplified, three-stitch open tip suture technique. Part I: Primary rhinoplasty. Plast Reconstr Surg 103:1491-1502, 1999.

Daniel RK. Rhinoplasty: a simplified, three-stitch open tip suture technique. Part II: Secondary rhinoplasty. Plast Reconstr Surg 103:1503-1512, 1999.

Daniel RK. Rhinoplasty: creating an aesthetic tip. A preliminary report. Plast Reconstr Surg 80:775-783, 1987.

Daniel RK. Secondary rhinoplasty following open rhinoplasty. Plast Reconstr Surg 96:1539-1546, 1995.

Davidson TM, Murakami WT. Tip suspension suture for superior tip rotation in rhinoplasty. Laryngoscope 93:1076-1080, 1983.

Dayan SH, Kempinars JJ. Treatment of the lower third of the nose and dynamic nasal tip ptosis with Botox. Plast Reconstr Surg 115:1784-1785, 2005.

de la Fuente A, Martin del Yerro JL. Calibrated nasal tip: review of 100 cases. Aesthetic Plast Surg 18:357-361, 1994.

Duarte A, Atilano J, Cuenca R. Apex columellar cartilage graft. Aesthetic Plast Surg 12:217-222, 1988.

Ellis DA, McDonald GA. Narrowing of the wide nasal tip. J Otolaryngol 13:55-57, 1984.

Fanous N. The "light reflex" tip-plasty—a new theory in tip esthetics and tip correction. J Otolaryngol 10:162-168, 1981.

Fanous N. The "light reflex" tip-plasty: surgical application of a new theory in tip esthetics. Laryngoscope 92:310-313, 1982.

Farina R, Cury E, Ackel IA. S-shaped nasal wings: rhinopteroplasty. Case reports. Aesthetic Plast Surg 7:177-178, 1983.

Farina R, Cury E, Ackel IA. The prominent nasal tip. Aesthetic Plast Surg 8:141-144, 1984.

Farkas LG, Kolar JC. Anthropometrics and art in the aesthetics of women's faces. Clin Plast Surg 14:599-616, 1987.

Farkas LG, Munro IR. Anthropometric Facial Proportions in Medicine. Springfield, IL: Charles C. Thomas, 1986.

Foda HM. Management of the droopy tip: a comparison of three alar cartilage-modifying techniques. Plast Reconstr Surg 112:1408-1417, 2003.

Fredricks S. Tripod resection for "Pinocchio" nose deformity. Plast Reconstr Surg 53:531-533, 1974.

Friedman WH, Biller HF. Evaluation of nasal tip surgery. Laryngoscope 85:1539-1549, 1975.

Garcia-Velasco J, Garcia-Velasco M. Tip graft from the cartilaginous dorsum in rhinoplasty. Aesthetic Plast Surg 10:21-25, 1986.

Ghavami A, Janis JE, Guyuron B. Regarding the treatment of dynamic nasal tip ptosis with botulinum toxin A. Plast Reconstr Surg 118:263-264, 2006.

Ghilardi C. An approach to nasal tip remodeling. Aesthet Surg J 21:345-348, 2001.

Giunta SX. Nasal tip surgery—a simple technique to aid in symmetry. Laryngoscope 94:974-976, 1984.

Goldman IB. The importance of the mesial crura in nasal-tip reconstruction. AMA Arch Otolaryngol 65:143-147, 1957.

Goode RL, Ross J. Columellar advancement for nasal tip elevation. Laryngoscope 83:1123-1127, 1973.

Gruber RP, Friedman GD. Suture algorithm for the broad or bulbous nasal tip. Plast Reconstr Surg 110:1752-1764, 2002.

946

Gruber RP, Grover S. The anatomic tip graft for nasal augmentation. Plast Reconstr Surg 103:1744-1753, 1999.

Gruber RP, Nahai F, Bogdan MA, et al. Changing the convexity and concavity of nasal cartilages and cartilage grafts with horizontal mattress sutures: Part I. Experimental results. Plast Reconstr Surg 115:589-594, 2005.

Gryskiewicz JM. The "iatrogenic-hanging columella": preserving columellar contour after tip retroprojection. Plast Reconstr Surg 110:272-277, 2002.

Guerrero-Santos J. Cosmetic repair of the acute columellar-lip angle. Plast Reconstr Surg 52:246-249, 1973.

Gunter JP. The tripod concept for correcting nasal-tip cartilages. Aesthet Surg J 24:257-260, 2004.

Gunter JP, Friedman RM. Lateral crural strut graft: technique in clinical applications in rhinoplasty. Plast Reconstr Surg 99:943-952, 1997.

Gunter JP, Rohrich RJ. Correction of the pinched nasal tip with alar spreader grafts. Plast Reconstr Surg 90:821-829, 1992.

Gunter JP, Rohrich RJ. External approach for secondary rhinoplasty. Plast Reconstr Surg 80:161-174, 1987.

Guyuron B, Behmand RA. Nasal tip sutures part II: the interplays. Plast Reconstr Surg 112:1130-1145, 2003.

Guyuron B, Poggi JT, Michelow BJ. The subdomal graft. Plast Reconstr Surg 113:1037-1040, 2004.

Ha RY, Byrd HS. Septal extension grafts revisited: 6-year experience in controlling nasal tip projection and shape. Plast Reconstr Surg 112:1929-1935, 2003.

Hamra ST. Crushed cartilage grafts over alar dome reduction in open rhinoplasty. Plast Reconstr Surg 92:352-356, 1993.

Hamra ST. Repositioning the lateral alar crus. Plast Reconstr Surg 92:1244-1253, 1993.

Hinderer UT. Relationship between the protrusion of the nasal tip and the dorsum in rhinoplasty. Aesthetic Plast Surg 8:201-212, 1984.

Hoefflin SM. Geometric sculpturing of the thick nasal tip. Aesthetic Plast Surg 18:247-251, 1994.

Hubbard TJ. Exploiting the septum for maximal tip control. Ann Plast Surg 44:173-180, 2000.

Ishida LC, Ishida J, Henrique Ishida L, et al. Total reconstruction of the alar cartilages with a partially split septal cartilage graft. Ann Plast Surg 45:481-484, 2000.

Janeke JB, Wright WK. Studies on the support of the nasal tip. Arch Otolaryngol 93:458-464, 1971.

Johnson CM, Toriumi DM. Open structure rhinoplasty: featured technical points and long term follow-up. Facial Plast Surg Clin North Am 1:1-22, 1993.

Kamer FM, Churukian MM. Shield graft for the nasal tip. Arch Otolaryngol 110:608-610, 1984.

Kamer FM, Churukian MM, Hansen L. The nasal bossa: a complication of rhinoplasty. Laryngoscope 96:303-307, 1986.

Kridel RW, Konior RJ, Shumrick KA, et al. Advances in nasal tip surgery. The lateral crural steal. Arch Otolaryngol Head Neck Surg 115:1206-1212, 1989.

Kuran I, Tümerdem B, Tosun U, et al. Evaluation of the effects of tip-binding sutures and cartilaginous grafts on tip projection and rotation. Plast Reconstr Surg 116:282-288, 2005.

Larabee WF Jr. The tripod concept. Arch Otolaryngol Head Neck Surg 115:1168-1169, 1989.

Mavili ME, Safak T. Use of umbrella graft for nasal tip support. Aesthetic Plast Surg 17:163-166, 1993.

McCollough EG, English JL. A new twist in nasal tip surgery. An alternative to the Goldman tip for the wide or bulbous lobule. Arch Otolaryngol 111:524-529, 1985.

McCollough EG, Mangat D. Systematic approach to correction of the nasal tip in rhinoplasty. Arch Otolaryngol 107:12-16, 1981.

McKinney P. Management of the bulbous nose. Plast Reconstr Surg 106:906-917, 2000.

McKinney P, Stalnecker M. Surgery for the bulbous nasal tip. Ann Plast Surg 11:106-113, 1983.

Micheli-Pellegrini V. Archivio Italiano di Otologia, Rinologia e Laringologia, Revista Italiana Di Chirurgia Plastica, 1975.

Micheli-Pellegrini V. Cause D'Insuccesso Nella Chirurgia Estetica Del Naso, Revista Italiana Di Chirurgia Plastica, 1974.

Micheli-Pellegrini V. LaTecnica Per Correggere la Punta Durante La Rinoplastica, Revista Italiana Di Chirurgia Plastica, 1990.

Millard DR Jr. Corrective rhinoplasty and augmentation mentoplasty. In Grabb WC, and Smith JR, eds. Plastic Surgery: A Concise Guide to Clinical Practice. Boston: Little Brown, 1968, p 510.

Mir y Mir L. Dissection of the medial crura as a standard procedure in rhinoplasty: case studies. Aesthetic Plast Surg 11:203-205, 1987.

Mischkowski RA, Kübler AC. Correction of congenital nasal hypoplasia associated with Kallmann syndrome using self-inflating injectable tissue expander pellets. Plast Reconstr Surg 118:1147-1452, 2006.

Mittelman H. A more precise technique of tip rhinoplasty with a cartilage-splitting incision. Arch Otolaryngol 107:425-427, 1981.

Mocella S, Bianchi N. Double interdomal suture in nasal tip sculpturing. Facial Plast Surg 13:179-196, 1997.

Muti E. Treatment of alar cartilages: should the "domes" be interrupted? Aesthetic Plast Surg 17:193-198, 1993.

Nagel F. Tip surgery and functional rhinoplasty. Facial Plast Surg 11:191-203, 1995.

Neu BR. Reduction of nasal tip projection with medial rotation of alar cartilages. Plast Reconstr Surg 108:763-770, 2001.

Ortiz-Monasterio F, Olmedo A, Oscoy LO. The use of cartilage grafts in primary aesthetic rhinoplasty. Plast Reconstr Surg 67:597-605, 1981.

Papel ID. A graduated method of tip graft fixation in rhinoplasty. Arch Otolaryngol Head Neck Surg 121:623-626, 1995.

Papel ID, Mabrie DC. Deprojecting the nasal profile. Otolaryngol Clin North Am 32:65-87, 1999.

Parkes ML, Kamer FM, Merrin ML. "Practical suggestions on facial plastic surgery—how I do it." Modifications of the Fomon technique in the approach to the lower lobule. Laryngoscope 87:1774-1778, 1977.

Peck G. The difficult nasal tip. Clin Plast Surg 4:103-110, 1977.

Peck GC. The onlay tip graft for nasal tip projection. Plast Reconstr Surg 71:27-39, 1983.

Pensler JM. The septal strut for nasal projection following closed rhinoplasty. Aesthet Surg J 26:275-279, 2006.

Petroff MA, McCollough EG, Hom D, et al. Nasal tip projection. Quantitative changes following rhinoplasty. Arch Otolaryngol Head Neck Surg 117:783-788, 1991.

Pitanguy I. Revisiting the dermocartilaginous ligament. Plast Reconstr Surg 107:264-266, 2001.

Pitanguy I, Salgado F, Radwanski HN, et al. The surgical importance of the dermocartilaginous ligament of the nose. Plast Reconstr Surg 95:790-794, 1995.

Psillakis JM. O papel da crus medial nas rhinoplastias. Folha De Cirurgia Plastica 80:6, 1980.

Rafaty FM. Correction of the over-projecting nasal tip by the suture technique. Arch Otolaryngol 103:361-364, 1977.

Randall P. The direct approach to the "hanging columella." Plast Reconstr Surg 53:544-547, 1974.

Raspall G, González-Lagunas J. Management of the nasal tip by open rhinoplasty. J Craniomaxillofac Surg 24:145-150, 1996.

Rees TD, LaTrenta GS. Aesthetic Plastic Surgery, 2nd ed. Philadelphia: WB Saunders, 1994, pp 159-244.

Regalado-Briz A. Aesthetic rhinoplasty with maximum preservation of the alar cartilages: experience with 52 consecutive cases. Plast Reconstr Surg 103:671-680, 1999.

Regalado-Briz A. Cephalo-crural suture: a new way to deal with supratip fullness. Aesthet Surg J 25:481-488, 2005.

Rich JS, Friedman WH, Pearlman SJ. The effects of lower lateral cartilage excision on nasal tip projection. Arch Otolaryngol 117:56-59, 1991.

Ricketts RM. Divine proportion in facial esthetics. Clin Plast Surg 9:401-422, 1982.

Rohrich RJ, Adams WP Jr. The boxy nasal tip: classification and management based on alar cartilage suturing techniques. Plast Reconstr Surg 107:1849-1863, 2001.

Rohrich RJ, Griffin JR. Correction of intrinsic nasal tip asymmetries in primary rhinoplasty. Plast Reconstr Surg 112:1699-1712, 2003.

Rohrich RJ, Gunter JP, Adams WP Jr, eds. Graduated approach to tip projection in rhinoplasty. In Dallas Rhinoplasty: Nasal Surgery by the Masters. St Louis: Quality Medical Publishing, 2002, pp 333-358.

Rohrich RJ, Gunter JP, Friedman RM. Nasal tip blood supply: an anatomic study validating the safety of the transcolumellar incision in rhinoplasty. Plast Reconstr Surg 95:795-799, 1995.

Rohrich RJ, Janis JE, Kenkel JM. Male rhinoplasty. Plast Reconstr Surg 112:1071-1085, 2003.

Rohrich RJ, Muzaffar AR, Gunter JP. Nasal tip blood supply: confirming the safety of the transcolumellar incision in rhinoplasty. Plast Reconstr Surg 106:1640-1641, 2000.

Rubin FF. Controlled tip sculpting with the morselizer. Arch Otolaryngol 109:160-163, 1983.

Safian J. The split-cartilage tip technique of rhinoplasty. Plast Reconstr Surg 45:217-220, 1970.

Sheen JH. Achieving more nasal tip projection by use of a small autogenous vomer or septal cartilage graft. A preliminary report. Plast Reconstr Surg 56:35-40, 1975.

Sheen JH. Middle crus: The missing link in alar cartilage anatomy. Perspect Plast Surg 5:31-53, 1991.

Sheen JH. Tip graft: A 20-year retrospective. Plast Reconstr Surg 91:48-63, 1993.

Sheen JH, Sheen AP. Aesthetic Rhinoplasty, 2nd ed. St Louis: CV Mosby, 1987.

Smith GA. Tip refinement in upturned noses. Ear Nose Throat J 62:14-23, 1983.

Smith RA, Smith ET. A new technique in nasal-tip reduction surgery. Plast Reconstr Surg 108:1798-1804, 2001.

Smith TW. Thoughtful nasal tip surgery. Arch Otolaryngol 97:244-246, 1973.

Spina V, Kamakura L, Psillakis J. A new method for correction of the prominent nasal tip. Plast Reconstr Surg 51:416-420, 1973.

Tardy ME, Cheng E. Transdomal suture refinement of the nasal tip. Facial Plast Surg 4:317-326, 1987.

Tardy ME Jr, Patt BS, Walter MA. Transdomal suture refinement of the nasal tip: long-term outcomes. Facial Plast Surg 9:275-284, 1993.

Tasman AJ, Helbig M. Sonography of nasal tip anatomy and surgical tip refinement. Plast Reconstr Surg 105:2573-2579, 2000.

Tebbetts JB. Letter to the editor. Plast Reconstr Surg 95:772-773, 1995.

Tebbetts JB. Rethinking the logic and techniques of primary tip rhinoplasty: a perspective of the evolution of surgery of the nasal tip. Otolaryngol Clin North Am 32:741-754, 1999.

Tebbetts JB. Shaping and positioning the nasal tip without structural disruption: a new systematic approach. Plast Reconstr Surg 94:61-77, 1994.

Uhm KI, Hwang SH, Choi BG. Cleft lip nose correction with onlay calvarial bone graft and suture suspension in Oriental patients. Plast Reconstr Surg 105:499-503, 2000.

Vuyk HD. Suture tip plasty. Rhinology 33:30-38, 1995.

Webster RC, Davidson TM, Rubin FF, et al. Nasal tip projection changes related to cheeks and lip. Arch Otolaryngol 104:16-21, 1978.

Webster RC, White MF, Courtiss EH. Nasal tip correction in rhinoplasty. Plast Reconstr Surg 51:384-396, 1973.

Williams JE. Pinched nasal tip. Clin Plast Surg 4:41-45, 1977.

CHAPTER 16

Exceptions to the Usual

Through tattr'd clothes small vices do appear;
Robes and furred gowns hide all. . . .

WILLIAM SHAKESPEARE
King Lear

A few naturalists . . . who have already begun to doubt
upon the immutability of species, may be influenced by
this volume; but I look with confidence to the future,
to young and rising naturalists, who will be able to
view both sides of the equation with impartiality. . . .

CHARLES DARWIN
On the Origin of Species by Means of Natural Selection

They don't make mirrors like they used to. . . .

TALLULAH BANKHEAD

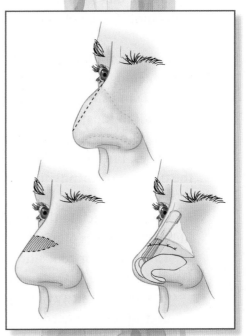

The Traumatized Nose

There is no nasal deformity for which prioritization is more important than the traumatized or crooked nose. The traumatized nose is already damaged—its skeleton is deformed and potentially unstable, and its soft tissues are scarred. Scarring of the soft tissues is important for both patients and surgeons to remember, because some soft tissue changes may have become irreversible. Every type of nasal trauma, whether surgically deliberate or accidental, precipitates a wound-healing cascade, part of which involves soft tissue changes. Even if the surgeon could magically replace every bit of cartilage and bone where it ideally belonged, the patient's soft tissues may be incapable of following those changes. Thus soft tissue deformity might remain even if skeletal deformity does not.

But it is worse than that, because only rarely can the surgeon place every skeletal structure where it belongs—the skeleton itself has often undergone irreversible changes. Although surgeons and patients may be acutely aware of the problems associated with correcting septal deviation and overcoming "cartilage memory," trauma may have created additional abnormal stresses in the upper or lower lateral cartilages, making symmetry difficult to achieve even if those structures were radically mobilized, positioned, and fixed by sutures or wires.

Finally, although not always discussed, the more aggressive techniques for septal straightening can be hazardous. Surgeons who fracture, score, or cut the dorsal septal strut, and surgeons who resect the entire septum, divide and reassemble it, and replace it in the midline, have reported impressive results. However, the complications of those techniques are not often described in the same vigorous detail as the successes, but they do occur, even in expert hands, and range from recurrence of the original deformity to complete septal collapse.

My own approach to the traumatized crooked nose is based on the principles used in the many cases of nasal asymmetry already described in this book:
1. Remove or reposition deviated or deformed skeletal parts that either obstruct the airway or mar the desired aesthetic result.
2. Clear the airway of septal obstruction.
3. Harvest the needed augmentation materials.
4. Graft to reestablish function, nasal equilibrium, proportion, and symmetry.

In planning these surgeries, my priorities are always safety, predictable function, and aesthetics, in that order, even though a patient's presenting complaint may be only cosmetic. In proposing and explaining my plan to a patient, I demonstrate the deformities that the previous trauma has created and discuss the surgical alternatives. I indicate that I cannot weaken or move every asymmetrical structure, because some of them are supporting the nose. I explain my priorities, and in doing so I reassure patients that, in following them, the chances of septal collapse or other catastrophe are quite remote, that nasal function will be maximized, and that I will try to create the best possible shape, *but that some asymmetry will probably remain.* Most patients readily understand (and support) the logic of a highly safe operation, even if it leaves residual asymmetry.

In that regard, when a concavity must be camouflaged by augmentation, I have learned to undercorrect rather than overcorrect. Patients accept a residual asymmetry to which they have become accustomed over a more symmetrical nose that has now become much wider.

Finally, it is important to remember that asymmetrical noses require asymmetrical strategies. When performing analysis and setting a plan, it is easiest to divide the crooked nose into thirds (bony vault, upper cartilaginous vault, and lower cartilaginous vault and caudal septum), as in the table below.

Strategies for Correcting an Asymmetrical Nose

Nasal Area	Basic Technique	Ancillary Techniques
Upper third Bony vault	Unilateral osteotomy	Lateral onlay graft (preferably ethmoid) Dorsal onlay graft
Middle third Upper cartilaginous vault	Unilateral spreader graft Unequally thick spreader grafts	Lateral onlay graft Dorsal onlay graft
Lower third Lower cartilaginous vault	Realign lateral crura Asymmetrical tip grafts	Onlays to lateral crura/alar walls
Caudal septum	Resect and replace caudal septum	Columellar grafts for contour

BONY VAULT

If the bony vault is shifted, bilateral osteotomies narrow the upper nose but the shift remains. A unilateral osteotomy (on the outfractured side) coupled with an onlay to the depressed side usually works better.

Bony vault onlays must be flawless; the unyielding bed is unforgiving. Deformities become obvious, and eyeglasses become uncomfortable. Choose your graft wisely: ethmoid is excellent, ear cartilage (solid or crushed) is not.

UPPER CARTILAGINOUS VAULT

A surgeon must remember the functional deficit manifested by sidewalls distorted by septal deviation. Unilateral or asymmetrically thick spreader grafts correct the functional and aesthetic abnormalities.

The most common combination for the upper and middle vaults (the middle third) is therefore a unilateral osteotomy (on the outfractured side), combined with a substantial spreader graft for the contralateral collapsed middle vault (adding onlays as needed).

Depending on dorsal height, it may also be helpful to place a dorsal onlay graft over the upper and middle thirds to camouflage underlying asymmetries.

LOWER CARTILAGINOUS VAULT AND CAUDAL SEPTUM

Realign the lateral crura if they are asymmetrical, place onlay grafts to fill the sidewall depressions and support the external valves, place multiple tip grafts asymmetrically to create a balanced tip, and resect and replace a deflected caudal septum, adding additional onlay columellar grafts for contour. (These techniques are detailed in Chapters 11 and 12.)

The exact shape of the nasal skeleton—asymmetrically resected, rotated, supported, or camouflaged—is irrelevant as long as it creates a stable, open airway and an attractive nasal shape.

The following cases are presented in order of asymmetry (other cases are presented in Part V, Secondary Rhinoplasty).

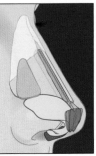

PATIENT STUDY ONE

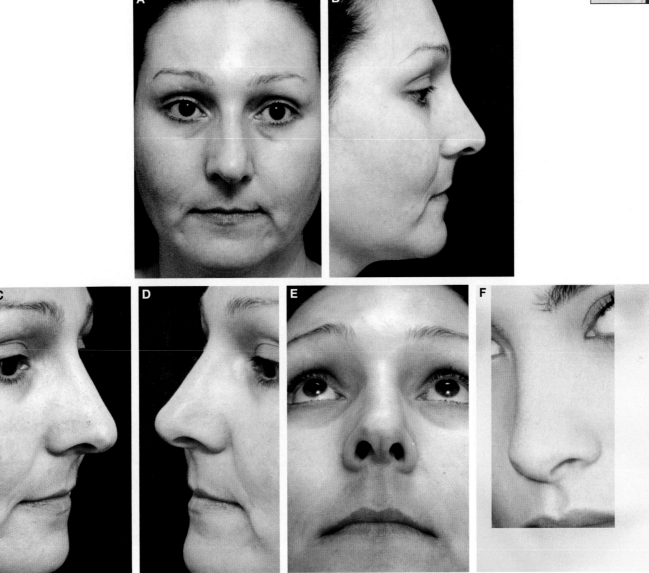

In this young woman, the most striking asymmetry is located in the middle third, accompanying the high septal deviation toward the left. The bony vault is almost midline and the caudal septum is centered.

However, notice the position of the lateral crura on the frontal and the oblique views: the left lateral crus is malpositioned (cephalically rotated), whereas the right lateral crus is orthotopic. Notice also the tip lobular configuration imparted by this asymmetry: the left side of the tip is inadequately projecting *(C)*, whereas the right side is adequately projecting *(D* and *E)*. The patient requested a slightly lower dorsum and symmetrical, adequate tip projection *(F)*.

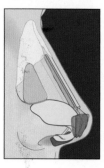

SUMMARY OF THE SURGICAL PLAN

1. Minimal skeletonization

2. Slight reduction of cartilaginous dorsum; no reduction of bony vault

3. Retrograde reduction of right orthotopic lateral crus

4. Dissection and relocation of left malpositioned lateral crus as flap

5. Transfixing incision, slight shortening of membranous septum

6. Septoplasty

7. Asymmetrical spreader grafts (a curved, thinner graft on the left with convexity facing toward the right, and a straight, thicker graft on the right)

8. Three crushed tip grafts

9. Columellar graft for contour

10. Left osteotomy

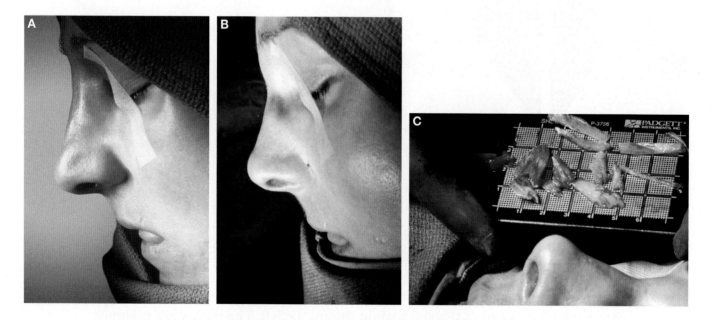

After relocating the left lateral crus and a slight dorsal reduction, the tip was brought into relief *(B)*. Septoplasty yielded excellent building materials *(C)*.

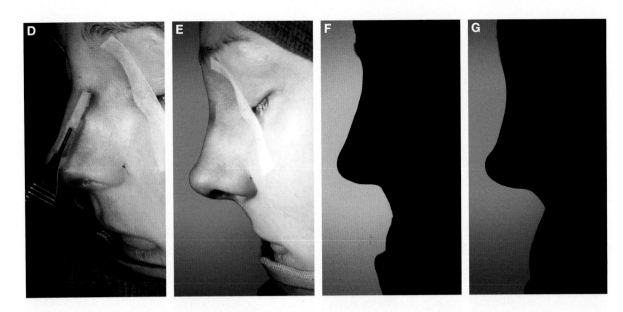

The curved piece in the upper right of the grid will form a large spreader graft to force the high septal deviation toward the right *(D)*. Tip and columellar grafts added support, symmetry, and contour *(E and G)*.

Postoperative Analysis

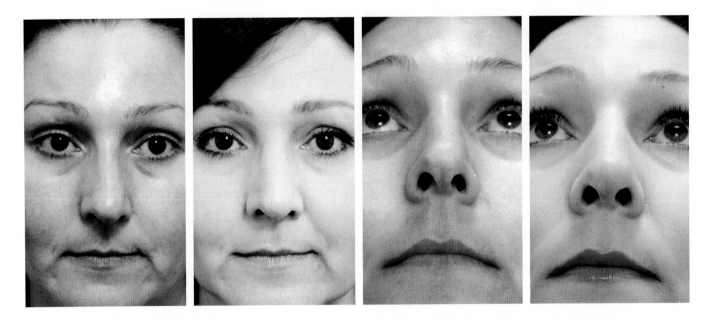

Five years after surgery, and without an onlay graft, spreader grafts have realigned the high septal deviation. The left osteotomy has repositioned the bony vault. Slight dorsal reduction and tip grafts have altered the nasal profile slightly, adding tip projection but leaving a straight dorsum. The lateral crura are now symmetrical, confirmed on frontal and oblique views, and the oblique views are now symmetrical.

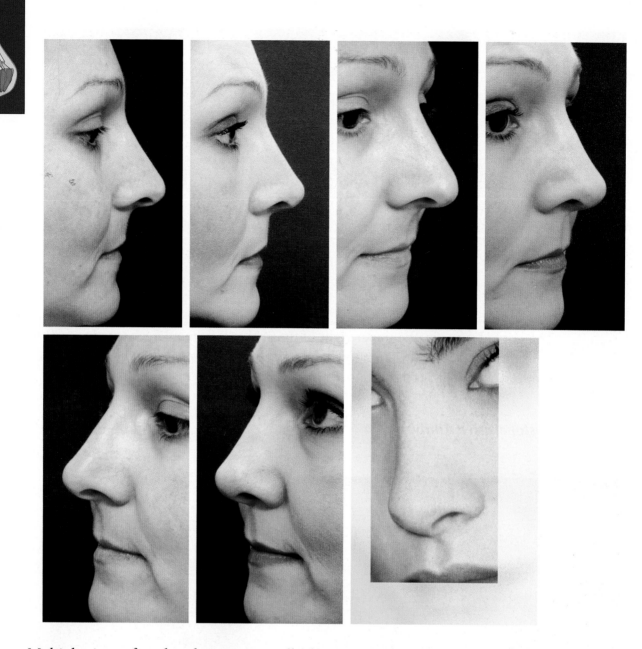

Multiple tip grafts, placed asymmetrically, have augmented the right side more than the left. Geometric mean postoperative airflow increased 12.5 times over preoperative values.

The oblique views demonstrate the relative positions of the bony vault, middle vault, and tip better than any others, but they differ when the nose is asymmetrical. Postoperative obliques therefore demonstrate how much symmetry—or residual asymmetry—exists.

PATIENT STUDY TWO

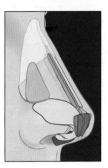

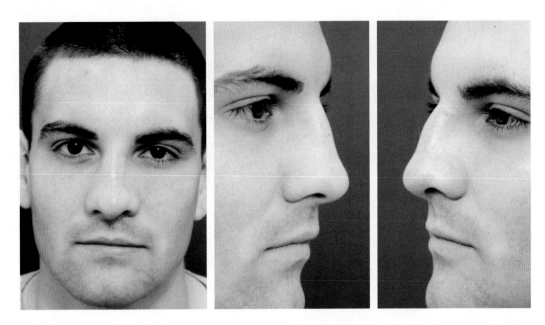

In this patient, whose tip is symmetrical and adequately projecting, previous sports injuries have displaced the bony and cartilaginous vaults toward the right. Because the bony vault has shifted, the dorsal hump seems higher on the patient's right compared with his left. Although the caudal septum is not dislocated, the columella is soft and will be supported by an onlay graft.

SUMMARY OF THE SURGICAL PLAN

1. Minimal skeletonization
2. Bony vault reduction with rasp, deepening high radix
3. Cartilaginous dorsal reduction with knife
4. No modification of alar cartilages
5. Septoplasty
6. Left spreader graft
7. Columellar graft (unsupported caudal septum)
8. Tip grafts
9. Right osteotomy

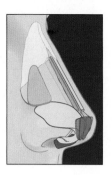

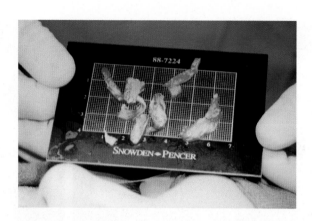

Septoplasty yielded a specimen that was largely calcified and distorted, which is the result of the patient's previous trauma. Fortunately, not many grafts are required.

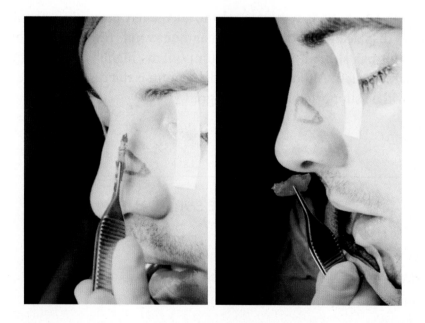

A thick left spreader graft was placed. Notice that the middle vault depression was marked before the procedure, denoting the location for an onlay graft. The best remaining piece supports the columella.

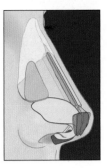

Postoperative Analysis

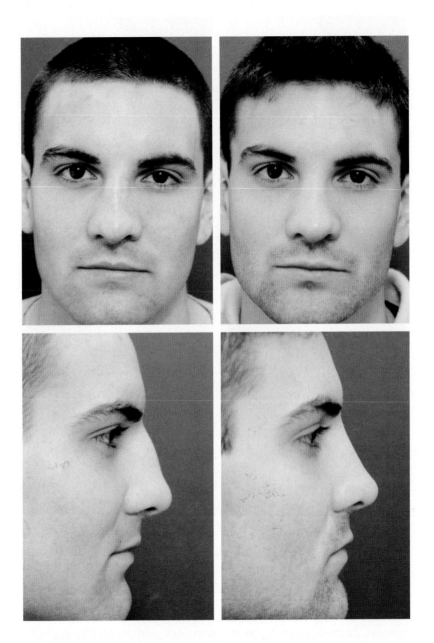

When the septum has been displaced to this degree, it is almost impossible to bring the bony vault to the midline, because the displaced septum blocks movement of the right sidewall. For a young, athletic man who intends to remain highly active in competitive contact sports, I leave a dorsal strut that is 25 to 30 mm wide for future protection. Because the airstream flows along the floor and over the middle turbinate, the dorsal strut does not block airflow. The postoperative dorsum is straight, and the tip is more refined.

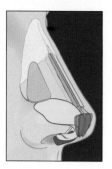

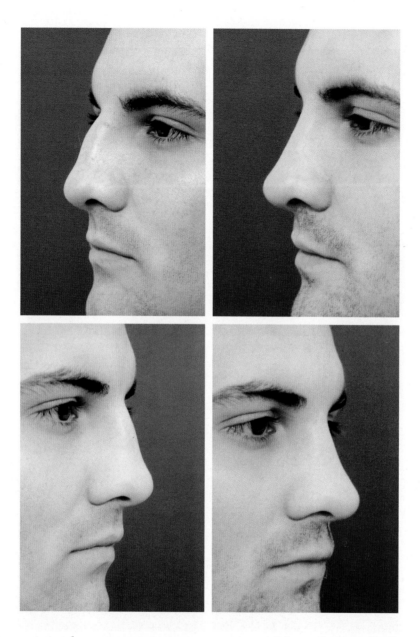

The oblique views demonstrate greater symmetry, although the right bony vault is still slightly higher than the left, and the left middle vault is slightly more concave than the right. Both airways are now widely patent, and the nose is stable for all of the patient's future athletic activities.

PATIENT STUDY THREE

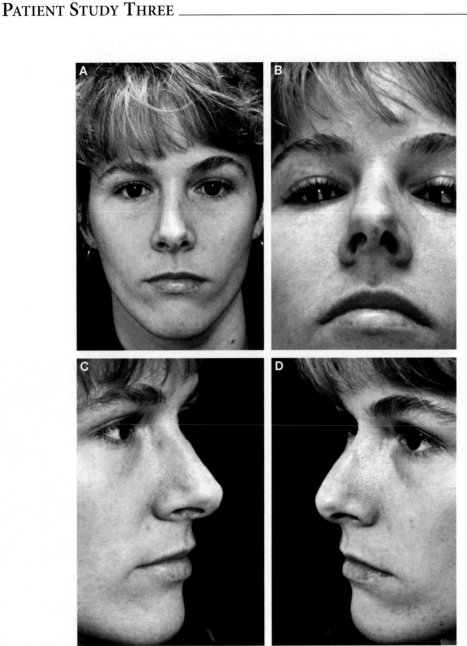

Unlike the previous patient, this woman's radix is low and her tip is inadequately projecting. Notice the difference in nasal contour. The base seems disproportionately large. The nose seems to arch downward, particularly in the left oblique view. The caudal septum is deflected into the right airway and therefore must be resected and replaced *(B).* Notice the asymmetry in the matching oblique views. Finally, notice the axes of the cephalically rotated lateral crura and the alar hollows that they create. Because the malpositioned cartilages are not deforming, they will be left in position, but their functional and cosmetic effects will be corrected.

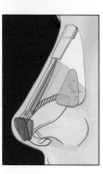

SUMMARY OF THE SURGICAL PLAN

1. Minimal skeletonization
2. Reduction of bony and cartilaginous dorsa
3. Resection of dislocated caudal septum and replacement as free graft
4. Retrograde reduction of alar cartilage lateral crura
5. Septoplasty
6. Left unilateral spreader graft
7. Left onlay graft
8. Radix graft
9. Multiple tip grafts
10. Right osteotomy

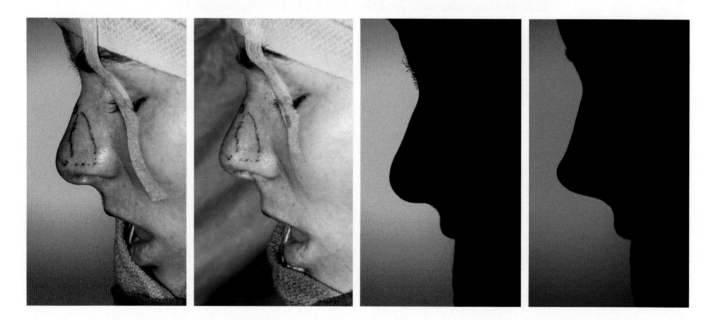

Notice that after the dorsal and tip resections, the nasal configuration has changed very little. This is typical of the low radix–inadequate tip projection combination. The nose cannot assume a new shape until the radix and tip have been supported.

Silhouettes dramatize the effect of dorsal and tip reduction, and radix and tip grafts, on nasal balance. The postoperative nose seems smaller and less bottom heavy.

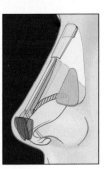

Postoperative Analysis

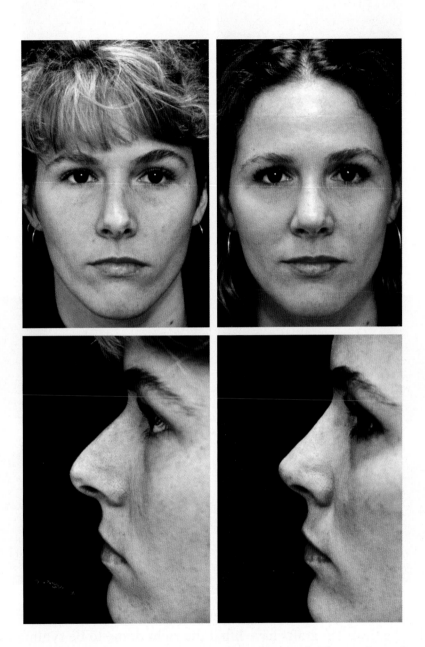

Two years postoperatively, the nose remains symmetrical. The unilateral osteotomy has created bony vault symmetry. The left spreader graft and onlay have created middle vault symmetry.

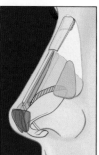

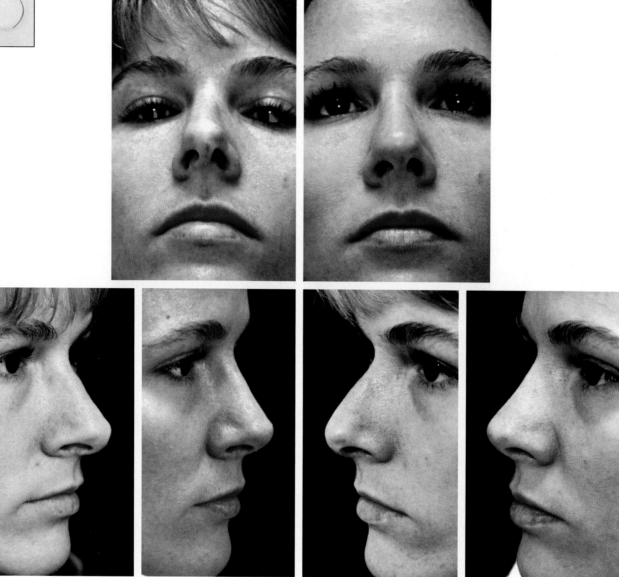

Despite significant preoperative asymmetry, the matching postoperative obliques are nearly identical. Tip grafts have lifted the right dome to be symmetrical with the left; the radix graft has reduced apparent nasal base size; and dorsal reduction, left spreader grafts, and onlay grafts have improved middle vault symmetry and camouflaged the high septal deviation. Slight lateral crural reduction, tip grafts, and caudal septal relocation have created nasal base (lower-third) symmetry. Remember that a small size without proportion or contour delicacy is not a victory.

966

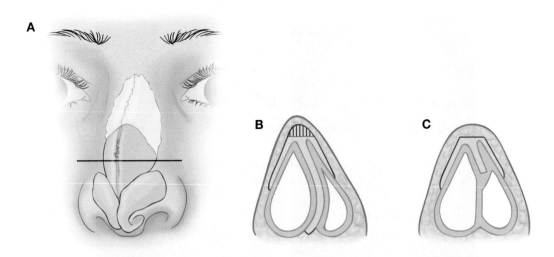

As this figure shows, dorsal resection favors a straighter nose. When the deviated nose has a convex bridge *(A)*, the nasal hump is often its most asymmetrical part *(B)*. By reducing bridge height, the surgeon also removes the area of greatest deflection and therefore makes a straighter nose even before performing other maneuvers *(C)*.

Conversely, when the nasal dorsum is low and asymmetrical relative to a large nasal base, the surgeon can frequently achieve more symmetry by camouflaging the deflection with a straight dorsal graft or by aligning the anterior septal edge with spreader grafts. The strategy for achieving symmetry therefore depends in part on whether the nasal dorsum is convex or concave, and therefore on the relationship of nasal bridge height to nasal base size.

Deflection of the septal angle is another frequent cause of malalignment, particularly of the nasal base. Septal angle resection releases soft tissues of the nasal tip, allowing them to move toward the midline. However, septal angle or dorsal resection sufficient to correct an asymmetry may simultaneously produce a nasal bridge that is now too low and therefore requires augmentation to reestablish postoperative balance and middle vault support. Asymmetrically thick spreader grafts can also align a deflected caudal septum or septal angle.

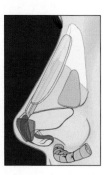

PATIENT STUDY FOUR

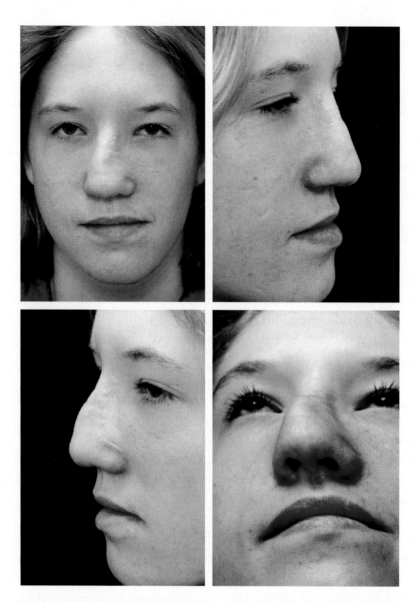

Some cases of previous trauma present unique problems. This young woman had sustained multiple injuries as a young child. The significant deviation of her bony and upper cartilaginous vaults is obvious. The caudal septum was dislocated, resulting in a retrusive maxillary arch and retracted columella. Her skin is scarred, and the oblique views are grossly different.

In this case, significant dorsal reduction is needed just to remove the deformity. The surgeon also can anticipate that a septum that is so scarred, calcified, and criss-crossed with fracture lines is unlikely to yield a good dorsal graft. Spreader grafts cannot align such a crooked nose. The approach, therefore, is to reduce the dorsum enough to decrease the deformity, and then to rebuild the dorsum, tip, columella, and maxillary arch by augmentation.

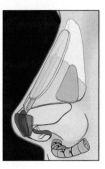

SUMMARY OF THE SURGICAL PLAN

1. Harvest calvarial bone graft
2. Harvest ear cartilage
3. Gore-Tex maxillary augmentation
4. Dorsal reduction
5. Septoplasty to clear the airway
6. Calvarial bone dorsal graft
7. Onlay graft of calvarial bone to left middle vault
8. Ear cartilage caudal support graft
9. Multiple tip grafts

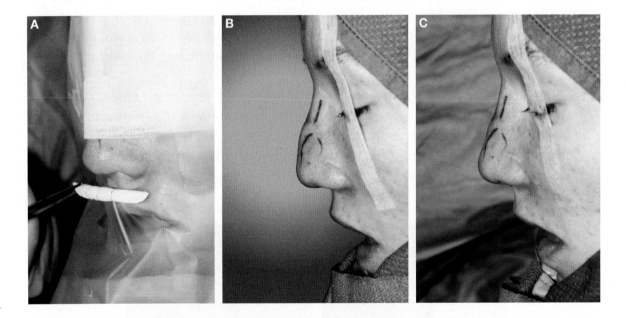

Gore-Tex was rolled into an implant to be placed through an incision in the right nasal floor into a subperiosteal pocket at the base of the piriform aperture. Before insertion, the patient's eyes were protected with gauze and the nasal base was isolated from the skin with a plastic drape *(A)*. My hands did not touch the patient's skin before I inserted the implant. Immediately on placement, the upper lip and nasal base moved forward (*B* and *C*).

969

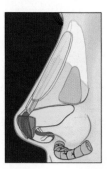

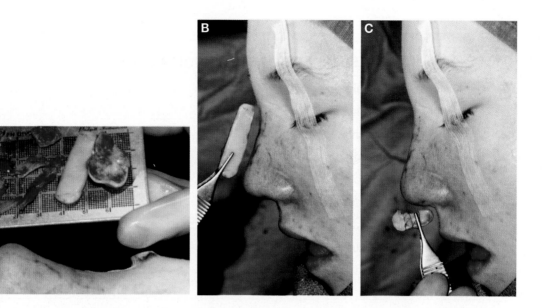

Dorsal reduction reduced the deformity, but the nose was small and soft, and the soft tissues were unsupported. The septal specimen can be seen the left side of the grid *(A)*; notice that most of the pieces were distorted or bony. Ear cartilage (right of grid) was used to support the base and tip. A calvarial graft was sized, and its edges were lightly beveled *(B)*. After placement, dorsal length was appropriate.

A boot-shaped graft was constructed from ear cartilage to replace the absent caudal septum (destroyed by trauma), according to Sheen's method *(C)*. This graft was placed through an incision in the membranous septum, replacing the caudal septum to the septal angle. In doing so, the graft moved the nasal base forward and provided normal support and firmness to the columella.

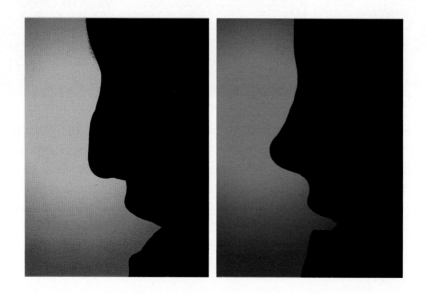

Silhouettes dramatize the changes in nasal proportion and shape that occurred.

Postoperative Analysis

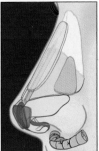

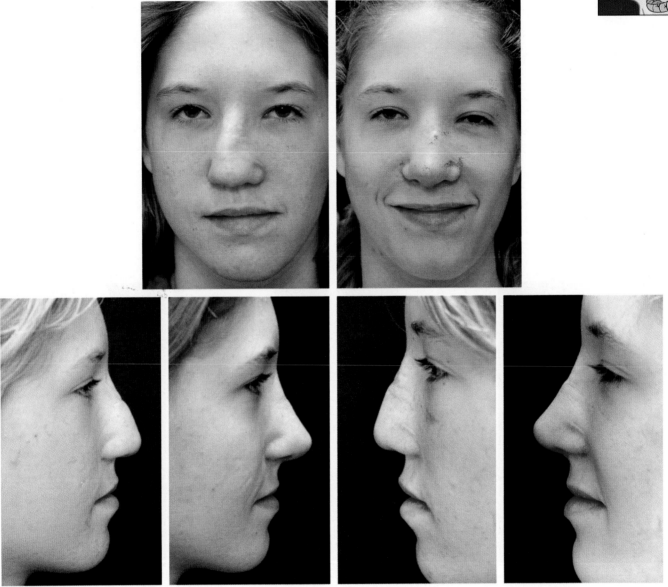

One year postoperatively, the nose remains straight. Although the dorsal skin is laced with scars, the dorsal line is smooth, the tip is adequately projecting, the upper lip is vertical, and the tip is projecting and contoured.

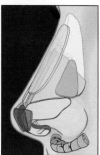

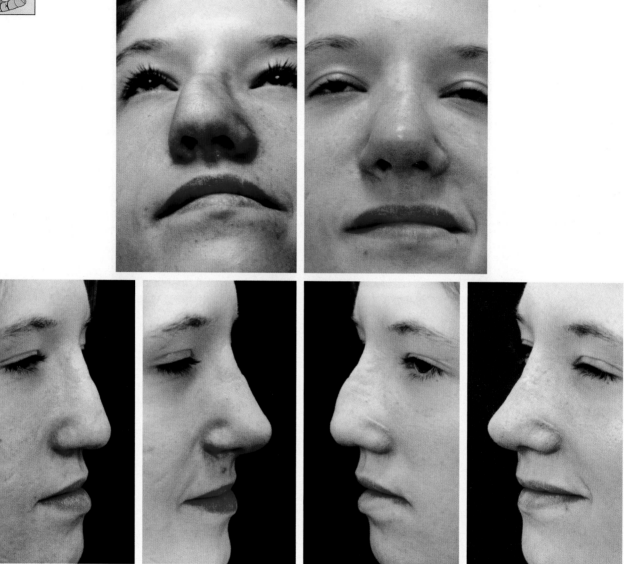

The oblique views now match much more closely. Normal tip projection, columellar support, and the restored vertical position of the upper lip combine to reduce the stigmata of previous damage. Geometric mean postoperative airflow increased 3.2 times over preoperative values.

PATIENT STUDY FIVE

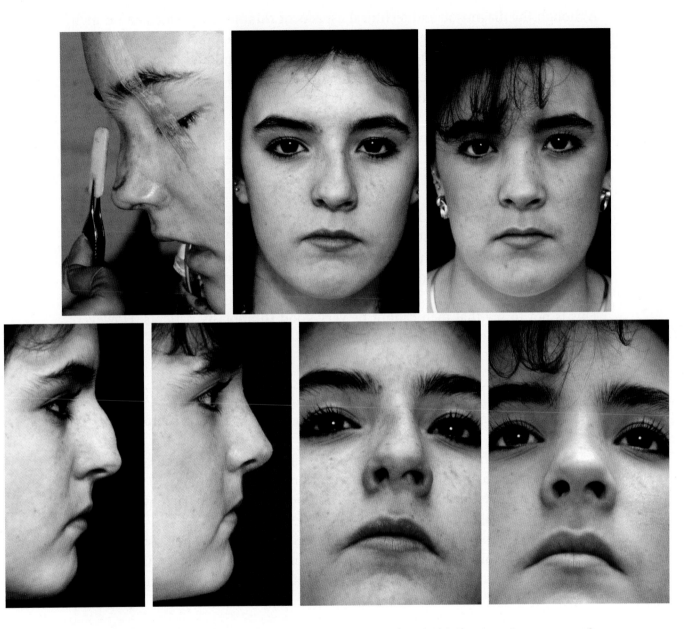

When noses have been significantly traumatized, the deviation may be too significant to camouflage, and the septal skeleton may be too distorted and calcified to form acceptable grafts. Retaining an intact L-shaped septal skeleton, the nose can still be rendered straight by resecting the deformity and placing a camouflaging dorsal graft of septal cartilage (if available), calvarial bone, or rib. The postoperative views are at 3½ years.

When treating the traumatized nose, attention must be paid to nasal analysis in thirds, and to evolving a strategy whose order of priorities is always safety, function, and then aesthetics.

Rhinoplasty in Men

Although the diagnostic and technical aspects of rhinoplasty performed on men do not differ from those performed on women, there are other differences. As a rule, men have larger frames, heavier bones, thicker skin, and historically have been more likely to involve themselves in contact sports and in work with high physical demands (though this is less true today).

We have already seen that men are judged to be most attractive when they represent their phenotype—that is, when they "look male": defined jaws, strong foreheads, and larger noses (see Chapter 7).

It is also true that men can have turbulent postoperative courses. In one group of 1000 consecutive rhinoplasty patients, men represented 30% of the disruptive or needy patients and 40% of patients with body dysmorphic disorder, even though men only represented 22% of the total population in that study (see Chapter 20).

This is not to say that men cannot be very good rhinoplasty patients. However, some generalities almost always apply.

- Men tolerate larger noses than women; that is, shape is more important than size.
- Bridge height is important. Most men prefer a straight (or even convex) dorsal line to one that is concave with retroussé.
- Men want noses that "look male"—not too short, not too narrow, and not too small.
- Secondary patients who have had significant reductions often complain that something is missing, even if they cannot articulate what it is.
- Whereas some women say, "I don't care how well I breathe as long as my nose is pretty," men expect excellent postoperative airways.

Each of the men on p. 975 brought a photograph to illustrate what he thought was wrong with his nasal contours. Notice that none of the presented noses are small or short; all of them have strong, high bridge contours. The third man, who had already undergone two rhinoplasties, could not easily articulate what was wrong; he just knew that something was missing from his nose. The fourth man, also a secondary patient, wanted to restore the high bridge seen in his high school photograph. In each case, maintaining contour and size (or, for the last two patients, rib graft reconstruction) was necessary to fulfill their conscious and unconscious expectations.

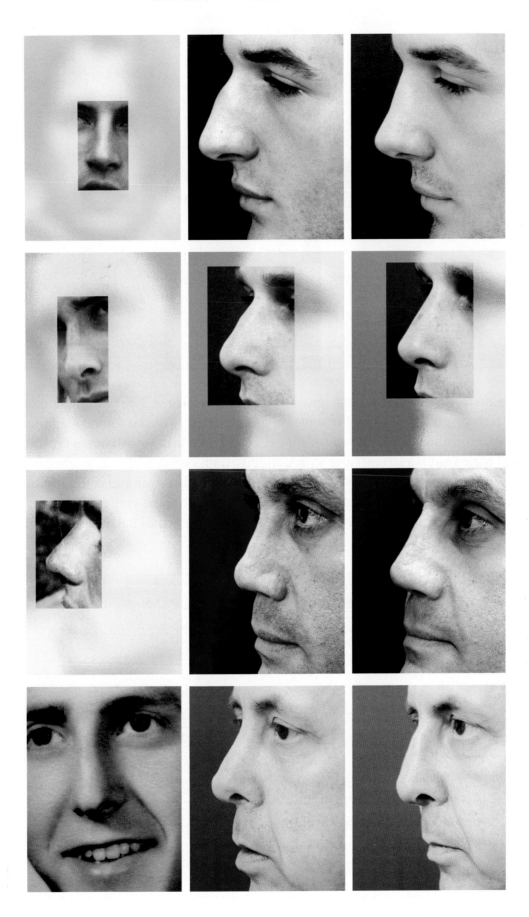

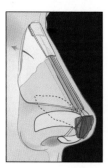

PATIENT STUDY ONE

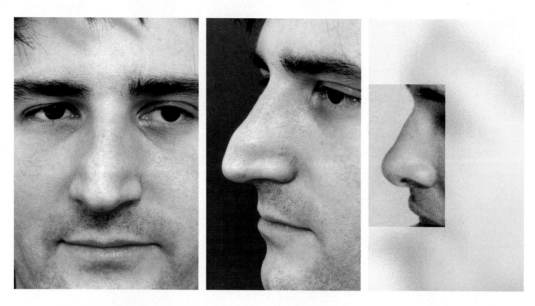

This is a large man with a large nose and a large skin sleeve. The tip is inadequately projecting and hangs from the septal angle. His nose will not tolerate significant reduction without losing airway or shape. The patient brings with him a typical desired male result: a strong nose with a slightly high dorsum and adequate tip projection. Although the patient's own nose is significantly larger and could not be reduced to duplicate the size of the nose in his illustration, the contrast provides the opportunity to discuss tip projection, radix height, and nasal balance.

SUMMARY OF THE SURGICAL PLAN

1. Limited skeletonization over bony vault, wide skeletonization over upper cartilaginous vault

2. Reduction of bony and cartilaginous dorsa

3. Relocation of alar cartilage lateral crura to strengthen external valves

4. Submucosal shortening of caudal ends, upper lateral cartilages (3 mm)

5. Transfixing incision; reduction of caudal and membranous septa, shortening the nose

6. Septoplasty

7. Asymmetrical spreader grafts (thicker on the left)

8. Upper dorsal graft, thicker at the radix and tapering into the middorsum

9. Multiple tip grafts

10. Right osteotomy

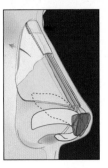

Postoperative Analysis

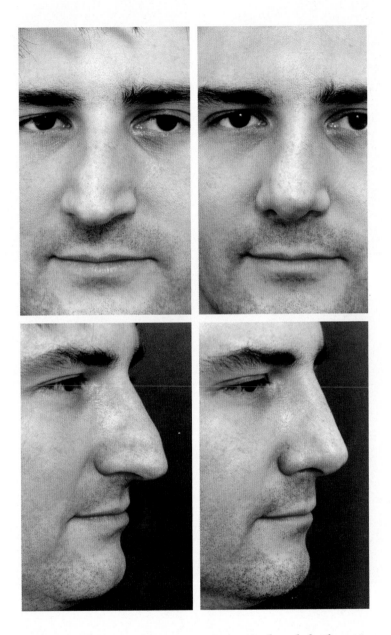

One year after surgery, the nose is more symmetrical and the base is appropriately wider. The patient no longer flares his nostrils to support his airway. Relocation of the lateral crura has favorably altered nostril contour. The tip no longer hangs from the septal angle. Although the skin remains thick, the nose has not lengthened again, because dorsal support is greater.

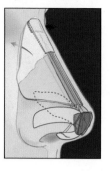

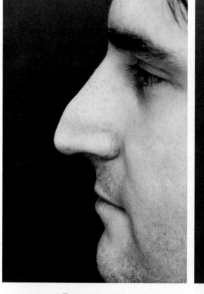

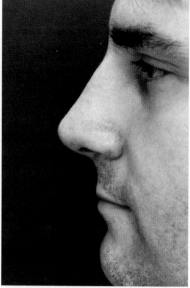

Preoperative   1 month postoperatively

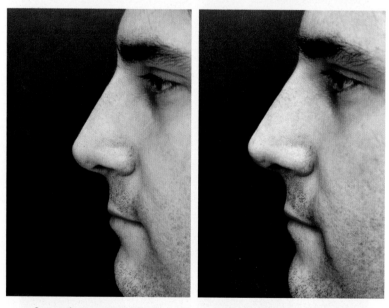

6 months postoperatively   12 months postoperatively

Notice the changes that occur from the preoperative nose at 1 month, 6 months, and 12 months postoperatively. As edema resolves, the nose lengthens slightly and then stabilizes after 6 months. Nasal balance has changed significantly. The nose is no longer bottom heavy, and postoperative airflow has increased 3.4 times over preoperative measurements.

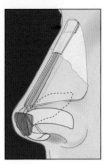

PATIENT STUDY TWO

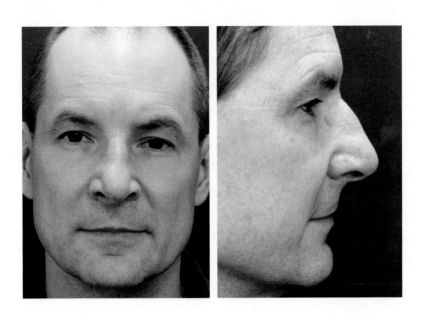

It is obvious that this man cannot breathe easily; notice that the nostrils flare to support his airways. The nasal bones are short, leaving an unsupported hollow that begins approximately 12 mm below the nasal radix, with high septal deviation toward the right (note the light reflex). The lateral crura are convex and malpositioned, leaving defects in the alar walls, parentheses that frame the tip, and unsupported external valves. The dorsum is strong and high, and the tip is blunt and inadequately projecting.

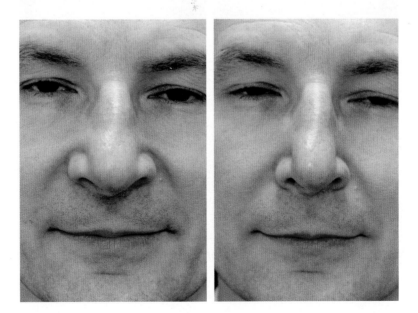

Valvular incompetence is confirmed by watching the patient breathe.

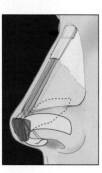

SUMMARY OF THE SURGICAL PLAN

1. Limited skeletonization over bony and upper cartilaginous vaults

2. Reduction of bony and cartilaginous dorsa

3. Resection and replacement of alar cartilage lateral crura through infracartilaginous incisions

4. Transfixing incision with trim of membranous septum; no nasal shortening

5. Septoplasty

6. Asymmetrical spreader grafts, thicker on the left

7. Radix graft

8. Tip grafts with buttress

9. No osteotomy

Postoperative Analysis

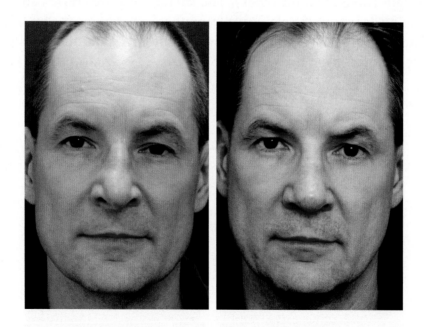

One year postoperatively, the nose is more symmetrical, the valves are stable, and the patient no longer flares his nostrils.

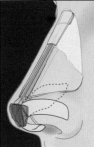

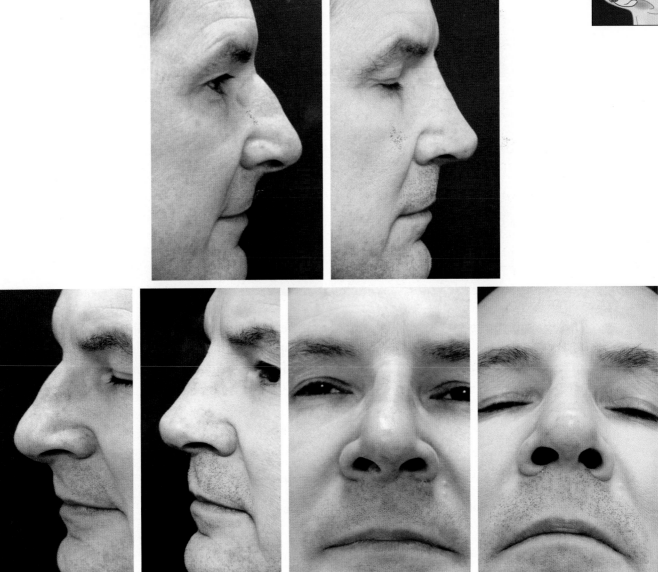

The nose has been rebalanced by the radix graft, reducing the required dorsal resection. Lateral crural relocation has ablated the alar hollows. The tip is adequately projecting and the nostril contour seems proportionately shorter, because tip lobular length has increased slightly. Lateral crural repositioning and tip grafting have favorably altered nostril contour and axis.

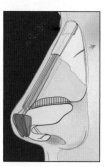

PATIENT STUDY THREE

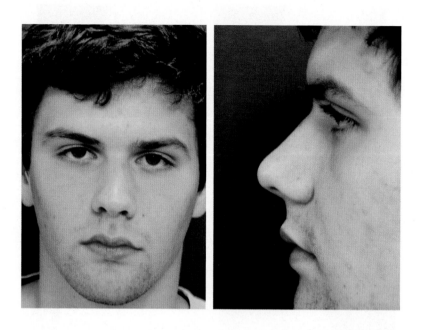

This is a tall young man with a left-sided high septal deviation and bilateral airway obstruction. Each nasal third (the bony vault, upper cartilaginous vault, and nasal tip) is asymmetrical. The dorsum is straight, and no net bridge reduction should be performed.

SUMMARY OF THE SURGICAL PLAN

1. Limited skeletonization over the bony and upper cartilaginous vaults

2. 2 mm trim of the cartilaginous dorsum

3. Retrograde reduction of lateral crura, 2 mm

4. Resection of ellipse, membranous and caudal septa, posterior third only

5. Septoplasty, leaving 20 mm dorsal and 15 mm caudal struts

6. Asymmetrical spreader grafts, right thicker than left

7. Upper dorsal graft, thicker at radix and tapering distally

8. Crushed tip grafts with ethmoid buttress

9. Left unilateral osteotomy

Postoperative Analysis

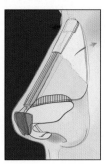

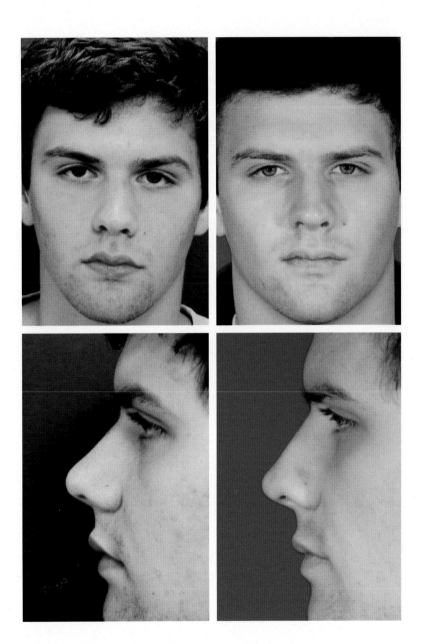

Postoperatively, radix and tip grafts have lengthened the dorsal line. Upper nasal augmentation and slight dorsal reduction have reduced the nasofacial angle and decreased base size.

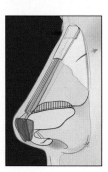

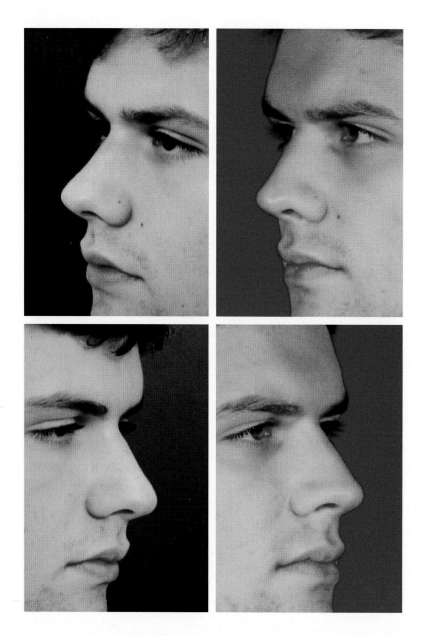

Asymmetrical spreader grafts have corrected the high septal deviation. Use of an ethmoid buttress has established a new angle of tip rotation, and the crushed grafts anterior to it have improved tip symmetry.

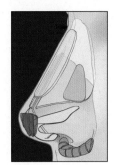

Patient Study Four

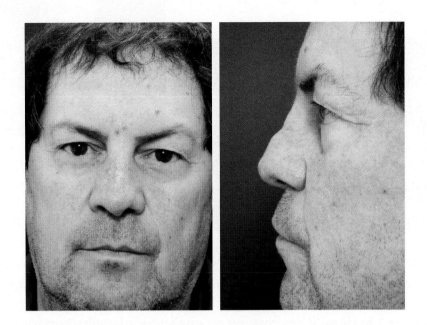

Multiple previous surgeries, including an iliac bone graft, had failed to correct this man's traumatic deformity. The bone graft had partially absorbed, leaving an irregular remnant along the dorsum.

Note also the degree of upper lip retrusion and the sunken subnasale, a common characteristic in secondary patients. Perhaps because of soft tissue thickness, the degree of lip lengthening and retrusion often seems greater in males than in similarly affected females.

SUMMARY OF THE SURGICAL PLAN

1. Minimal skeletonization
2. Remove old bone graft
3. Harvest rib cartilage
4. Rib cartilage maxillary augmentation
5. Dorsal graft
6. Tip grafts
7. Lateral wall grafts
8. Columellar grafts

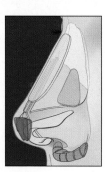

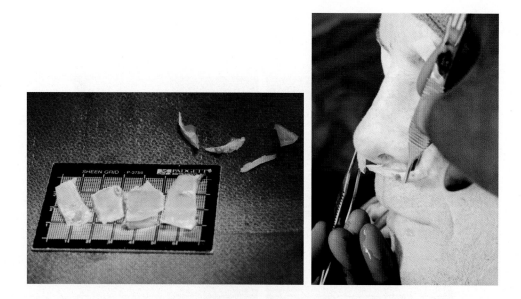

Rib was harvested and split tangentially. Notice the yellowness of the cartilage, typical of a patient this age. The slices are arranged with the outer rib edges at each end of the grid. Multiple areas of calcification (visible as white spots) prevent rib distortion, even in those strips covered on one surface by perichondrium. One of the rib strips was cut to create a two-piece maxillary augmentation. Independent pieces allow common asymmetries to be individually addressed, and seem to be more comfortable than a single rigid graft.

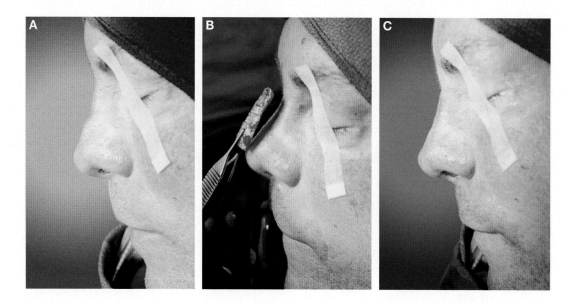

One of the perichondrially covered slices was trimmed and scored to lessen its distorting forces. It was designed to extend from the radix into the supratip, but not into the tip lobule *(B)*. Once dorsal and tip grafts were placed, contour improved and the nose lengthened *(C)*. Note the change in upper lip position provided by the maxillary augmentation.

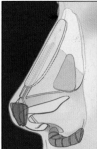

Postoperative Analysis

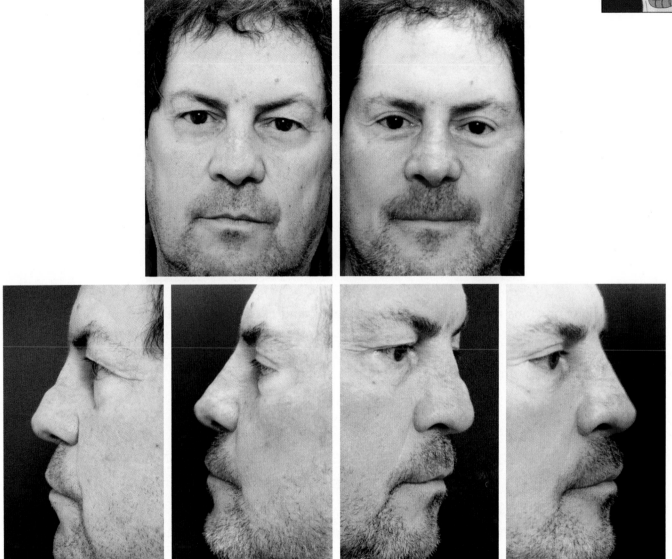

Two years postoperatively, the nasal contours have a smooth and natural appearance—properties gained partially by graft quality and the patient's thick, soft tissues. The multiple preoperative irregularities are gone, and the dorsum is straight, leveled by the rib graft. Notice that the patient's preoperative skin was heavily scarred and would have adapted poorly to a simple reduction of the supratip dorsum. His columella and maxillary arch have been braced, moving the nasal base anteriorly. Postoperative airflow increased 2.4 times over preoperative measurements.

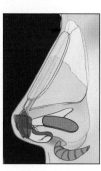

PATIENT STUDY FIVE

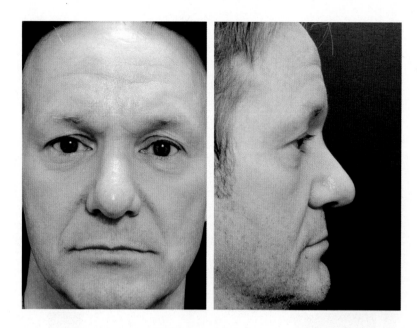

Four previous rhinoplasties, including septal and ear cartilage grafts and an allo-plastic implant to support the airway, had not corrected the patient's other problems: convex, cephalically rotated lateral crura, and an imbalance caused by a low, straight dorsum ending in a large, blunt nasal base.

SUMMARY OF THE SURGICAL PLAN

1. Harvest rib cartilage

2. Resect and replace cephalically rotated lateral crura

3. Rib cartilage for:
   a. Maxillary augmentation
   b. Dorsal graft
   c. Caudal support graft
   d. Tip grafts
   e. Alar wall grafts

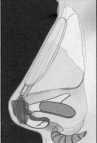

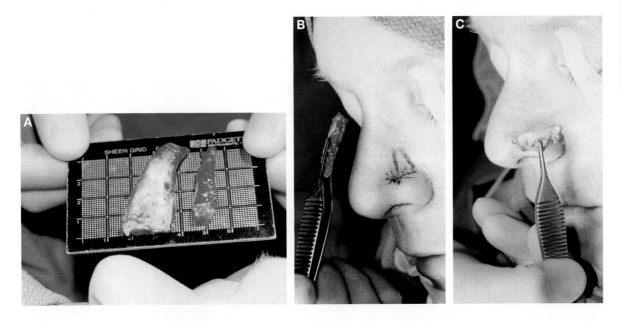

Segments of the eighth and ninth ribs were removed for the reconstruction *(A)*. The tip of the ninth rib was used for maxillary augmentation. Sections of the eighth rib were trimmed, scored, and fashioned into a laminate by suturing the periphery with 6-0 nylon interrupted sutures (the knots were buried between the rib slices) *(B)*. Additional slices were trimmed to support the alar walls, patterning their shape according to the deficient areas *(C)*.

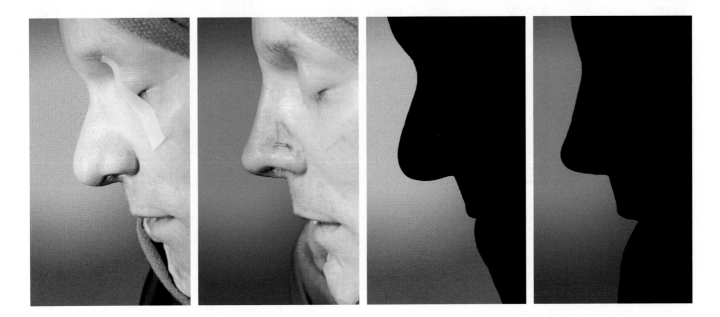

After removing the deformity and resupporting with grafts, the effect of rearrangement became visible. Percutaneous sutures coapted the external and vestibular skin after resection of the malpositioned lateral crura.

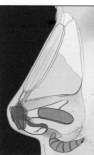

Postoperative Analysis

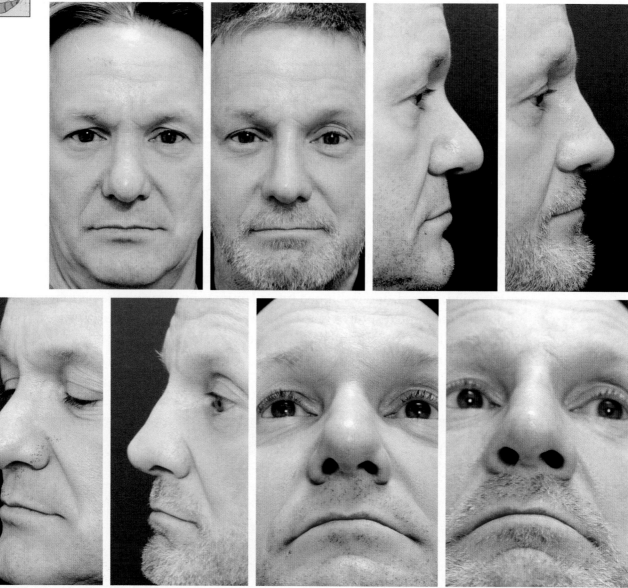

Three-year postoperative views show a nose that is narrower because of increased dorsal height—osteotomies were not performed. Tip lobular width has diminished after lateral crural replacement. The dorsum remains straight and the tip is supported. The maxillary arch is less retrusive. Both dorsal and alar wall grafts have improved valvular function. Alar wall grafts support the rims. Alar hollows have disappeared.

Ethnic Rhinoplasty

Beauty is subjective. Throughout this book we have seen patients whose private aesthetics were quite specific, and patients who simply wanted the surgeon to remove the bump and restore the airway. I have shown examples of Asian, Jewish, Italian, Armenian, Scandinavian, Mediterranean, Hispanic, and African noses, discussing their treatment in terms of function and patient aesthetic. So what is *ethnic rhinoplasty?*

The answer is that ethnic rhinoplasty does not differ from any other type of rhinoplasty. Nature's laws do not change when one crosses borders or changes passports. Middle vaults collapse and unsupported soft tissues contract everywhere in the world. Perhaps even the term *ethnic rhinoplasty* could be improved, because who is not ethnic?

The point that I believe Sheen and Sheen were making when they brought attention to the topic is an important one: for some patients, ethnic background helps determine their aesthetic goals. This determination can work two ways: some patients wish to retain the ethnic characteristics of their noses, and other patients want to lose them. *But the surgeon must ask.*

The principles of forming and performing the surgical plan, however, do not differ. The surgeon trying to correct a low, broad dorsum and a large nasal base covered by thick soft tissue, faces the same imbalances and the same technical challenges whether the patient is of African or eastern European descent. Donor sites may differ (for example, the septum of an African or Asian may be smaller than the septum of a Caucasian, with a higher percentage of ethmoid bone), but if the aesthetic goals are the same, the surgical strategy must be the same. Even though the surgeon must be aware of particular ethnic characteristics, it is the interaction with each patient that sets the plan.

> In one sense there is no such thing as ethnic rhinoplasty. Throughout this book, we have seen examples of different ethnic backgrounds in patients with a wide span of surgical objectives. Some patients have wished to retain their ethnicity, and others have not. It is important for a surgeon to determine the importance of ethnicity to the patient *so that all changes are intentional* and reflect the patient's aesthetic and ethnic sensibilities.

PATIENT STUDY ONE

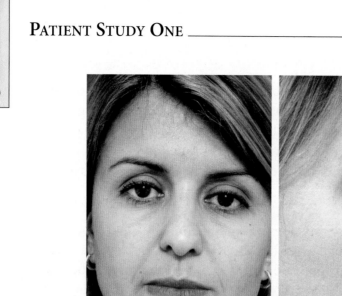

This woman illustrates a number of characteristics typical of the Latino patient: a broad face with a proportionally small nose, medium to thick soft tissues, a short columella, a small tip lobule with soft alar cartilages, an acute nasolabial angle, a retrusive upper lip, and a sharp subnasale. The treatment to produce any desired result is the same for a patient of any ethnicity possessing these characteristics. Patients must individually decide how much change they desire. This particular patient wanted a nose that seemed shorter and straighter, and a narrower tip that "turned up instead of down" (an appearance created by the combination of a low radix, high dorsum, convex supratip, indistinct tip-defining point, acute nasolabial angle, and sharp subnasale).

SUMMARY OF THE SURGICAL PLAN

1. Gore-Tex maxillary augmentation
2. Limited skeletonization
3. Reduction of the bony and cartilaginous dorsa
4. Resection and replacement of alar cartilage lateral crura
5. Transfixing incision, shortening membranous septum only
6. Septoplasty
7. Spreader grafts
8. Radix grafts
9. Multiple tip grafts
10. No osteotomy

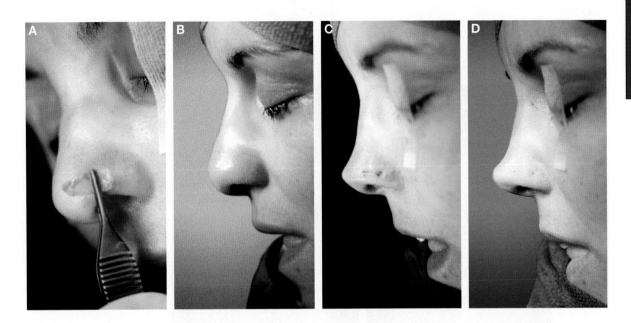

After maxillary augmentation and dorsal reduction, the lateral crus is resected and trimmed *(A)*. It is shown here before replacement along the alar rim.

After dorsal reduction and maxillary augmentation, a single, solid tip graft was placed *(C)*. Because the graft supports the tip along only one edge, it looks artificial and would not provide a satisfactory long-term result. Notice the change in the vertical plane of the upper lip after maxillary augmentation. With the addition of lightly crushed grafts anterior to the buttress, the lobule became less angular *(D)*.

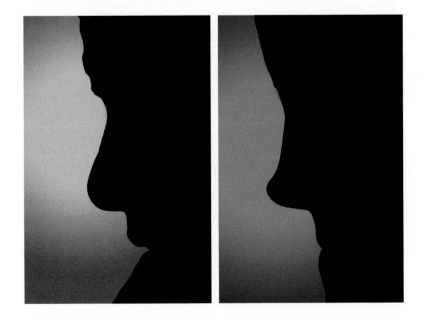

Compare the blue silhouette here with the postoperative lateral view on p. 995.

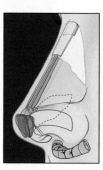

Postoperative Analysis

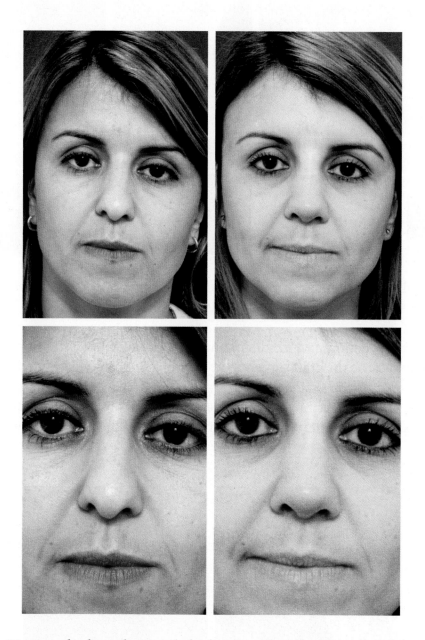

By repositioning the lateral crura (which can widen the base slightly) and even without osteotomy, nasal width is now appropriate for the patient's face. Maxillary augmentation has corrected the upper lip retrusion and softened the subnasale.

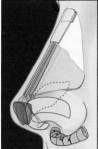

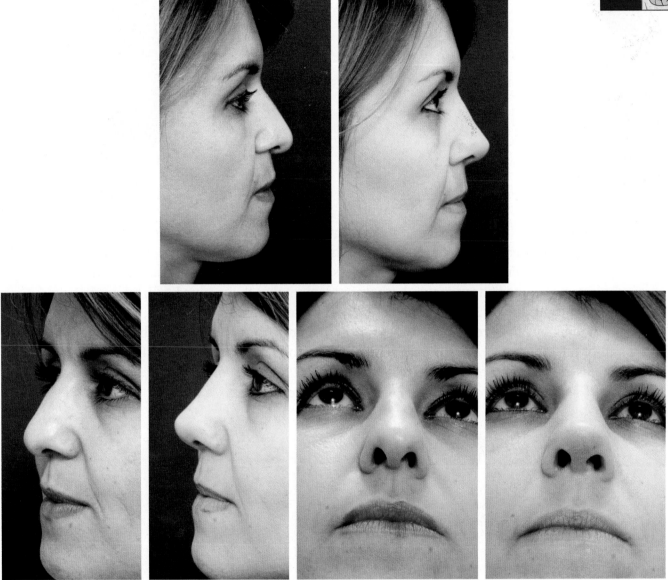

The dorsum is now straight, the nose is shortened, and the tip is supported above the septal angle, but the appearance has changed slightly from the blue silhouette as the tip lobule has contracted. Such expected changes can only be learned from sequential intraoperative and postoperative photographs. Maxillary augmentation improved the nasolabial angle. The nasal base remains unscarred, and the tip lobule is slightly narrower.

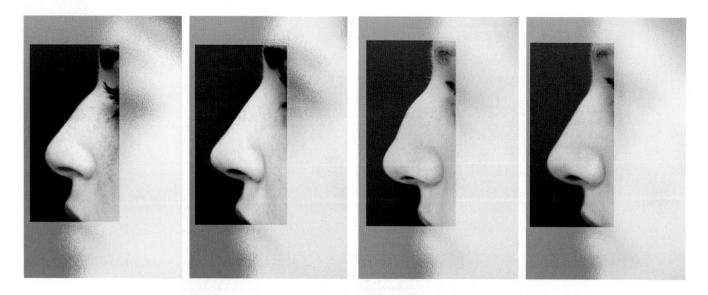

Maintaining bridge height and nasal length is an important surgical goal for many Middle Eastern and Mediterranean patients. Although both of these Jewish women (whose surgeries are detailed in Chapters 8 and 9, respectively) desired more delicate noses and better airways, both were adamant that they wanted to preserve dorsal height. In each case, dorsal contour was maintained but modified, in the first patient by dorsal reduction and a radix graft, and in the second patient by resection of the hump and a long dorsal graft. Notice also that the tip was modified in both cases, increasing refinement and contour. *A straight dorsum is not necessary for an elegant nose, but good tip aesthetics are always necessary.*

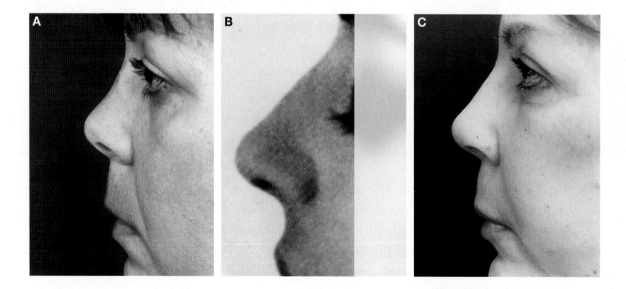

In contrast, this woman had undergone a previous rhinoplasty that she believed had cost her ethnic identity: her nose was too short, and the bridge was too low. Her objective *(B)* was a longer nose with a suggestion of dorsal convexity. This was achieved using multiple dorsal, tip, and composite grafts *(C)* (see Chapter 2).

PATIENT STUDY TWO

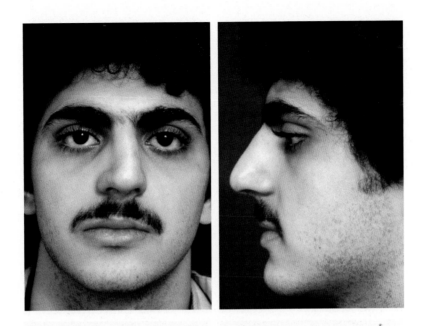

Maintaining dorsal height and length is just as critical in men as it is in women. This young Egyptian man, on whom I operated 3 years into my practice, had a high radix, a straight dorsum, inadequate tip projection, and a nose that was shifted toward his left from previous trauma. The septum protrudes from the left side of the columella. The soft tissues are moderately thick, and nasal contours are blunt, even at this size. How could I straighten this nose without reducing the dorsum excessively? The answer, I concluded, was to resect the dorsal deformity and camouflage the asymmetry with a dorsal graft.

SUMMARY OF THE SURGICAL PLAN

1. Limited skeletonization
2. Reduction of the bony and cartilaginous dorsa
3. No modification of tip cartilages
4. Hemitransfixing incision with resection and replacement of caudal septum as free graft
5. Septoplasty
6. Dorsal graft
7. Tip graft
8. Left osteotomy

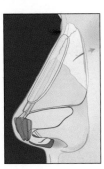

Postoperative Analysis

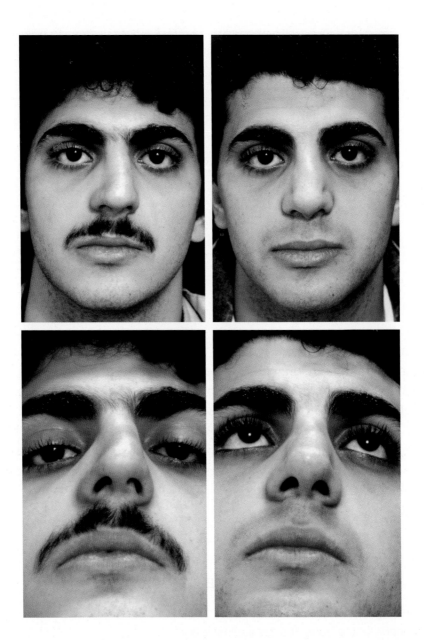

Four years after surgery, the nose is straighter, and the dorsal graft has camouflaged many of the remaining underlying asymmetries. The dorsum is strong and straight, with a suggestion of height over the bony vault. Notice the profound change wrought by a slight change in dorsal height combined with adequate tip projection: although not smaller, the nose seems more refined, slightly shorter (a result of the change in tip lobular shape), and more elegant.

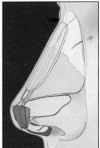

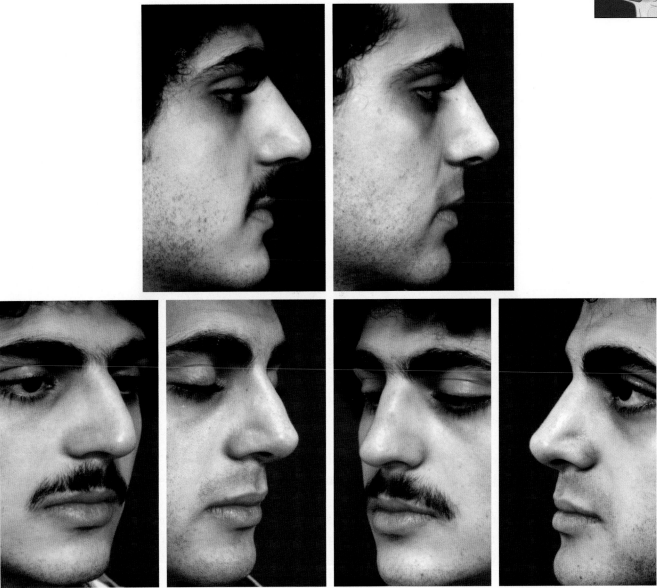

The patient's oblique views now match more closely. A slight depression between the dorsal graft and the tip graft sets the tip apart from the bridge. The supratip depression is not created by thinning the skin or suturing soft tissue to the skeleton, but by adequate dorsal height and tip projection and by separating dorsal and tip supports. An L-shaped framework will not provide the same contour. The base is unscarred, and the nostrils are equally sized.

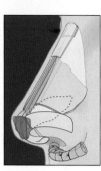

PATIENT STUDY THREE

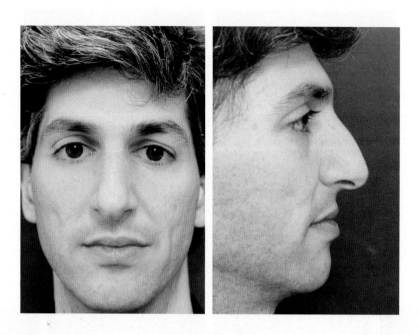

This young Armenian man wanted a shorter nose without a dorsal hump, but retroussé or a highly angular tip would be inappropriate for his face. On the frontal view, the upper lip seems flattened and retrusive, and the lateral crura are convex and cephalically rotated. The lateral view reveals a low radix with an inadequately projecting tip slung from a high dorsum.

With the heavier tissues that men have, shortening the nose always requires maintaining support. If dorsal reduction is planned, where can a surgeon add support?

This is the time to look for relative low spots or weak areas. The radix is slightly low relative to the large nasal base. The middle crura are weak, reducing tip support. The maxillary arch is slightly retrusive, which allows the nasal base to fall posteriorly and caudally. The skin is moderately thick, so shortening by soft tissue contraction cannot be assumed. This nose must be rebalanced and supported so that it holds its new shape without lengthening again.

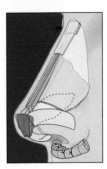

SUMMARY OF THE SURGICAL PLAN

1. Gore-Tex maxillary augmentation
2. Dorsal reduction
3. Resection and relocation of alar cartilage lateral crura
4. Submucosal shortening upper lateral cartilages, 3 mm
5. Transfixing incision, shortening the caudal and membranous septa
6. Septoplasty
7. Dorsal graft of septal cartilage
8. Multiple tip grafts
9. No osteotomy

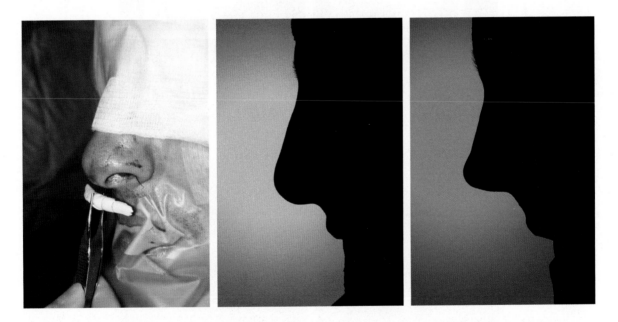

Before beginning the rhinoplasty, a piece of 1 mm Gore-Tex sheeting was rolled and placed in a subperiosteal pocket high over the maxillary arch through a short incision in the right nasal floor.

In examining the silhouettes, notice that the dorsum is lower and straighter, and it is now separated visually from the tip lobule. The tip is adequately projecting, and the upper lip is more vertical.

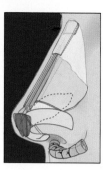

Postoperative Analysis

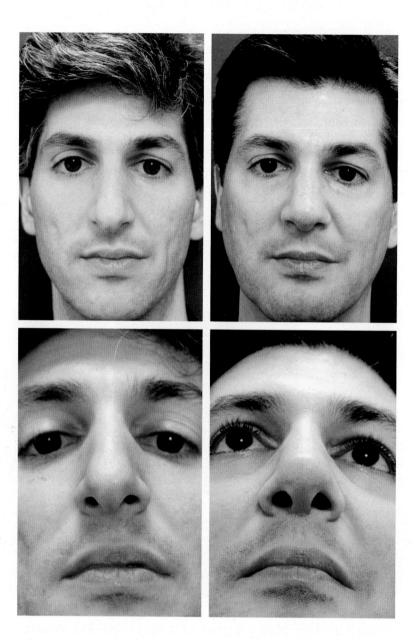

Eight years after surgery, the nose is shorter, more symmetrical, and stable. The widths of the upper nose and the lower nose are appropriate for each other.

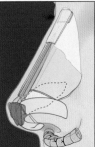

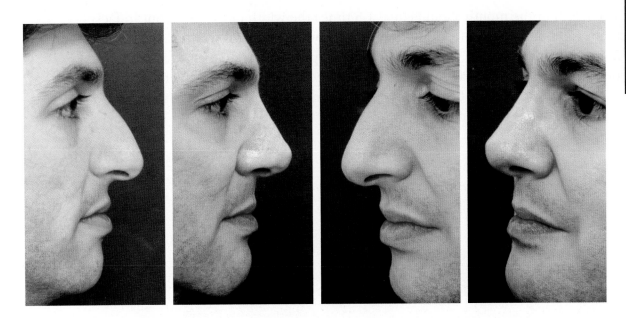

The radix is slightly higher, the dorsum is straight, and the tip is differentiated from the dorsum. The upper lip remains vertical, and the base is supported. Resection and replacement of the lateral crura flattened the supratip and ablated the alar hollows. Geometric mean nasal airflow increased 4.2 times over preoperative values.

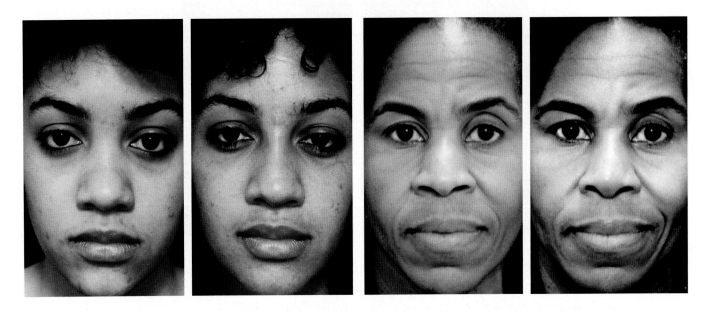

Before operating on black patients, it is worth remembering how infrequently the neoclassical canons apply not only to Caucasians and Asians, but to those of African heritage in particular (see Chapter 7).

Consider these young black women shown preoperatively and postoperatively. Although aesthetic norms theoretically require that the intercanthal distance equal the interalar distance, that rule applies in only 3% of blacks.

The width of the mouth should equal 1.5 times the width of the nose, but in fact, that canon only applies to 1% of the black population. Nasal width should equal 25% of total facial width, but that rule never applies to black patients. Imagine the poor result that would have been created by the surgeon who attempted to narrow this patient's nose, nasal tip, and nasal base to equal her intercanthal distance or to equal 25% of her total facial width.

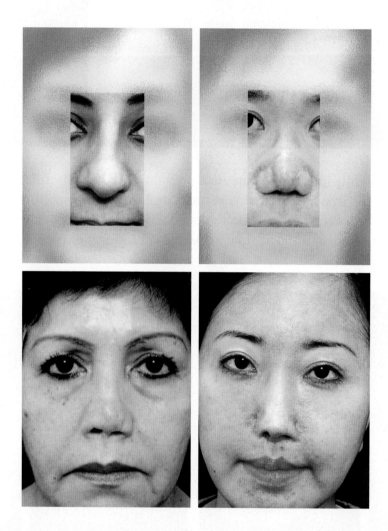

The surgeons treating each of these patients were apparently influenced by the neo-classical canons without recognizing their practical limitations. The canons do not apply to most human beings—not even to most Caucasians.

The only goals that a surgeon has any realistic chance of achieving are trying to match each patient's aesthetic goals, preserving or increasing function, and creating noses that appear balanced and attractive *unto themselves*.

PATIENT STUDY FOUR

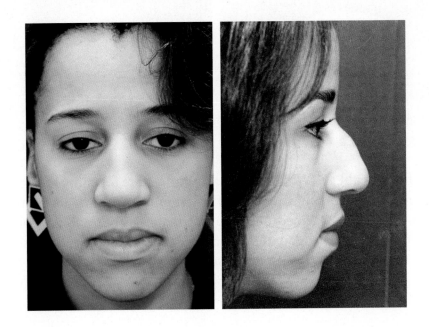

This young black woman dramatizes the two themes we have just discussed: the impracticality of abstract aesthetics and the importance of the patient's perception of beauty. Her skin is somewhat thin, her bony vault is slightly narrow, her septal curvature turns to the right. Her low radix and dorsal hump are exaggerated by inadequate tip projection, and her upper lip is retrusive. The patient's tip lobular width exceeds her intercanthal width. She desires a straight dorsum and an angular, projecting tip.

SUMMARY OF THE SURGICAL PLAN

1. Gore-Tex maxillary augmentation

2. Minimal skeletonization

3. Dorsal reduction, right more than left

4. 3 mm reduction of alar cartilage lateral crura, retrograde

5. Septoplasty

6. Asymmetrical spreader grafts, left thicker than right

7. Layered radix graft

8. Tip grafts

9. Columellar graft

10. Right unilateral osteotomy

11. No alar wedge resections

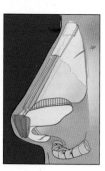

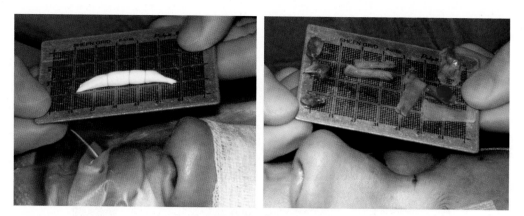

Before performing the rest of the rhinoplasty and before touching the skin with my gloved hands, I formed a maxillary augmentation from 1 mm Gore-Tex sheeting. The patient's septum provided only modest material, but enough for spreader, radix, and tip grafts. Spreader grafts are in the center of the grid, the resected nasal skeleton is to the left, and the rest of the septal specimen is to the right. Notice that half of it is bony.

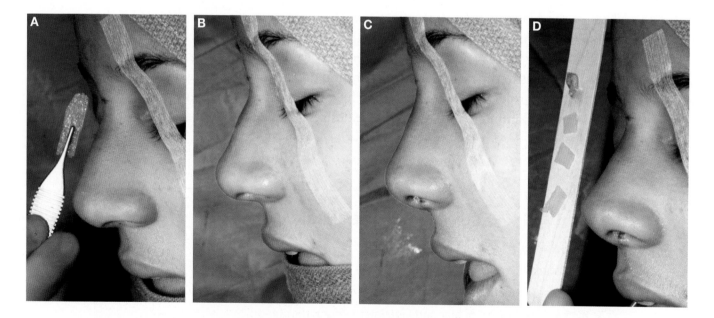

A radix graft was fashioned, crushed, and layered to conform to the defect. The graft is longer than the actual defect and tapers at its distal end to integrate with the nasal skeleton (A). The dorsum was reduced (B), enough to form a straight line after the radix graft placement (C). The remaining cartilage was cut into tip grafts (D). Notice that none of the grafts qualify as a standard shield graft. Shape is not as important as graft substance, pocket position (high in the lobule, to maximize effect), and the use of multiple grafts to avoid asymmetry and to produce a natural lobule.

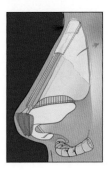

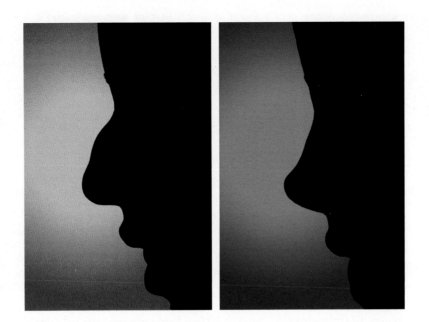

At the conclusion of the procedure, nasal contour has been significantly altered but function has been preserved. The tip now supports itself independent of dorsal height, and maxillary augmentation has moved the upper lip anteriorly. Columellar grafts (for caudal repositioning, not struts) have strengthened the medial crura.

Postoperative Analysis

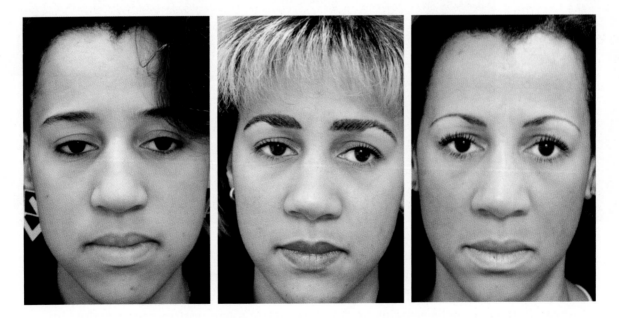

The patient is shown preoperatively and at 1 year and 12 years postoperatively (her interval postoperative sequence is shown in Chapter 2). Contours remain stable over time.

1007

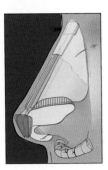

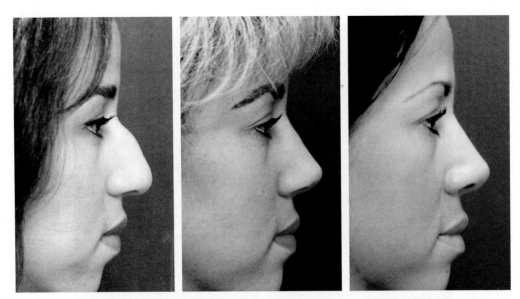

Minimal retrograde tip reduction and grafting have altered tip lobular contour significantly, without the variables associated with a more extensive dissection, permanent sutures, or struts. Grafts are smooth and impalpable. The tip remains adequately projecting.

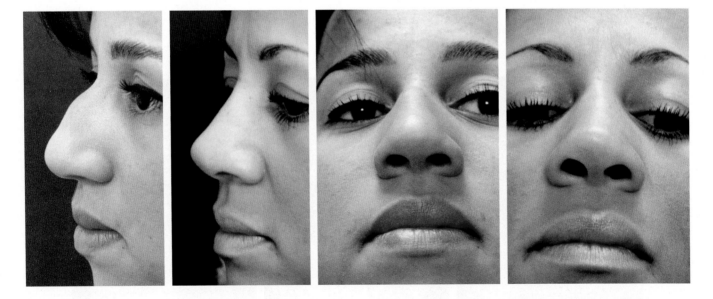

At 12 years, the effect of even small tip graft fragments, placed high in the lobule for maximum effect, is evident. The nasal base is unscarred, and the nostril axis is less horizontal because of increased tip support. Although tip projection has increased, the columella remains narrow. Geometric mean postoperative airflow increased 15.5 times over preoperative values.

Imagine the deformity that would have been created by alar wedge resections sufficient to narrow the base to the patient's intercanthal distance.

PATIENT STUDY FIVE

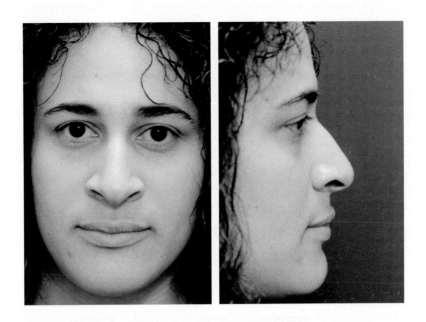

This patient is interested in a result that is "ethnically appropriate," by which she means a straight dorsum without retroussé, angular tip, or excessive narrowness. She had seen numerous plastic surgeons, some of whom would not operate and others who proposed aggressive nasal base narrowing.

This nose is full of traps: balance problems, aesthetic puzzles, and anatomic variants. On the frontal view, the bony vault is narrow, but the nasal base is excessively wide. In addition, the alar walls flare outward like a skirt. The lateral crura are flat but malpositioned, visible only by their internal reflections. The nasal base is large, the tip is flat and inadequately projecting, and the maxillary arch is slightly retrusive, particularly in the perialar areas. The dorsum is high, and the radix is low.

Her tissues are thin but unforgiving, and they have a soft, inelastic, "fluffy" quality; they do not easily coapt the skeleton that she has. Augmentation is essential but must be understated, and septal cartilage may be inadequate for long grafts.

The alar walls are a problem by themselves. Simulating alar wedge resection with my fingers, I still could not duplicate the shape that I wanted, because the rims still everted. I decided that the best approach would be to relocate the lateral crura, hoping that they would brace and invert the rims, so that alar wedge resections could narrow the base appropriately.

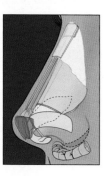

SUMMARY OF THE SURGICAL PLAN

1. Gore-Tex maxillary augmentation (two pieces, right side more than left)
2. Alar cartilage relocation as flap
3. Wide skeletonization
4. Submucosal shortening of caudal ends, upper lateral cartilages
5. Transfixing incision, shortening membranous septum only
6. Slight dorsal reduction
7. Septoplasty
8. Single-layer radix graft
9. Spreader grafts
10. Multiple tip grafts with buttress
11. Alar wedge resection, removing external and vestibular skin

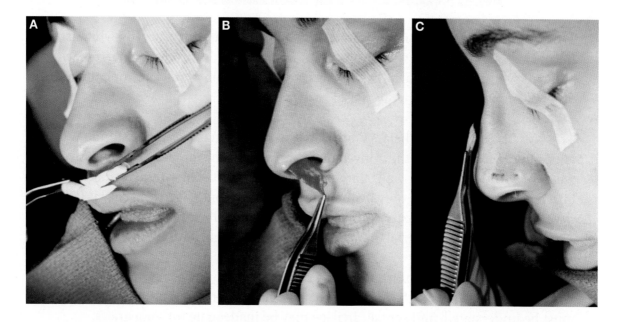

Two Gore-Tex implants were made by rolling 1 mm Gore-Tex sheeting *(A)*. Each implant was fed through the same incision in the right nasal floor and placed so that the widest end determined the amount of perialar augmentation, and the midline overlap determined the degree of central augmentation.

Each lateral crus was dissected free from its external and vestibular skin through an incision 3 mm above the rim *(B)*, and the crus was rotated at the lateral genu and fixed by catching the edge of the cartilage in the wound closure. A percutaneous suture coapted the skin and lining for 48 hours. The bony vault was rasped and the cartilaginous dorsum was resected 2 mm *(C)*.

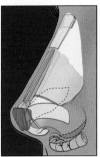

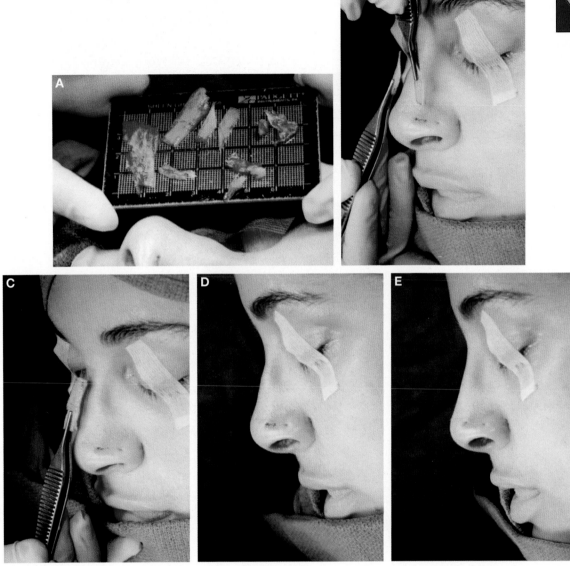

The septum produced an excellent specimen *(A)*. Spreader grafts were cut and placed to support the narrow middle vault, which had been weakened by dorsal resection *(B)*. The best piece of septal cartilage was trimmed, beveled, and lightly crushed to make a conforming dorsal graft *(C)*. Compare the appearance before and after radix grafting *(D* and *E)*, and note the change in dorsal contour and apparent nasal base size.

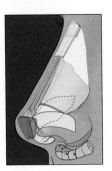

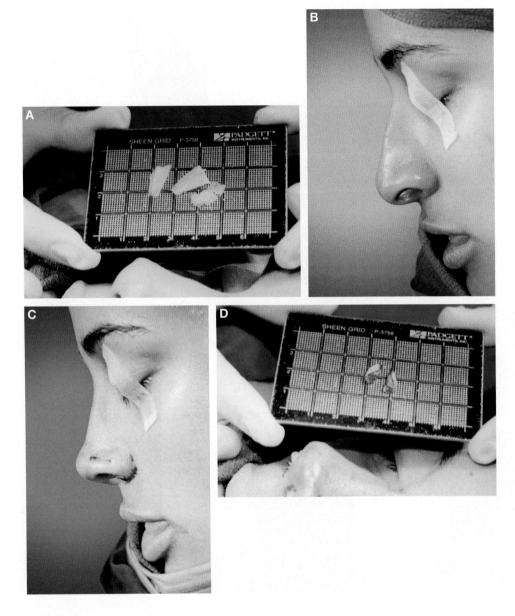

The operation was completed by placing tip grafts, both solid (center of grid) and lightly crushed *(A)*. Radix augmentation, nasal shortening, and tip grafting altered the dorsum–tip relationship. Note the change in alar rim contour produced by moving the lateral crura closer to the rims (*B* and *C*). From each side, 3 mm of external skin and 2 mm of vestibular skin were removed *(D),* preserving a medial flap on the nasal floor to avoid notching.

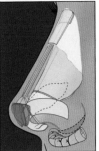

Postoperative Analysis

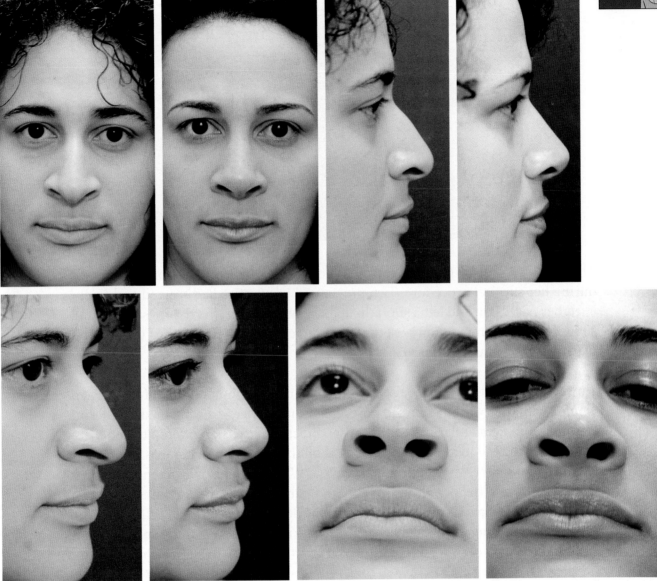

Postoperatively, the nose is better balanced and the nasal base deformity has improved. The base is still wide, but it is appropriate for the patient's face, and the nose is balanced within itself. Maxillary augmentation has improved upper lip retrusion, which can best be seen in the frontal view. Despite tip grafting, radix augmentation has improved nasal balance and reduced apparent nasal base, as has nasal shortening. The tip is in line with the dorsum, and the alar walls remain flat. Preservation of the medial flap and closure without tension have created alar base scars that are almost imperceptible.

PATIENT STUDY SIX

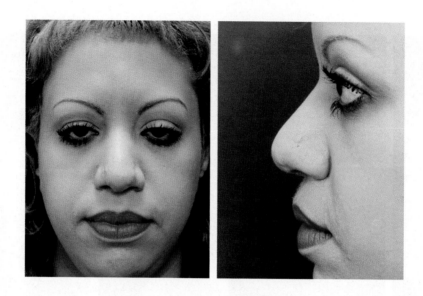

This black secondary patient presented a cosmetic quandary that only deepened during her surgical procedure. Two previous rhinoplasties had scarred and thickened her nasal skin and left a supratip deformity. However, the tissues seemed well supported by the remaining skeleton, and the septum was intact; thus the surgical plan appeared straightforward.

However, to illustrate her goals, the patient brought photographs of Caucasian women with narrow, thin-skinned noses that were shorter and contained significant retroussé and tip angularity. For this nose, direct skin excision offered the only avenue to absolute reduction; however, based on the condition of her existing scars, I believed that direct skin excision was unwise. With this type of difference between the expected and the practical, surgeon and patient must come to an explicit understanding of what can really be done; and the determined course of action must be capable of satisfying the patient's goals. We were able to come to such an agreement (a straighter, narrower dorsum with retroussé, if possible), so surgery proceeded.

SUMMARY OF THE SURGICAL PLAN

1. Maxillary augmentation
2. Minimal skeletonization
3. Septoplasty
4. Dorsal graft
5. Tip graft
6. Left lateral wall graft

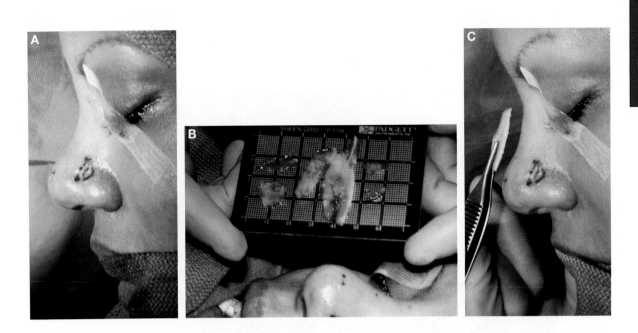

What could not be accurately palpated was the degree of previous skeletal resection. After skeletonization, a deep upper dorsal defect appeared *(A)*; compare this image to the preoperative lateral image. I proceeded with the septoplasty, which yielded only a thin specimen (notice the translucence of the largest piece in the center of the grid) *(B)*. I inserted a single dorsal graft from that piece *(C)*, but it had almost no effect.

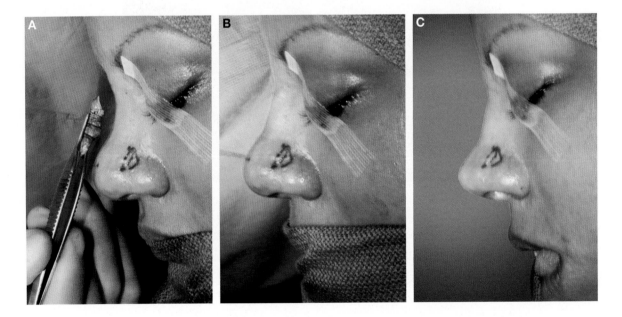

Accordingly, I rolled and fixed ear cartilage circumferentially with 5-0 nylon sutures, filling the undersurface with cartilage scraps according to Sheen's method *(A)*. The thicker graft elevated the dorsum and produced a surface difference *(B)*. Tip grafts completed the reconstruction *(C)*.

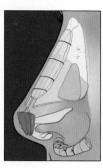

Postoperative Analysis

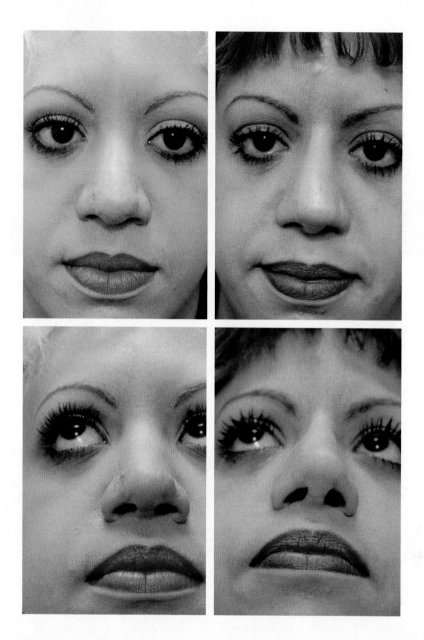

Six years postoperatively, the dorsum remains straight and narrower because of augmentation. Skin-sleeve volume has not changed. Maxillary augmentation has softened the perialar retrusion without moving the nasal base forward.

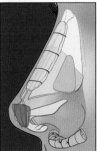

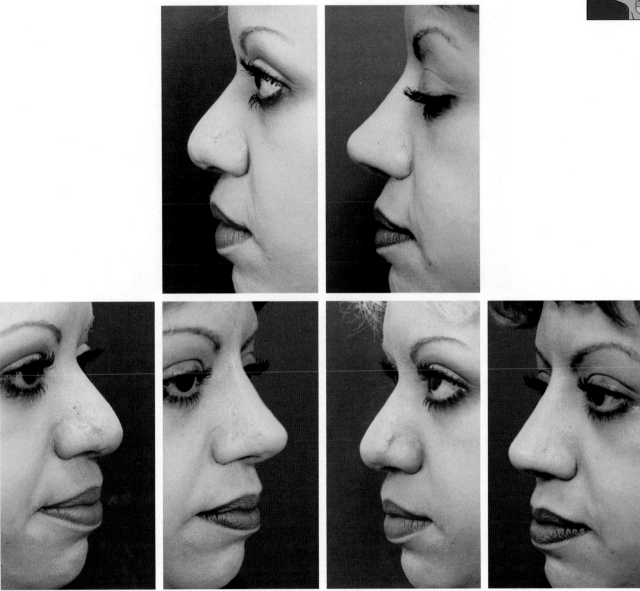

Although the nose is still large, its mass has been redistributed cephalad so the nasal base seems less dominating. Tip grafts created a slight degree of retroussé as desired, narrowed the tip lobule, and produced a more angular tip. Geometric mean postoperative airflow increased 2.7 times over preoperative values.

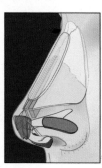

PATIENT STUDY SEVEN _____

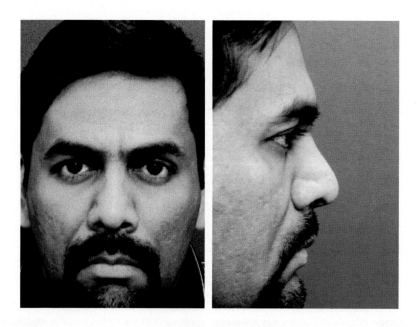

This man from southern Asia had undergone a rhinoplasty that not only failed to change his nasal appearance but also created a new airway obstruction. The dorsum was still low, the supratip was still high, and the tip cartilages were soft. The only perceptible change was a new airway obstruction, evident on inspection when the patient flared his nostrils to support his airway. Typical of this racial group is medium-thickness soft tissues, a distally located dorsal convexity, a low radix, a soft tip, and thin tip cartilages. The patient desired a straight dorsum, more tip shape, and a patent airway. As an engineer, he was distressed by the undulations of his nasal sidewalls.

SUMMARY OF THE SURGICAL PLAN

1. Harvest ear cartilage
2. Minimal skeletonization
3. Rasping bony vault for graft adherence
4. Septoplasty
5. Spreader grafts
6. Dorsal graft
7. Grafts to alar creases
8. Multiple tip grafts

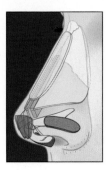

The entire operation was performed through three short incisions. The first was an intercartilaginous incision carried around the septal angle and provided access for dorsal and spreader grafts. The dorsum was rasped for bony vault adherence.

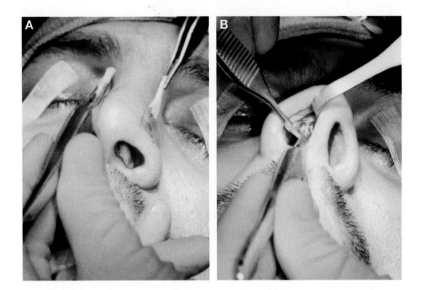

Spreader grafts were cut from the septal specimen and placed into each tunnel. Both grafts are visible in *B, where the tip of the forceps indicates the caudal septum.*

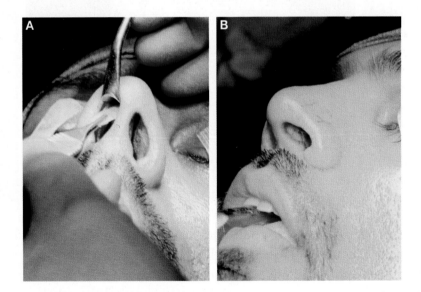

The best septal piece was beveled on the edges and adjusted to fit the defect, with the thickest end going toward the root *(A).* Placed through the same intercartilaginous incision, the graft leveled the dorsum *(B).*

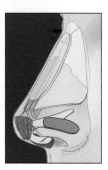

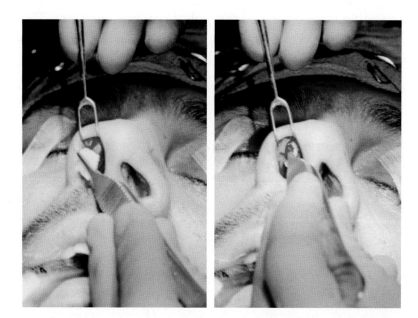

Through separate incisions approximately 3 mm above each alar rim and in separate pockets, trimmed ear cartilage was placed to re-create the lateral crura.

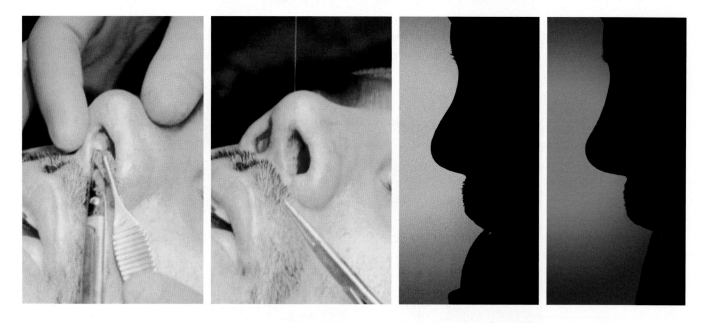

Tip grafts have been placed (see additional illustrations for this patient in Chapter 12). The medial crura are further strengthened by placing a columellar graft. Scissor tips hold open a short, left-sided columella incision so that the graft can slip into place and complete the reconstruction. Silhouettes reveal the rebalancing and alteration of the dorsum-tip relationships. No supratip skeleton was resected.

Postoperative Analysis

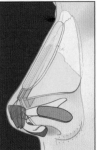

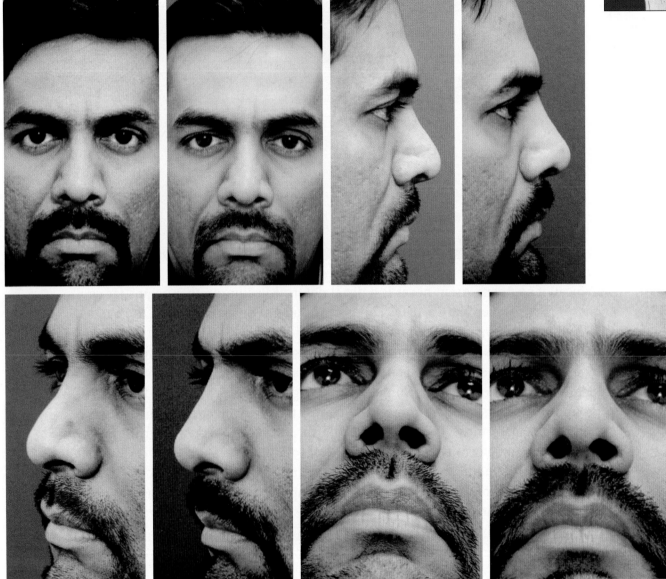

Postoperatively, the patient no longer flares his nostrils. The sidewalls are smooth and confluent, and the alar wall creases have softened. The dorsum is now straight, and the tip of the dorsal line and the middle vault are confluent with the upper and lower thirds. The inverted-V deformity and the alar wall shadows have ablated. Alar resections were not performed, but dorsal, alar wall, and tip augmentation have improved the contours. Retroussé would be ethnically inappropriate in this patient.

PATIENT STUDY EIGHT

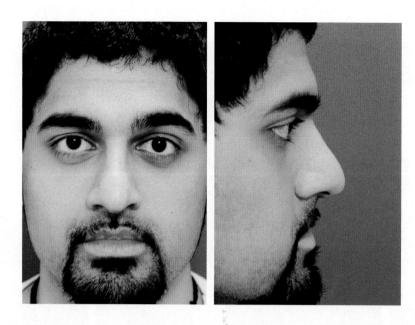

Typical of southern Asian noses is a distal deformity: a hump that begins far caudally, malpositioned alar-cartilage lateral crura, and a convex supratip. Often added to these characteristics is a long nose or, in this patient's case, a nose that seems longer than it is. Notice in the frontal view that some nostril is visible, yet the combination of a high supratip and poor tip lobular shape exaggerate the patient's nasal length. Notice also that the columella-labial angle is just less than 90 degrees. Although this nose should be shortened slightly, tip shape creates the most significant visible deformity. The steps involved in a standard reduction rhinoplasty would create a deformity essentially identical to the one seen in the previous patient: collapsed middle vault, deep alar creases and external valvular incompetence from resection of malpositioned lateral crura, supratip deformity, increased tip ptosis, and a new bilateral airway obstruction.

SUMMARY OF THE SURGICAL PLAN

1. Moderate skeletonization over upper cartilaginous vault, none over bony vault
2. Shortening caudal ends, upper lateral cartilages, submucosally
3. Transfixing incision, shorten membranous septum only
4. Relocate malpositioned lateral crura
5. Minimal trim of distal cartilaginous dorsum (not opening roof)
6. Septoplasty
7. Spreader grafts
8. Tip grafts

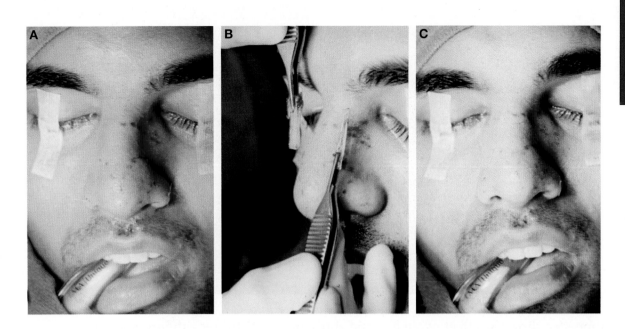

The patient's bony vault length measured only 5 mm (marked), leaving a long span of cartilaginous sidewall support. After skeletonization, the middle vault hollow became more obvious *(A)*. Spreader grafts, sized to span the sidewall from the bony arch to the supratip *(B)*, were slipped into submucoperichondrial tunnels. The change in middle vault support was visible externally *(C)*.

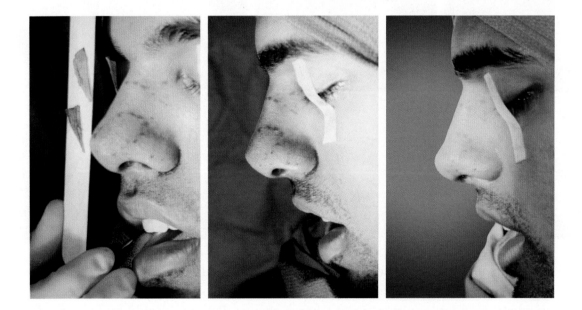

The first solid graft placed into the tip created the angle of rotation, but the lobule remained flat and the tip was unnaturally angular. Additional crushed grafts placed anterior to that graft rounded the lobule and completed the reconstruction.

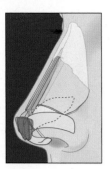

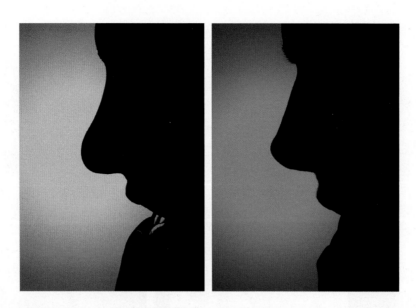

Silhouettes show the effect of slight nasal shortening and tip reconfiguration. No dorsal augmentation was performed.

Postoperative Analysis

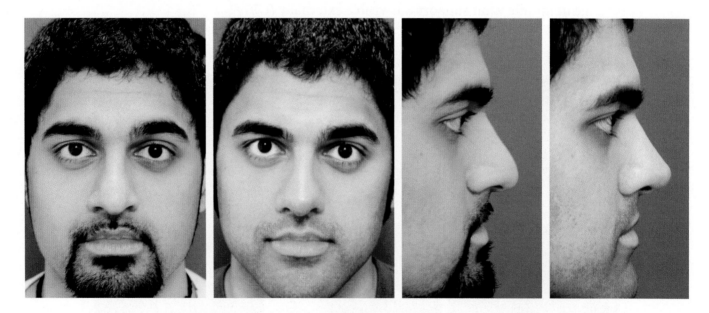

Two years after surgery, there is little change in frontal view. Although the lateral crura were resected and their previous bed now feels soft, the patient's tissues were unable to manifest any significant surface change. Patients should be forewarned of such tissue limitations. Tip lobular contour has improved: the supratip is flat, there is a defined point of tip projection, and the mass of the tip lobule is now caudad, rather than cephalad. The alar walls are slightly convex and supported, the hollows are ablated, and the nose seems shorter even without a significant change in the columella-labial angle.

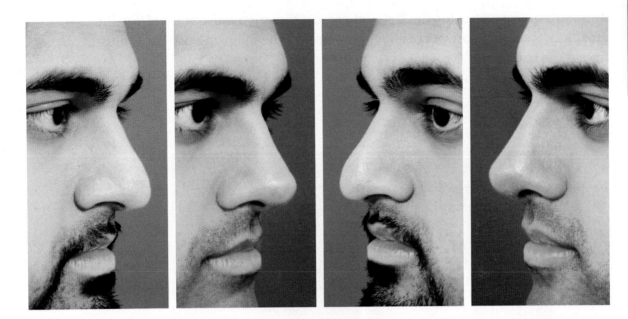

Similar to blacks, Asians share few of the neoclassical aesthetic canons. Nasal width constitutes 25% of total facial width in 51.5% of Asians (compared with 36.9% of Caucasians and 0% of blacks, as noted by Bashour). The distance between the eyes equals the interalar distance in 35.4% of Asians and 40.8% of Caucasians, but only 3% of African Americans.

As a rough generalization, many Asian faces have low nasal dorsa, medium-thickness subcutaneous tissues, retrusive upper lips, bimaxillary protrusion, short nasal septa (predominantly ethmoid), and thin, soft tip cartilages. Overall, the nose tends to be small, and so the Asian nose satisfies some of the neoclassical canons designed for Caucasians as well as or better than some Caucasians. Many Asians dwelling in the United States desire "Americanization," by which they mean a higher, narrower dorsum and a more angular tip.

Because the nose is small, surgeons must be wary of applying techniques slavishly without assessing nasal balance. For example, the low radix, which is helpful in altering nasal proportion in Caucasian noses, has much less relevance in Asian noses, where the base is generally so short that routine placement of the radix at the supratarsal fold or upper lash margin may produce a nasofacial angle that is too vertical.

In addition, donor sites are often an issue in Asian rhinoplasty, hence the common use of silicone implants throughout Asia and the United States. The conchae are typically small and deep, virtually never providing grafts of sufficient length for the nasal dorsum. For many years, before I became more comfortable with costal cartilage, I used calvarial bone for these patients. However, calvarial bone only supplies dorsal grafts, and perhaps lateral wall and columellar grafts; conchal cartilage

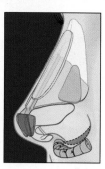

must still be harvested for the tip, and some alternative must be used for the maxillary arch. Rib grafts serve all of these needs. The following two cases illustrate these issues.

PATIENT STUDY NINE

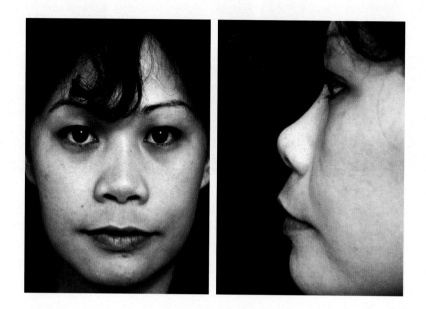

This young Thai woman wanted a nose that was as narrow and angular as possible. She had a broad, low dorsum, an obtuse nasolabial angle, and bimaxillary protrusion. The alar base was slightly flared, but the nose was not large.

SUMMARY OF THE SURGICAL PLAN

1. Harvest calvarial bone and ear cartilage grafts
2. Maxillary augmentation
3. Limited skeletonization through single cartilage splitting incision (better coverage for the dorsal graft)
4. No transfixing incision
5. Septoplasty
6. Dorsal graft, calvarial bone
7. Lateral wall graft, septal cartilage
8. Columellar graft, calvarial bone
9. Tip grafts, septal cartilage
10. Alar wedge resections, removing external and vestibular skin

---

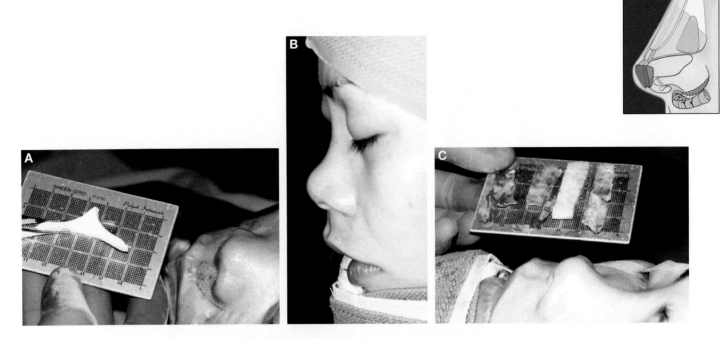

In 1988, when this surgery was performed, I was using Proplast (which is no longer available) for maxillary augmentation *(A)*. Although Proplast was successful in many ways, it was a rigid implant, unyielding in the sulcus. Notice the change in the vertical plane of the upper lip after maxillary augmentation *(B)*. The septal and cranial bone harvest is shown in *C*. Notice that the septal specimen was mostly thin ethmoid with only small cartilage fragments. This is typical of many Asian noses.

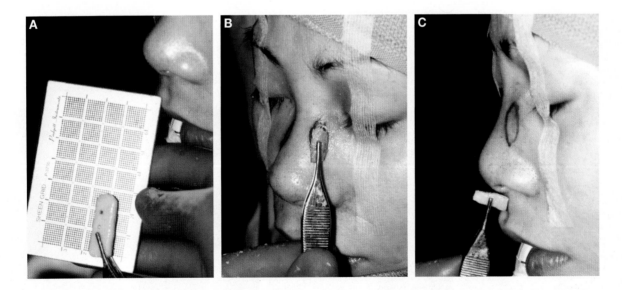

The calvarial graft was shortened and contoured to fit the defect; notice that it is only 3 cm long, but it is all that was required to fit this short dorsum. Once the dorsal graft was placed, remaining pieces of ethmoid or calvarial bone were used to fill the lateral walls *(B)* and columella *(C)*. When the dorsum is raised, lateral wall grafts are often necessary to reconstruct the dorsal pyramid, not only for contour but also to diffuse support and therefore camouflage the dorsal graft edges.

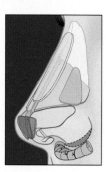

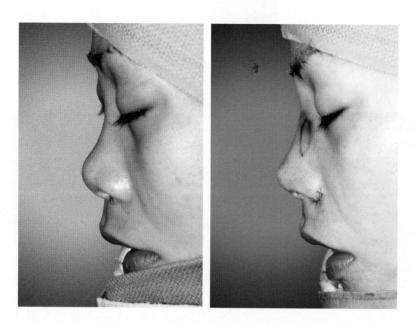

Profiles at the beginning and end of the procedure show the transformation. The dorsum is higher, the tip is more angular, and the nasal base is apparently smaller.

Postoperative Analysis

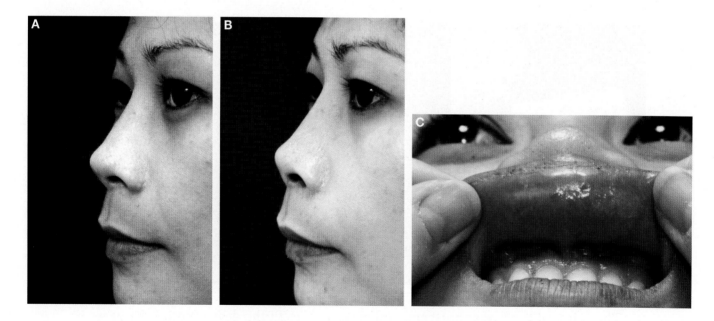

At 6 weeks the early postoperative course was benign *(A)*. At 5 months, however, she returned with upper lip swelling *(B)* and fluctuance in the upper gingivobuccal sulcus *(C)*. The Proplast was removed.

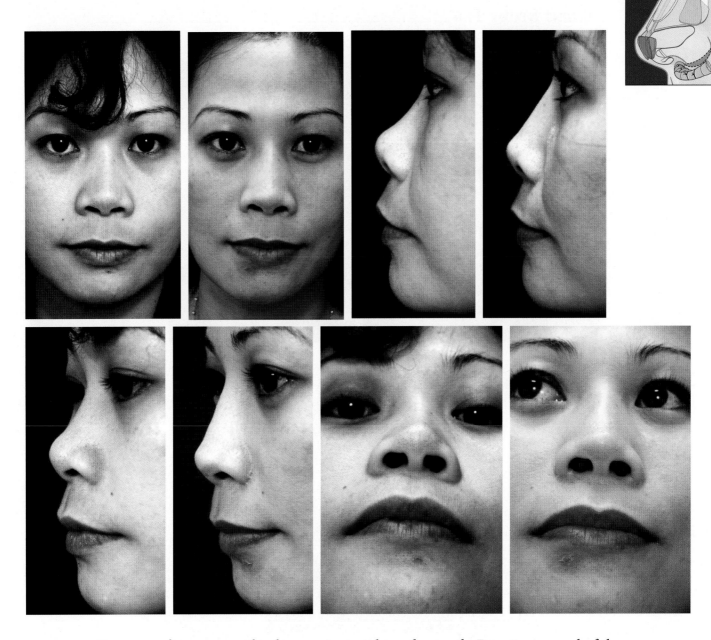

One year after surgery, the dorsum is straight and smooth. Despite removal of the Proplast, enough scar tissue remains to maintain lip position. The radix is slightly low in absolute terms (it is at the midpupillary level) but appropriately balanced for this nose. The alar base was narrowed, but closure without tension and preservation of the medial flap avoided notching.

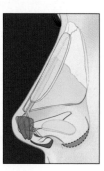

PATIENT STUDY TEN

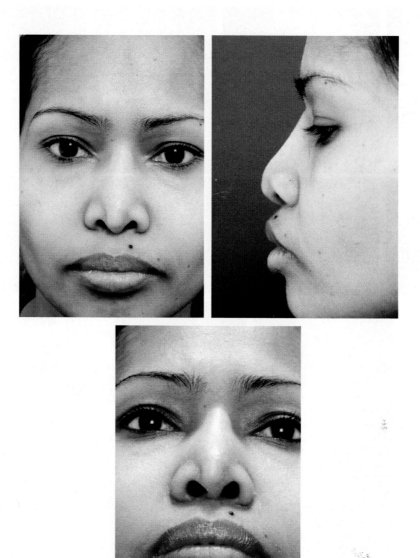

This patient presented with an L-shaped implant that threatened extrusion through the tip, and was already exposed intranasally at the septal angle. Notice the strange appearance of the high radix. Because there was no purulence or soft tissue infection, and because I wanted to preserve the space that the implant had created, I resected the distal portion of the implant, leaving just the segment along the dorsum, and closed the wound. Healing was uneventful.

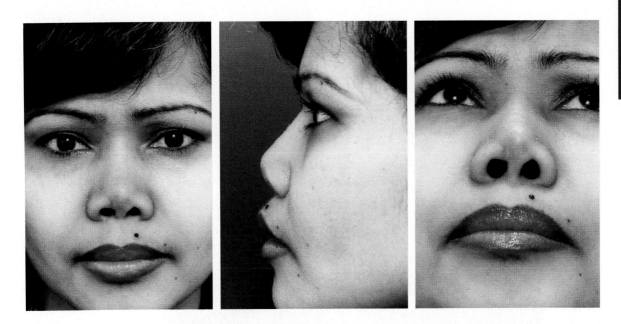

As healing progressed, the base collapsed proximally as the soft tissues contracted, but dorsal height was preserved. Aside from a crease in the right alar wall and some wound retraction on the left, the soft tissues survived nicely. Notice how nasal balance improved when the implant dropped distally at the radix once the columellar section had been removed. This is the proper height for the patient's radix.

A costal cartilage reconstruction was planned for the dorsum and tip. Alar wedge resections (external skin only) were to be used for composite grafts to correct wound retraction and to gain apparent nasal length (as a delayed, isolated procedure).

SUMMARY OF THE SURGICAL PLAN

1. Harvest rib cartilage

2. Skeletonization through a single cartilage-splitting incision

3. Removal of dorsal implant

4. Dissection under implant capsule, maintaining good soft tissue cover; rasp bony vault for graft adherence

5. Dorsal laminate of rib cartilage

6. Multiple tip grafts

7. Columellar grafts

8. No delivery of tip cartilages

9. No transfixing incision

10. No osteotomy

11. Alar wedge resection to rim transfer (composite graft) as a secondary procedure

---

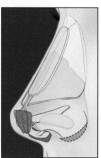

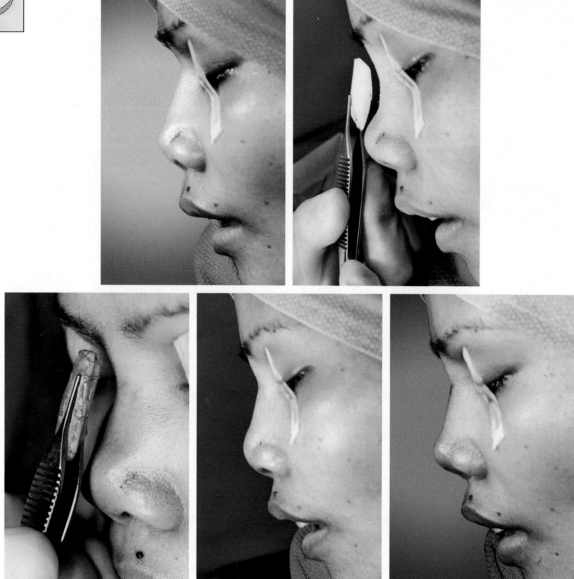

After the silicone implant was removed, notice how the nose shortened and the nasal base apparently enlarged. A laminate was fashioned from cartilage/perichondrial strips, leaving the perichondrial surfaces facing externally and burying the 6-0 nylon knots between the slices. Once the graft was in place, the nasal base apparently became smaller and the nose lengthened once again. Tip grafts completed the reconstruction.

Postoperative Analysis

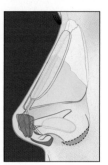

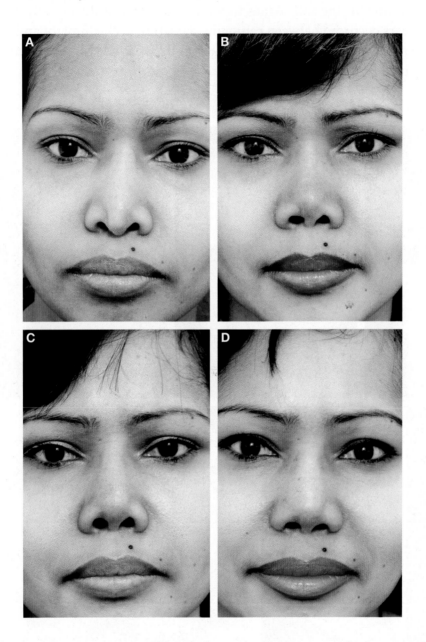

The patient is shown in stages during the reconstruction: with the extruding implant in place *(A)*, after partial implant removal *(B)*, after rib graft reconstruction *(C)*, and after coronally oriented composite grafts to the alar rims (using alar lobules as donor sites) *(D)*. After the final stage, the dorsum is smooth and stable, and the rib graft is impalpable. Cartilage and composite grafts have reconfigured the nasal base, correcting the peculiar deformity conferred by the implant.

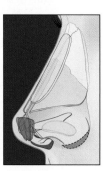

These procedures must be performed with appropriate waiting periods, giving sufficient time for the soft tissues to mature and recover from each step. In this case, 3 years occurred between removing a portion of the implant and the definitive rib reconstruction, and it was 8 months between the rib reconstruction and the composite grafts.

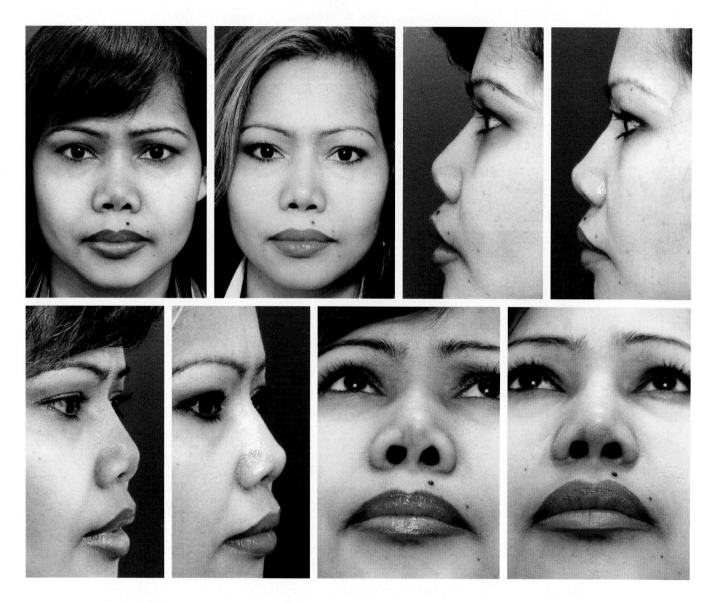

The patient is shown 3 years after reconstruction. The deformities caused by the implant are almost imperceptible, except for a slight depression in the right medial alar wall. Her nose is balanced between dorsal height and nasal base size, both aesthetically and appropriately for her ethnic group. Her tip projects above the dorsal line, but there is no exaggerated retroussé or angularity. Her reconstruction was autogenous and should therefore be permanent. Without a strut or open rhinoplasty dissection, the columella remains narrow. Geometric mean airflow increased 2.3 times over preoperative values.

Older Patients

Older, of course, is a relative term, like most things in rhinoplasty. Two important considerations for the older patient are (1) how long dissatisfaction with the nose has been present and (2) any particular structural characteristics that may require altering the surgical plan.

Older nasal bones are thinner and more brittle, and the bony arch must be able to support eyeglasses. Soft tissues have become atrophic and less elastic, and they tend to wrinkle instead of tighten, making some intraoperative judgments more difficult and contraction to a reduced framework less probable. Cartilages may have become more rigid, and many patients believe that their tips have grown larger with time. Whether this reflects actual cartilaginous growth, elongation or thinning of soft tissues, or even absorption of the bony vault creating a new imbalance is not yet known. Tips that were adequately projecting in prior years begin to hang from the septal angle, causing an apparent curvature in the lower nose.

It is therefore wise to inquire how long the patient has been unhappy with his or her nasal shape. For some patients, it has been since their teen years. These patients can undergo more fundamental surgical changes, but exotic alterations (such as too much dorsal reduction, too much retroussé, and excessive narrowing) should be avoided.

Alternatively, the patient whose unhappiness with his or her nasal shape is recent may simply be noticing aging changes. The surgeon's task in these cases is to restore the nose, insofar as possible, to its previous, more youthful appearance.

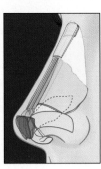

PATIENT STUDY ONE

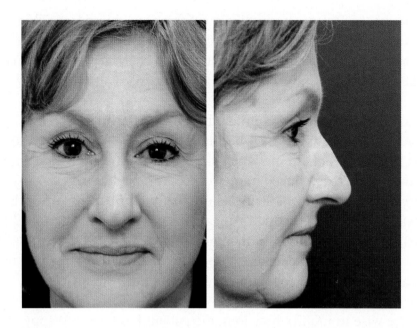

This woman had noticed that her nose had begun to lengthen and that it seemed to have grown larger at the base. However, the tissues were firm and of excellent quality, suggesting that some contraction was still possible. The lateral crura were malpositioned, and there was a high septal deviation toward the right.

SUMMARY OF THE SURGICAL PLAN

1. Resect and replace alar cartilage lateral crura

2. Wide skeletonization over upper cartilaginous vault, narrow over bony vault

3. Transfixing incision with trim of caudal and membranous septa, shortening the nose

4. Submucosal shortening of upper lateral cartilages retrograde 3 mm

5. Dorsal reduction, slightly greater on the left than the right

6. Septoplasty

7. Asymmetrical spreader grafts, thicker on the right than the left

8. Thin radix graft

9. Multiple crushed cartilage tip grafts

10. No osteotomy

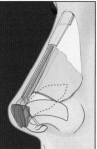

Postoperative Analysis

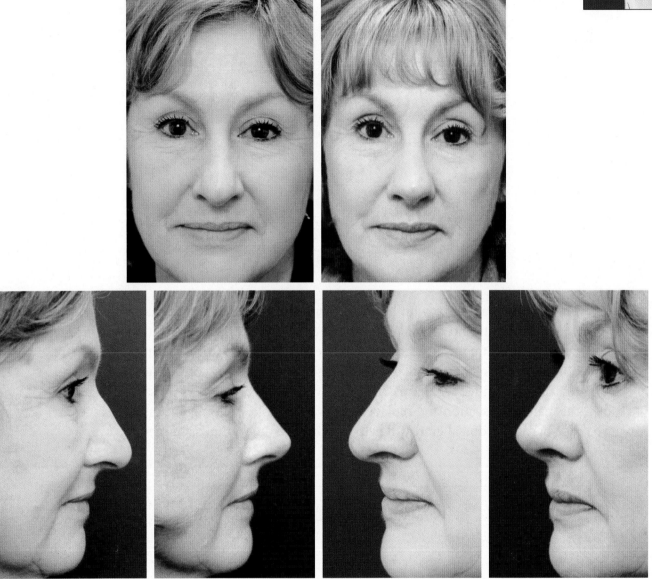

Two years postoperatively in the frontal view, there is very little change. The base is rotated slightly, and the right sidewall is now confluent. The nose is shorter in the lateral and oblique views, the radix is slightly higher, and the tip now ends in a defined point of projection.

Aging tissues cannot always be relied on to contract around a reduced framework. Although support assists balance and shortening at any age, it is particularly important in older patients to avoid postoperative elongation and disappointment.

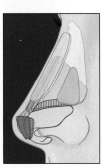

PATIENT STUDY TWO

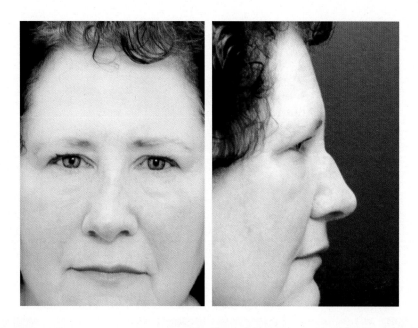

This patient was happy with her nasal contour until a recent trauma increased the dorsal convexity and created new frontal asymmetry. She has an undulating bridge with adequate tip projection. The two alternatives for creating a straight profile are dorsal resection alone (which will increase nasal base size), or dorsal resection and replacement with a septal cartilage graft (which will not increase nasal base size). In this patient, resection and replacement is preferable, not only for nasal balance but also because a dorsal graft will help camouflage the frontal asymmetry.

SUMMARY OF THE SURGICAL PLAN

1. Minimal skeletonization
2. Dorsal reduction
3. Retrograde reduction of the right lateral crus (preoperative asymmetry)
4. No transfixing incision
5. No nasal shortening
6. Septoplasty
7. Asymmetrical spreader grafts, much thicker on the left than the right
8. Onlay graft to the left middle vault
9. Dorsal graft
10. Minimal tip grafts for symmetry

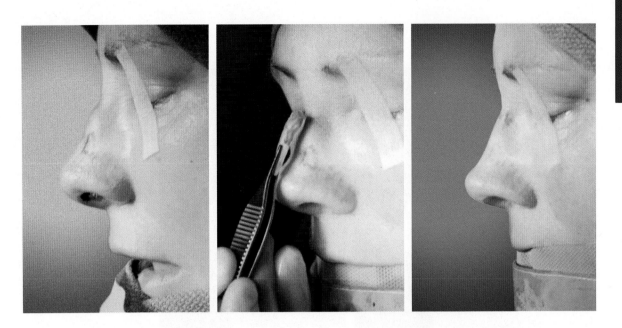

The septum fortunately yielded a perfect dorsal graft that was thicker at one end than the other. The graft edges were contoured and beveled distally to fit the defect. The remaining small cartilage scraps were placed into the superior tip lobule for contour and symmetry.

Postoperative Analysis

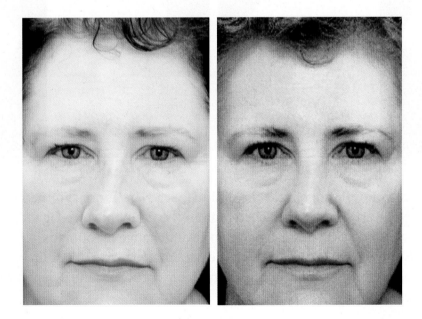

The patient is shown 6 months after surgery. The nose is significantly more symmetrical in the frontal view by virtue of the asymmetrical spreader and dorsal grafts. Nasal length has not changed.

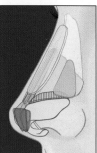

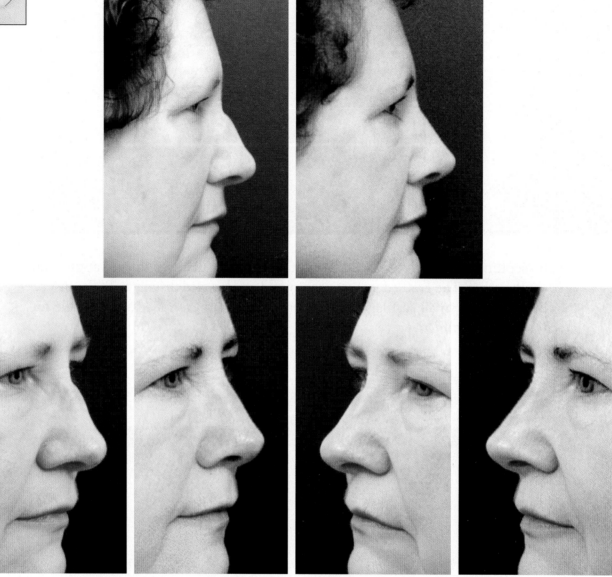

The dorsum is now straight and the oblique views are more symmetrical. A few crushed septal cartilage scraps placed high in the tip lobule (see Chapter 12) have improved symmetry without causing significant change in lobular size, tip projection, or nasal base volume. Notice that the patient's retrusive upper lip carriage has not changed, because neither a transfixing incision nor a caudal septal reduction was performed.

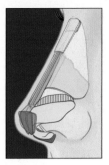

PATIENT STUDY THREE

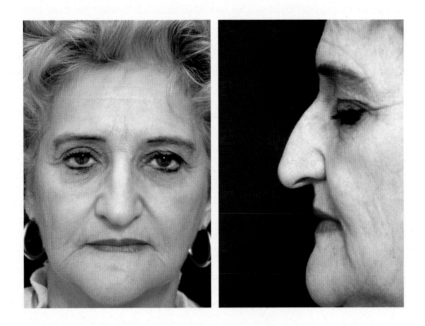

This French Canadian grandmother had decided it was time to do something about her lifelong nasal deformity. Length is a problem. The dorsum must be lowered and the base must be rotated, but any skeletal reduction will increase the patient's relative skin excess.

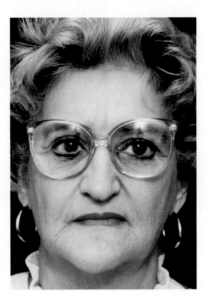

Accordingly, skin reduction was planned at the radix. The scar was less important in this case, because the patient's heavy eyeglasses would camouflage it. Much of the caudal septum would be preserved and sleeved between the medial crura as a tongue-in-groove, fixed with absorbable sutures only (see Chapter 11).

SUMMARY OF THE SURGICAL PLAN

1. Wide skeletonization over upper cartilaginous vault, narrow over bony vault

2. Dorsal reduction

3. Transfixing incision, shortening of caudal septum 2 mm and membranous septum 5 mm; sleeve caudal septum into columella as tongue-in-groove

4. Retrograde reduction of alar cartilage lateral crura, 3 mm

5. Reduction caudal ends, upper lateral cartilages, 4 mm

6. Septoplasty

7. Excision of upper nasal skin

8. Bilateral spreader grafts

9. Radix graft

10. Tip grafts

11. Columellar grafts

12. No osteotomy

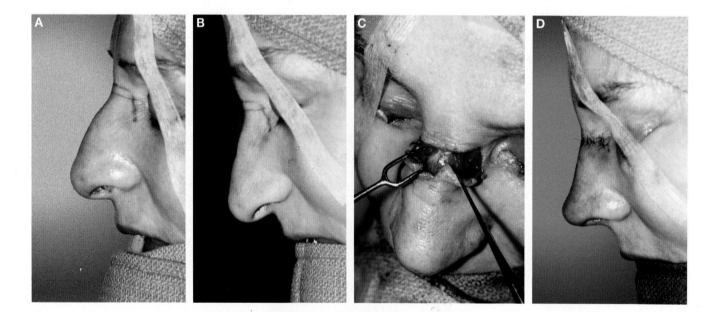

After dorsal reduction, notice that the nose lengthens *(B)*. This is typical not only of many long noses but also noses in which the hump is located distally. An incision was made as previously marked, extending across the radix, with back cuts along each side to absorb the dog-ears. Notice that, despite a significant dorsal reduction, the bony vault was still intact, and the cephalic part of the bony arch was quite dense *(C)*. The skin resection equilibrated the soft tissue and the skeleton *(D)*.

Postoperative Analysis

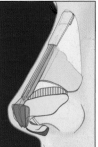

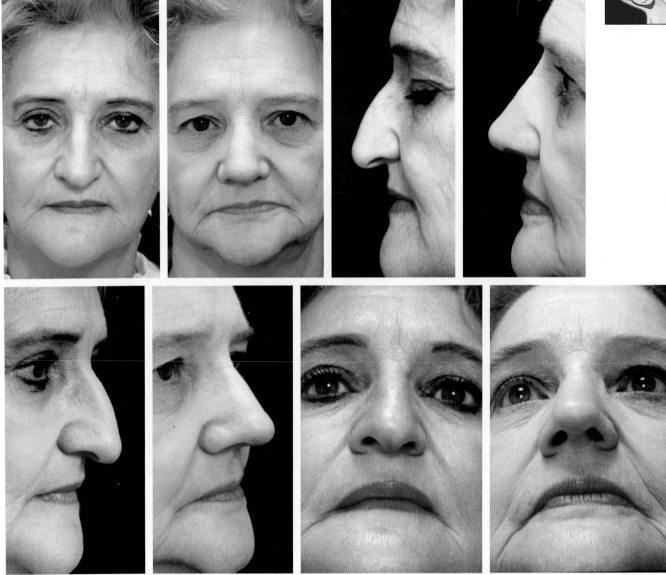

More than 4 years postoperatively, the nose remains shorter. Though the patient is 4 years older, dorsal reduction and nasal shortening have had a rejuvenating effect on her appearance (and her psyche, evidenced by her carrying her chin higher). The shortening has held, assisted by a skin excision and a firm caudal septal repair. Bony vault width and stability remain unchanged. Notice the persistent depressions caused by her heavy eyeglasses.

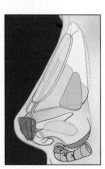

SECONDARY RHINOPLASTY IN OLDER PATIENTS

Secondary rhinoplasty in older patients requires the same precautions as in primary cases regarding anatomic variants, the soft tissue and skeletal changes that occur with aging, and the degree of change that patients expect or can tolerate. However, the surgeon must also cope with lost airway and support and with deficient donor sites.

PATIENT STUDY ONE

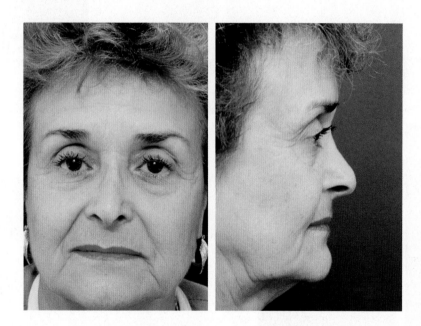

This patient had undergone two previous rhinoplasties that had diminished her airway (notice the nostril flare and the narrow middle vault). Lateral crural reduction has allowed the alar rims to retract cephalad. The tip lobule was essentially empty, hanging from the septal angle. This patient is an excellent example of someone with a large nasal base that is nonetheless inadequately projecting, indicating a large lower skin sleeve with deficient skeletal support. Septal cartilage was absent, and so rib cartilage was harvested for the dorsum and all other graft requirements. The septal partition was flaccid, and synechiae bound the septum to the inferior turbinate on one side.

SUMMARY OF THE SURGICAL PLAN

1. Harvest rib cartilage
2. Minimal skeletonization through single intercartilaginous incision
3. Divide synechiae between inferior turbinate and the septum
4. Thin rib cartilage maxillary augmentation
5. Rib cartilage dorsal graft
6. Rib cartilage lateral wall grafts
7. Rib cartilage alar wall grafts, left thicker than right
8. Multiple crushed tip grafts with solid rib cartilage buttress
9. Right alar wedge resection (lobule only), transferred to left alar rim as composite graft

Postoperative Analysis

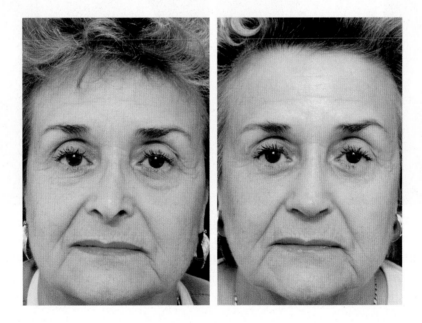

Two years postoperatively, the dorsum is straight. The dorsal graft has opened the middle vault, and lateral wall grafts have obscured the edges of the dorsal graft and smoothed the irregularities in the nasal sidewalls. Alar wall grafts have replaced the missing lateral crura. The transfer of the right lobule to the left rim has corrected the rim height asymmetry.

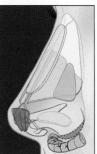

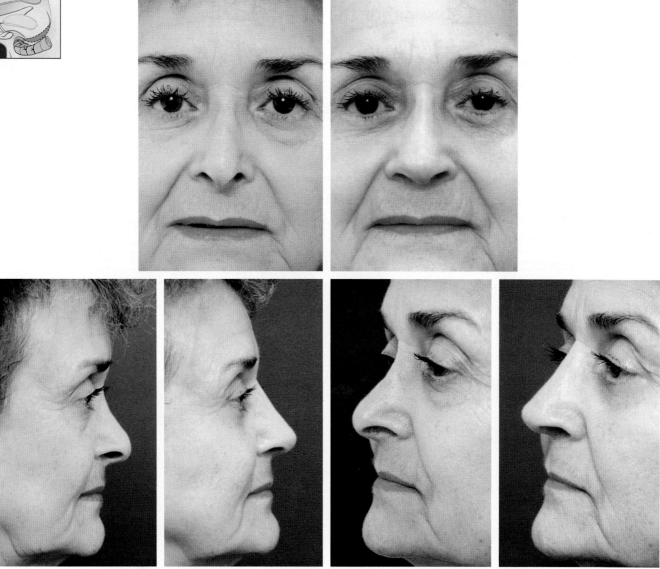

The dorsum is now correctly positioned, and the radix has moved from the lower lash margin to the level of the upper lash margin. The empty tip lobule has been expanded by grafts and now supports the tip above the level of the septal angle. The alar hollows have decreased.

PATIENT STUDY TWO

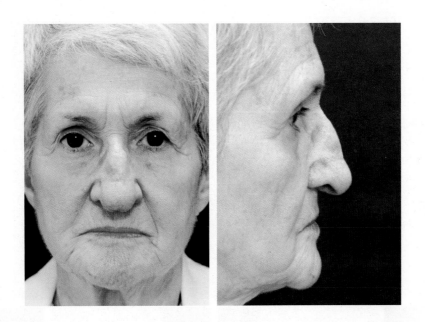

Although at first glance the dorsal hump may seem to be the most striking characteristic of this nose, examine also the nasal base. The maxillary arch is retrusive, and the entire base has rolled caudad and posteriorly. Despite strong alar cartilages, a previous septoplasty had included resection of the distal 25% of the septal partition, leaving nothing to support the base. A portion of the septum remained but was distorted. My plan was to reduce the dorsum, rotate the base, and then use the remaining septal and conchal cartilage to re-create caudal support and level the dorsum.

SUMMARY OF THE SURGICAL PLAN

1. Wide skeletonization over upper cartilaginous vault, narrow over bony vault

2. Resection of bony and cartilaginous dorsa

3. Submucosal shortening of upper lateral cartilages, 3 mm

4. Transfixing incision, shortening caudal and membranous septa

5. Delivery of alar cartilages as a bipedicle flap, reducing cephalic margin by 3 mm and resecting a 3 mm vertical wedge from each dome

6. Septoplasty

7. Harvest conchal cartilage

8. Unilateral spreader graft, right

9. Dorsal graft of septal cartilage

10. Ear cartilage graft to membranous septum, replacing caudal septum to the septal angle

11. No osteotomies

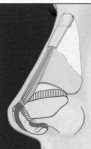

Postoperative Analysis

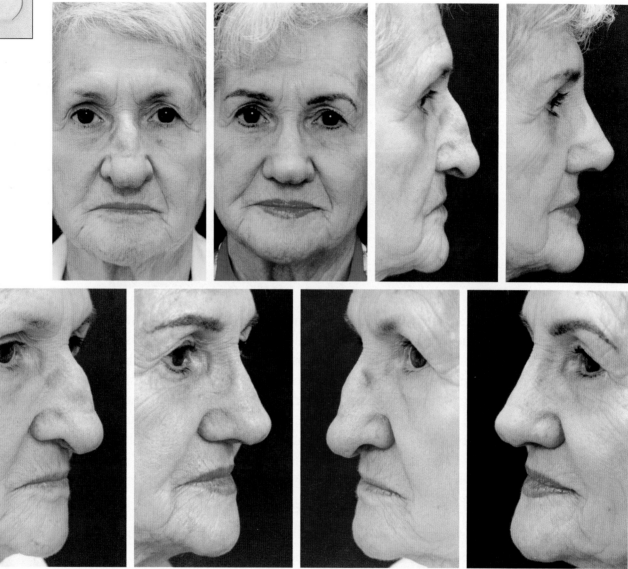

Postoperatively, the rejuvenating effect of a shorter nose is immediately obvious, not only in absolute aesthetic terms but in the patient's perception of her own attractiveness. The nasal base has been narrowed slightly by the domal resection, but skeletal reduction did not exceed soft tissue contractile limits. The nose is supported by increased middle vault width, maintenance of bridge height, and replacement of the caudal septum. No maxillary augmentation was performed to avoid pushing the large nasal base farther anteriorly.

Although some reduction was performed, a great deal of dorsal height and alar cartilage strength was maintained. The middle vault and the caudal septum were augmented, and osteotomy was avoided. Geometric mean nasal airflow increased 2.9 times over preoperative values.

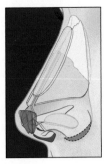

PATIENT STUDY THREE

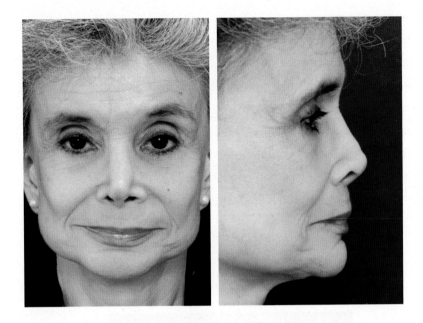

This patient had undergone four previous rhinoplasties, the last of which, 27 years earlier, had been a silicone dorsal augmentation. Although the silicone implant had been in place for many years, the patient was bothered by its movement and its sensitivity to winter cold.

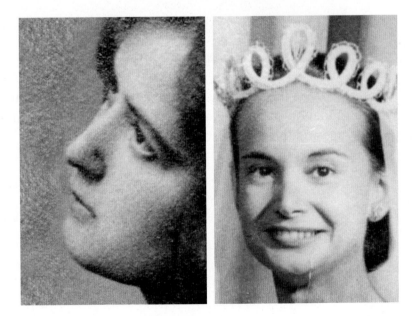

Photographs of the patient as a teenager and at her wedding show a high dorsum and a projecting tip without retroussé.

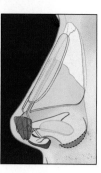

SUMMARY OF THE SURGICAL PLAN

1. Harvest rib cartilage
2. Minimal skeletonization through right-sided intercartilaginous incision
3. Remove silicone prosthesis
4. Skeletonize dorsum behind prosthetic capsule
5. Rasp bony vault for adherence
6. Rib cartilage dorsal graft
7. Rib cartilage alar wall grafts
8. Multiple tip grafts, placed on caudal side of lobule
9. Bilateral alar wedge resections, removing external and vestibular skin; transfer of alar wedge resection tissue to alar rims as composite grafts

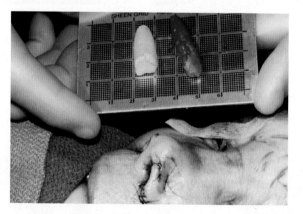

The old silicone prosthesis is shown next to its rib graft replacement, which is longer to facilitate caudal tip rotation. Note the color of the rib graft, highly calcified at this patient's age and therefore virtually impervious to warping.

Postoperative Analysis

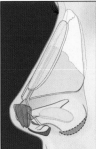

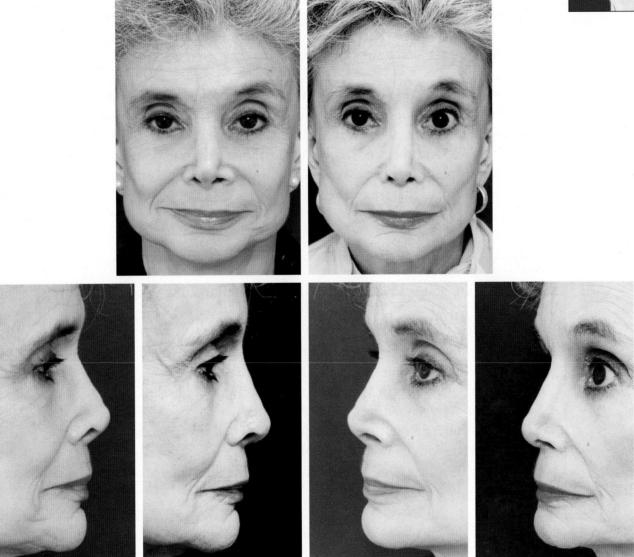

Three years after surgery, the dorsum remains stable and smooth. The rib graft, unlike the silicone implant, has firmly united to the bony arch. The nasal base is narrower, and the alar rim notches have softened. Because the alar resections were small, their transfer to the rims produced a negligible improvement. More significant changes in alar rim height could have been effected by conchal cartilage/skin composite grafts, which are stiffer than alar lobular skin but would have necessitated another donor site. The patient's soft tissue laxity, a bonus in this older tertiary rhinoplasty patient, allowed several millimeters of nasal base rotation caudally. Combined with an elevation of the radix by the dorsal graft, the increase in nasal length is noticeable. Geometric mean nasal airflow increased 4.3 times over preoperative measurements.

Thin Skin

The soft tissues and skeletons of patients with thin skin treat both patients and surgeons mercilessly. Thin skin reveals every underlying skeletal flaw and tightens around a reduced framework until it reaches its contractile limits, after which the skin begins to thicken and a supratip deformity develops.

However, it is not the skin alone that constitutes the problem in these patients—it is the underlying skeleton, particularly the alar cartilages, which are usually strong, convex, and full of internal stresses. Reduced excessively, alar cartilages knuckle. Resected, crushed, and replaced, they may heal unevenly, one bowing more than the other. Interrupted with vertical resections, the ends may curl outward, producing unattractive ridges that frame the tip.

The following points should be kept in mind when treating patients with thin skin:
- Give particular care to producing a smooth skeleton.
- Preserve enough alar cartilage arch to retain shape and avoid postoperative kinking and knuckling at the domes or elsewhere.
- Place spreader grafts to avoid any postoperative middle vault discontinuity, almost always visible in these patients.
- Use only softened or crushed cartilage dorsal and tip grafts, which provide support with a lower chance of visible edges.

Malpositioned alar cartilages and other anatomic variants are particularly noticeable in thin-skinned patients and must be treated to produce a normal result.

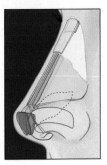

PATIENT STUDY ONE

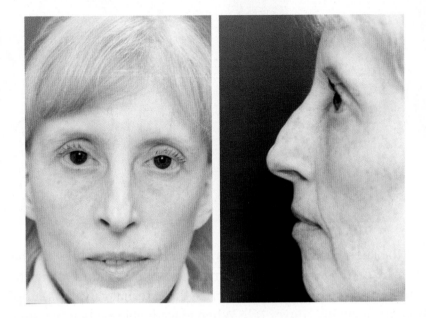

If this patient's skin were thicker, her malpositioned lateral crura would not be so obvious. Thin skin outlines the caudal end of the bony vault, the contour of the middle vault, the normal declivity between the alar cartilages, the tip of the septal angle, and the extended abnormal position of each lateral crus. The patient's flared nostrils manifest her poor airway.

SUMMARY OF THE SURGICAL PLAN

1. Resect and reposition alar cartilage lateral crura

2. Dorsal reduction

3. Transfixing incision, with 2 mm trim of caudal and membranous septa

4. Septoplasty

5. Bilateral spreader grafts, thicker on the left than right (preoperative asymmetry)

6. Thin radix graft

7. Multiple crushed cartilage tip grafts

8. Columellar grafts to smooth columellar/lobular contour

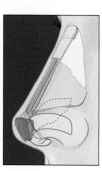

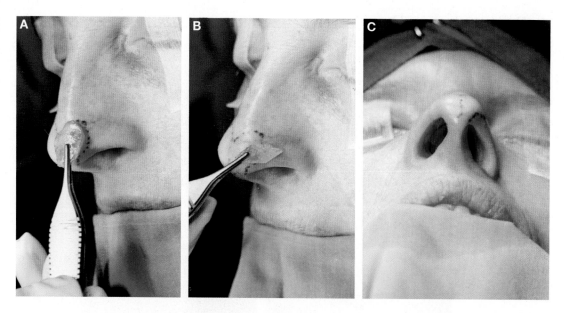

Notice that the lateral crural dimensions correspond exactly to what the skin had shown *(A)*. The cartilage was crushed, trimmed, and replaced along the alar rim *(B)*. After repositioning the right lateral crus, the external valve was supported and the rim became normally convex *(C)*. When placed where it belongs, anatomy creates the normal.

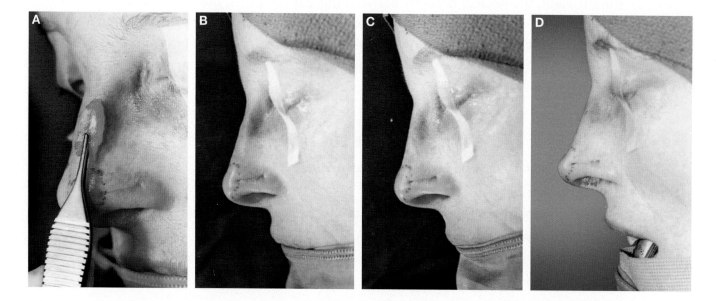

The resected roof, 2.5 mm thick, shows normal surface markings, with its central depression denoting the fusion line between the upper lateral cartilages and the anterior septal edge *(A)*. Compare the views before *(B)* and after *(C)* a single-layer radix graft, and notice the difference in dorsal contour and apparent nasal base size. At the conclusion of the procedure the dorsum was straight, the tip was adequately projecting, and all four valves had been reconstructed *(D)*.

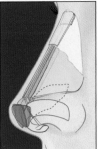

Postoperative Analysis

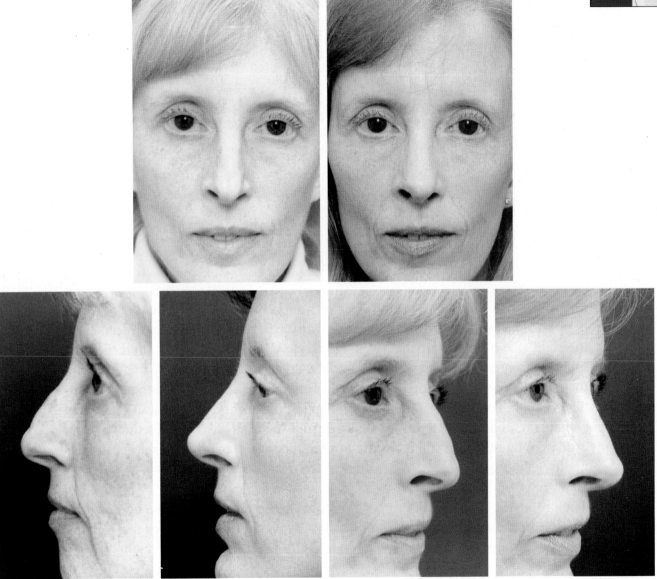

Eighteen months postoperatively, the dorsal lines are smooth and continuous. The bony vault is slightly narrower, the middle vault is appropriately wide and confluent with the upper and lower vaults, and the alar cartilages are repositioned, now with normal surface markings. The dorsum is straight, the septal angle is in line with the tip, and the tip itself has been recontoured by multiple soft grafts with edges that do not show. Correction of external valvular support alone doubles airflow in most patients.

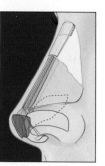

PATIENT STUDY TWO

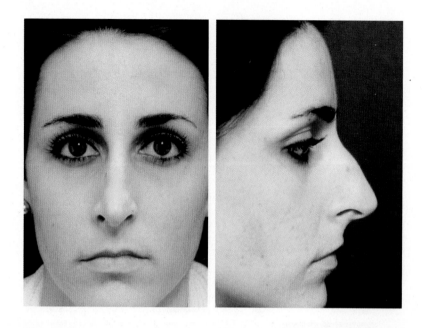

This woman's nose is an asymmetrical version of the previous patient's, although her narrow, excessively angular tip is more distorted and her septum projects from the right side of the columella, twisting the nasal base first one way and then the other. The entire nose is pencil-thin, and the dorsum is high and unbalanced (with the radix too low and the tip inadequately projecting). This is a tension nose, manifested by slitlike nostrils and a skeleton that seems too large for the skin sleeve that contains it, pulling the upper lip forward from the midface. Dorsal reduction and caudal septal resection will allow the nose to recess posteriorly and release the upper lip.

The problem here is not the upper lip musculature or an overactive or short depressor septi muscle. The problem is a skin sleeve that cannot cover the skeleton beneath it. When the skeleton is recontoured, the soft tissues will correct themselves.

SUMMARY OF THE SURGICAL PLAN

1. Resect and relocate malpositioned lateral crura
2. Minimal skeletonization over dorsum
3. Reduction of bony and cartilaginous vaults
4. Transfixing incision
5. Shorten caudal and membranous septa, 3 mm
6. Asymmetrical spreader grafts, thicker on right than left
7. Thin, layered radix graft
8. Multiple crushed cartilage tip grafts
9. No osteotomy

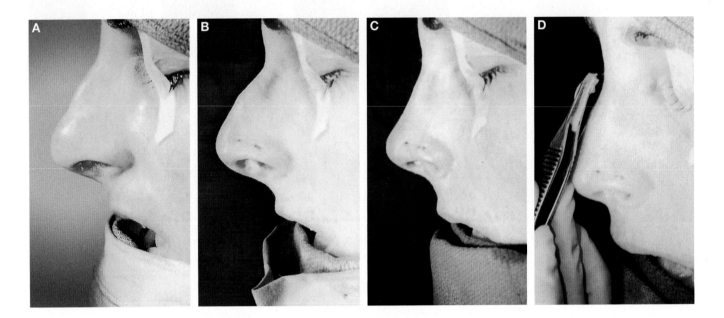

Compare the patient's appearance at the beginning of the case to her appearance after bony vault resection alone (*A* and *B*). Bony vault reduction further decreased the low radix, creating the illusion of an even larger nasal base. The tip rotated cephalad, raising the nostril rim and producing a relatively low caudal septum. After completing the dorsal reduction, the caudal septum required a compensatory adjustment (*C*). After dorsal, tip, and caudal septal reductions, notice the new upper lip position: the distortion self-corrected without any direct modification of the lip itself. A layered radix graft was used to improve nasal proportion (*D*).

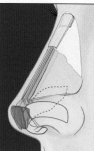

Postoperative Analysis

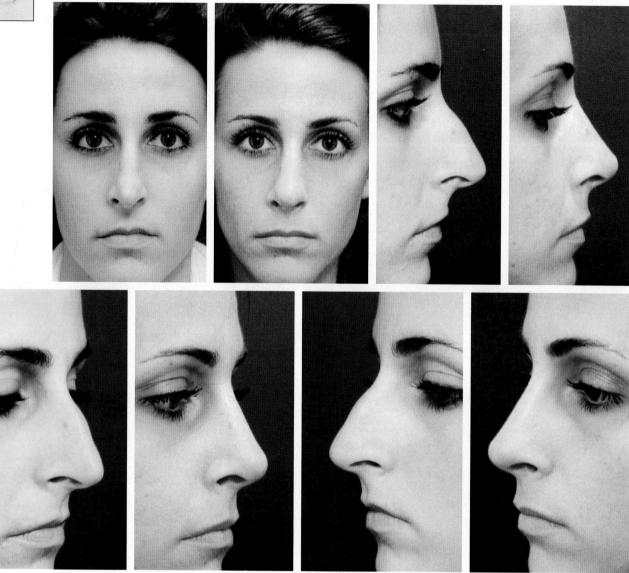

Eighteen months postoperatively, nasal contours are smooth and more symmetrical. Spreader grafts have improved the high septal deviation, but the patient's rigid, posttraumatic cartilage has resisted complete correction. Dorsal and caudal septal reductions have allowed the entire nose to recess so that it no longer dominates the patient's midface. Her upper lip contour is normal, without distortion at the subnasale. The radix is slightly higher, continuing into a straight dorsum and ending in a tip that is slightly higher but less severely narrow, according to the patient's wishes. The oblique views match more completely. Notice also the apparent diminution in nostril length (although no alar wedge resections were performed), which is the result of a better nostril-lobular proportion.

Thick Skin

The problem for surgeons treating patients with either thin skin or thick skin is that the surface cover does nothing to help. Thin skin shows everything; thick skin shows nothing. It was not so long ago that patients with thick skin were summarily rejected for rhinoplasty, because previous experience had shown that results for these patients were uniformly poor. And the results were poor when rhinoplasty was only a reduction operation, because nasal soft tissues do *not* have an infinite capacity to conform to the shape of any reduced skeleton (in contrast to False Assumption Number One [see Chapter 2]). Thick skin does not move much.

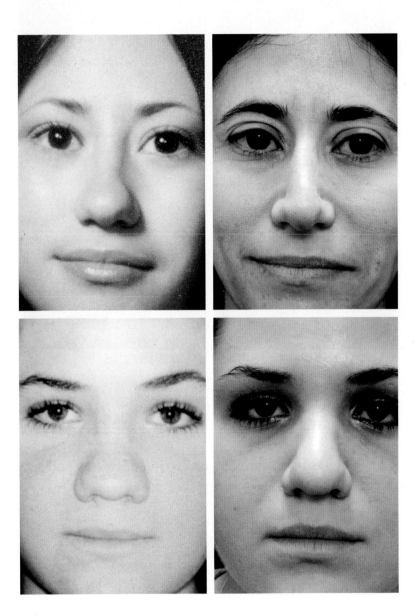

If thick soft tissues can move at all, they collapse and obstruct the airway when underlying support decreases.

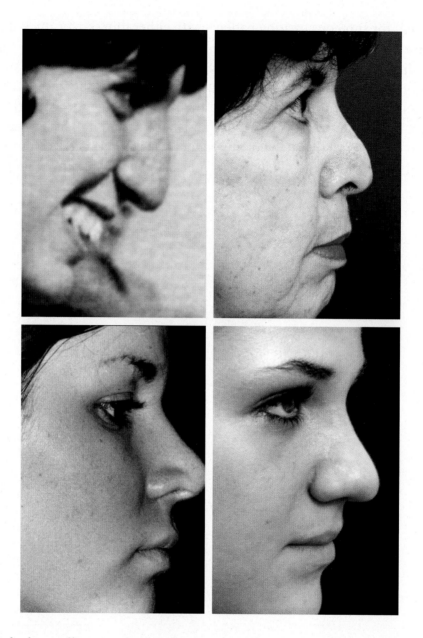

Or, if thick skin collapses posteriorly, tip projection decreases and supratip deformity is produced.

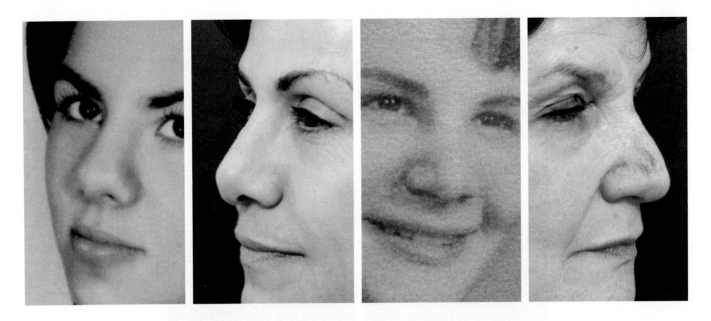

When malpositioned lateral crura have created a ball tip, skeletal reduction obstructs the external valves and costs tip shape and projection. The problem may be the skin, but the solution is not the skin. Dermal thinning is never effective.

Several ground rules are helpful when treating the thick-skinned nose:
- Thick skin conforms poorly to a reduced framework. Consider it a fixed parameter, not variable.
- To the extent that thick skin can contract and conform, it becomes even thicker, causing the nose to lose definition.
- The heavier the tissues, the more support is required.
- The heavier the tissues, the more substantial the grafts must be to produce a given surface effect.
- When the augmented skeleton projects and influences surface contour, the nose appears more refined.

PATIENT STUDY ONE

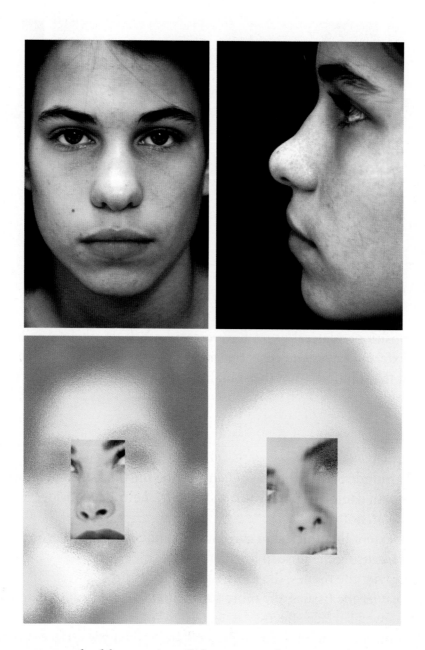

This young woman had been rejected for surgery by numerous prior physicians, who believed she was untreatable. They were right to assess this nasal configuration as difficult. Adding complexity to the procedure was the patient's surgical goal as pictured in the magazine photographs: a smaller, narrower nose with a slender, angular tip.

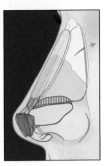

This type of consultation must be a journey into what is possible and what is not. I explained to the patient that the model's soft tissues and skeleton are entirely different from her own, and that such a transformation is not surgically possible by methods that I know. I then showed her photographs of thick-skinned patients with similar problems, explaining that these examples demonstrated the limits of what Nature would permit. I explained the logic of augmentation and the restrictions imposed by her tissues.

Some patients accept these limitations (as this young woman did) as the best of the available alternatives, even though they must reset their goals. Other patients are not willing to accept them, and they should seek treatment elsewhere.

This young woman's tissues are thick, and her contours are blunt. The dorsum is slightly low relative to the nasal base size, therefore giving room for dorsal augmentation (which should narrow the frontal view). Bony vault width equals base width. The lateral crura are bossed and broad, but the overlying soft tissues do not coapt the lateral crura that she has, indicating that they will not tighten around cartilages that are even smaller. However, modest tip reduction followed by lobular augmentation becomes a rearrangement rather than a reduction, allowing the tip to become more angular without the need to change volume.

SUMMARY OF THE SURGICAL PLAN

1. Limited skeletonization over bony and upper cartilaginous vaults

2. Rasp bony vault for graft adherence

3. Reduction of alar cartilage lateral crura through a delivery technique, leaving 8 mm; 3 mm vertical wedge taken from each lateral genu

4. Septoplasty

5. Dorsal graft of septal cartilage

6. Tip grafts

7. Bilateral osteotomies

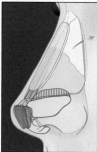

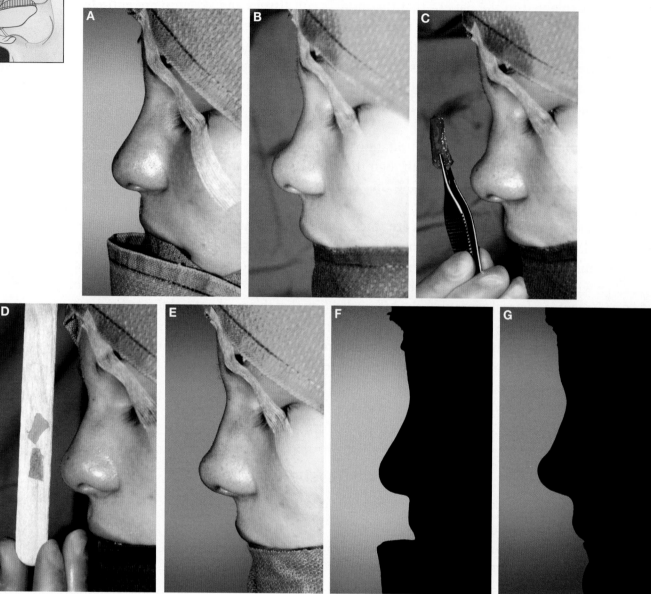

After alar cartilage reduction, dorsal contour changed very little, as expected *(B)*. The best piece of septal cartilage was beveled and trimmed for the dorsum *(C)*, and two firm pieces were selected for the nasal tip *(D)*. After dorsal and tip augmentation, the skeleton has better shape and angularity *(E)*.

Silhouette views document the increase in tip projection *(F and G)*. Dorsal height seems unchanged despite augmentation.

Postoperative Analysis

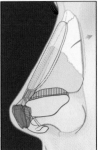

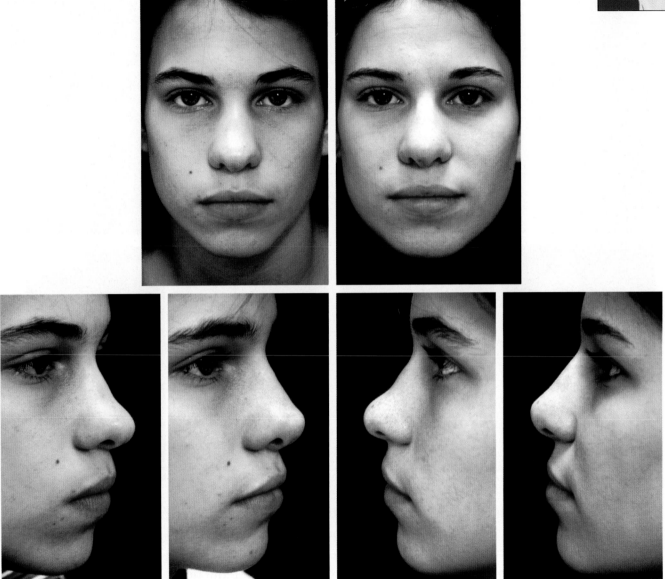

Two-and-one-half years after surgery, the frontal view is slightly narrower (the result of osteotomies and dorsal grafting), and the tip change is real but modest. Despite lateral crural reduction and dome resection, the tip lobule has only narrowed slightly. Lateral and oblique views show smooth, more angular contours with an apparent reduction in apparent nasal base size. The nose has a nonsurgical appearance. This patient was pleased with her outcome, largely because she had accepted a limited change preoperatively and redefined her goal.

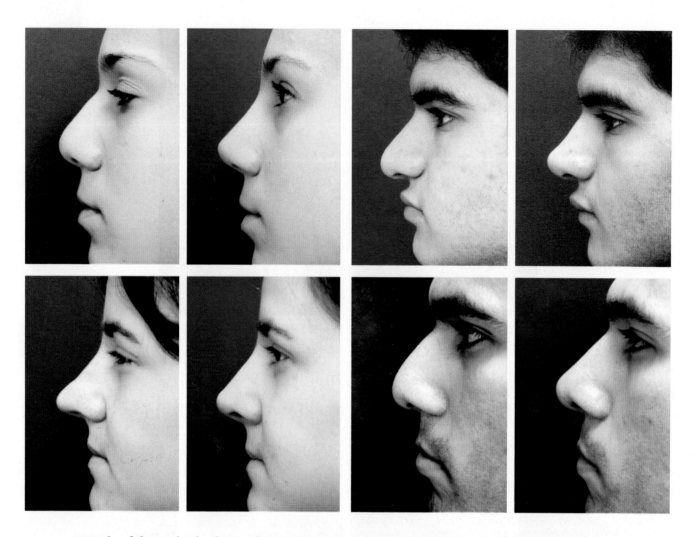

Each of these thick-skinned patients was treated in the same way: by conservatively reducing areas that were excessive and looking for areas that could be augmented and for places where angularity could be increased to provide the illusion of refinement. All patients received minimal dorsal and tip reductions, tip grafts, and either radix or dorsal grafts (depending on the configuration). When tip-grafting patients with thick skin, the firmer the grafts and the fewer their number, the more angularity they will produce (see Chapter 12).

Rhinophyma

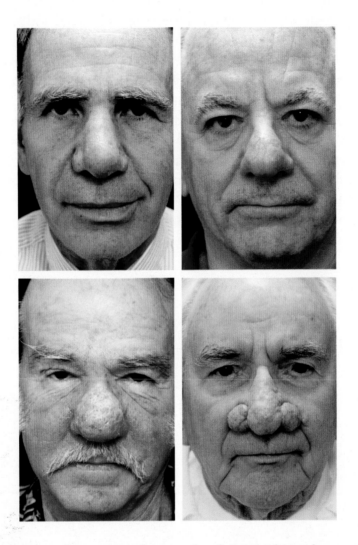

Rhinophyma is the perfect setting for a real reduction rhinoplasty mindset. All of the noses pictured here really are too large, distorted by sebaceous and vascular overgrowth, chronic inflammation, exudates, and sometimes grotesque excesses of nasal soft tissue.

There is no question that the soft tissue must be reduced, either by tangential excision or direct excision. As the excised surface heals, skin texture changes, sometimes becoming smoother and sometimes becoming scarred, depending on the depth of the excision. Patients must be forewarned of the latter possibility, but few patients object, because the deformity is so significant and so inaccurately associated with middle-aged ethanol abuse.

Three principles can guide the surgeon treating rhinophyma:

- Not every nose with rhinophyma was originally small and straight. Before beginning the excision, try to visualize the patient's real underlying contour, and obtain old photographs if possible. The objective is to reduce the nose but produce as little scarring as possible. An initial shape compromise may be necessary.
- Do not assume that every nose was well balanced before it became diseased: some had dorsal humps and low radices, some had inadequate tip projection, and some were already too long. Your patient may need a second rebalancing procedure; skin excision does not correct skeletal abnormalities.
- Plan excisions according to the nasal planes and aesthetic units to minimize distracting color and contour discontinuities.

PATIENT STUDY ONE

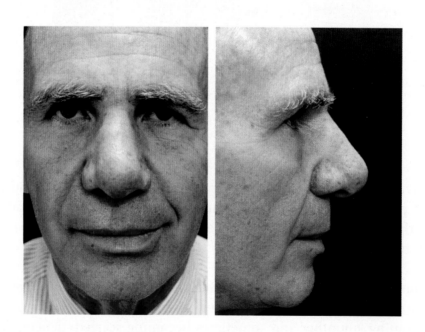

This physician had noticed a progressive, mild enlargement of his nose over the previous 3 years. His medial cheeks were similarly affected: the rubor and telangiectases of the nose, upper lip, and cheeks indicate acne rosacea.

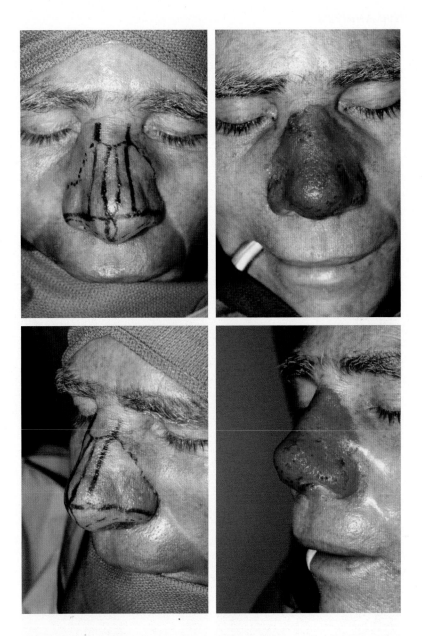

I began by outlining the nasal planes and light reflexes so that I would not lose my orientation during surgery. After local anesthesia infiltration, I worked from area to area with a scalpel, changing No. 15 blades frequently. I began with the dorsal reflex, extending down the sidewalls, and then carving the tip lobule. If the tissues permit, I try to narrow the middle vault slightly to show the demarcation of the caudal end of the bony arch and to highlight the point of maximum tip projection and the tip facets, all of which give the illusion of refinement to a thick nose. Notice that the soft triangles were spared to avoid retraction and nostril deformities.

Postoperative Analysis

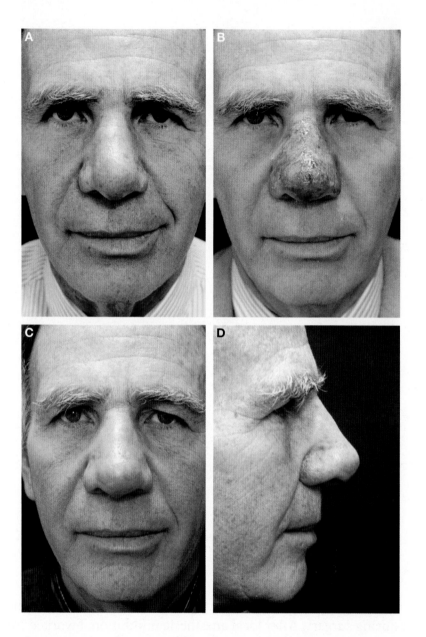

Four days after excision, the wound has the expected amount of exudate, but epithelization has already begun *(B)*. The tissues are protected with petrolatum. At 4 weeks, epithelization is complete and contour is good *(C* and *D)*.

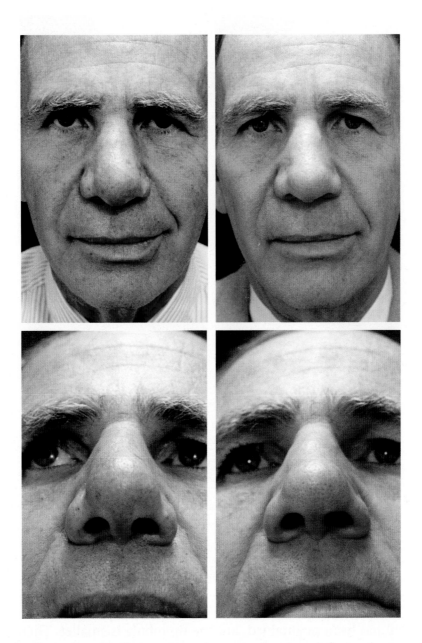

At 1 year, the frontal and inferior views show modest but definite changes. Excision has been sufficiently superficial to avoid scarring. The midnose and tip lobule are narrower, and alar rim contour has been preserved. The columella remains narrow.

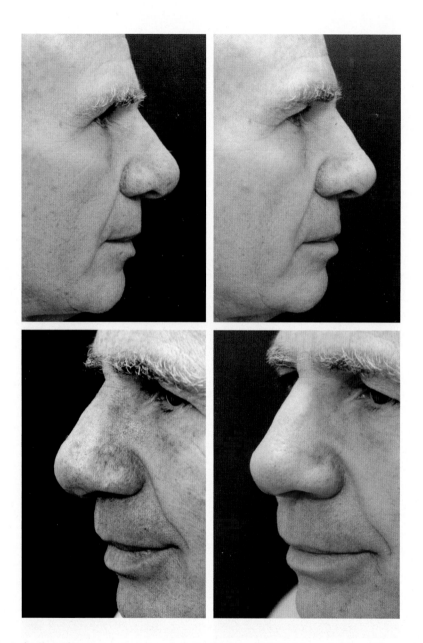

Dorsal height has been maintained, but the tip lobule is smaller. There is a slight concavity over the middle vault, and skin texture has been preserved. The skin has hypopigmented as expected, but it is confined to aesthetic units.

PATIENT STUDY TWO

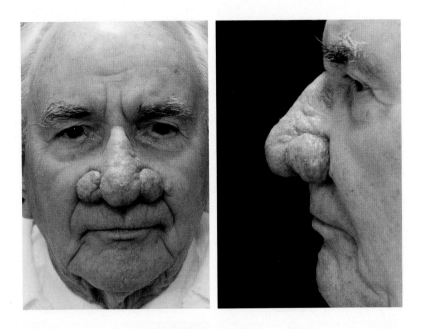

This man has a more severe manifestation of the same disease, with gross enlargement of the alar lobules and extension onto his medial cheeks. The nasal skin is pitted and filled with sebaceous secretions, and there are vascular ulcerations in the right alar lobule.

The treatment in this case is the same as the previous case, but visualization is more difficult. By palpation, it is obvious that the dorsum is not straight, and the tip lobule must therefore be sized appropriately for this nose. The same applies to the tip and alar lobules in the frontal view.

Disease of this depth requires excision into the upper dermis and middermis, which means that the texture and color of the healed skin will not be normal, but hypopigmented and scarred in some areas. Although patients must be forewarned, I have never seen a patient be discouraged by these possibilities.

Postoperative Analysis

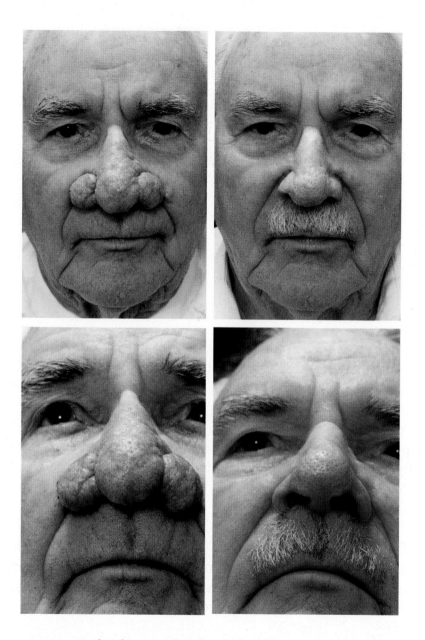

One year postoperatively, the nose has healed, and the skin is smooth but lightly scarred and hypopigmented. Nevertheless, the excised area blends well with the unoperated nasal skin. The alar walls are normally thin, and the tip lobular width is appropriate for the patient's frontal aesthetics. General dorsal contour—including the underlying hump—has been preserved, and tip and alar lobular aesthetics have improved.

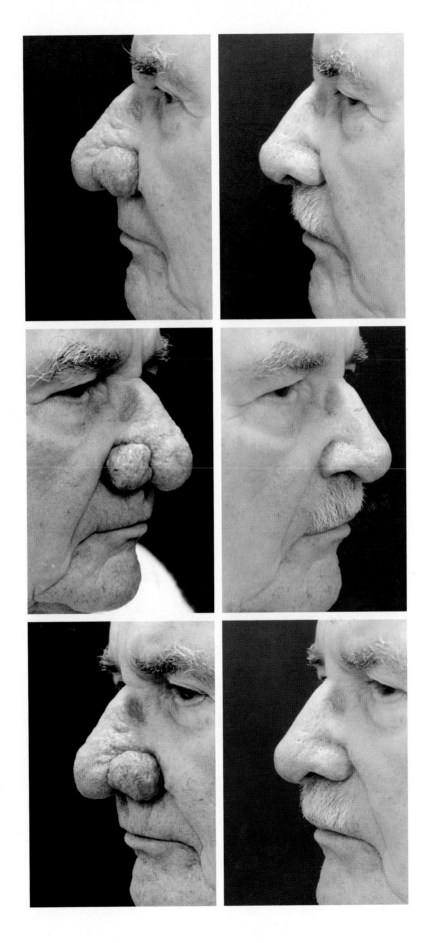

PATIENT STUDY THREE _____

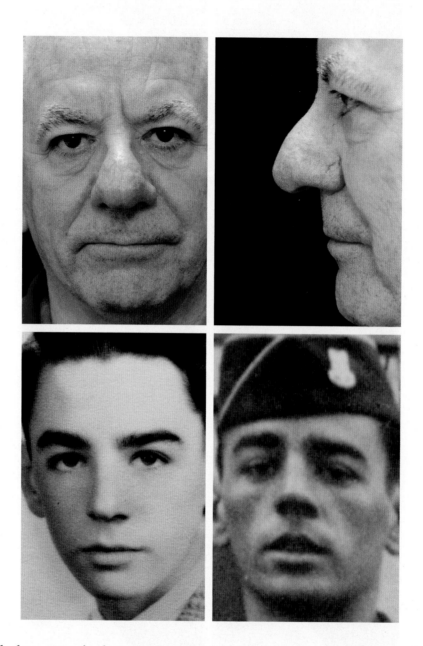

Although this patient's photographs of himself as a young man show much thinner skin, they do not give information about his profile. His preoperative lateral view reveals a significant imbalance between the upper and lower nose. The surgeon should not assume that beneath a thickened, rhinophymatous exterior lies a straight dorsum with adequate tip projection, because patients with dorsal humps, excessive tip projection, or low radix imbalance can all develop rhinophyma. In this particular case, correction necessitated two stages: shaving in the first stage, followed by skin excision and rebalancing in the second stage.

The patient had undergone a previous septoplasty but his airway was still obstructed. Although totally obscured by the skin cover, his internal valves were narrow and incompetent.

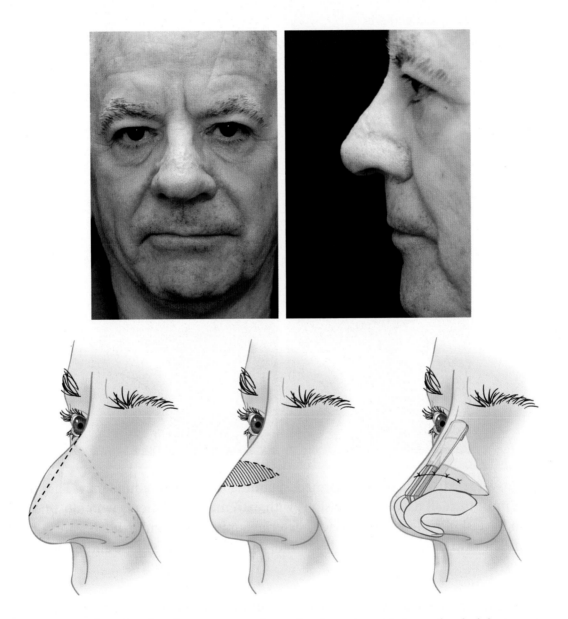

Three months after the shaving procedure, the dorsum and tip are healed, but some hypertrophic scarring has developed in the patient's midnose at the site of the most prominent disease. On the lateral view, the supratip convexity is still obvious. The nose remains slightly long, and the upper dorsum is slightly low relative to the nasal base size. A direct transverse excision is planned, which will lower the supratip and shorten the nose; spreader grafts will reconstruct the internal valves. As a necessary compromise, crushed ear cartilage will form a thin radix graft to improve nasal proportion.

SUMMARY OF THE SURGICAL PLAN

1. Transverse resection of supratip skin
2. Harvest ear cartilage
3. Bilateral spreader grafts
4. Cartilage graft to posterior columella for contour and support
5. Thin, crushed ear cartilage graft to upper dorsum

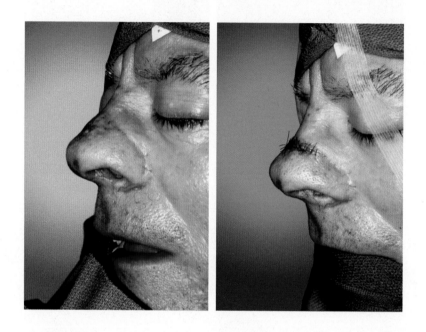

A transverse skin excision was planned, spanning the area of redundancy. The surgeon must treat all nasal skin excisions with extreme care. Patients who most need them have skin replete with surface bacteria. Suppuration and exudates are common. The skin cannot be resected, sutured, and left covered by tape and plaster for 7 days.

Place fine subcuticular sutures so that skin sutures may be removed early. I change the dressings myself daily and begin suture removal at 48 hours. The wound must be kept scrupulously clean. If proper attention is paid, then the scars, although not invisible, reach their potential best.

Postoperative Analysis

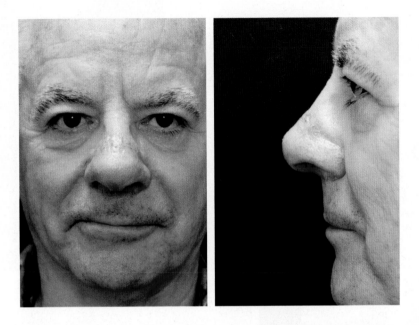

One week following the second procedure, the skin wound has healed primarily. The dorsum is straight, and the nose is slightly shorter.

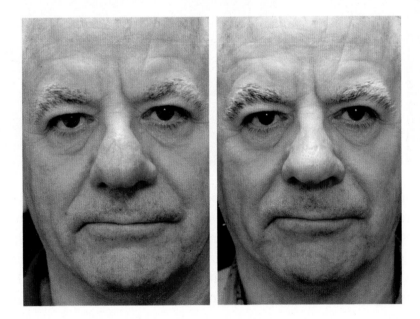

Fourteen months following the second procedure, nasal contours are smooth. The transverse excision has virtually disappeared within the area of hypertrophic scarring, which itself has matured.

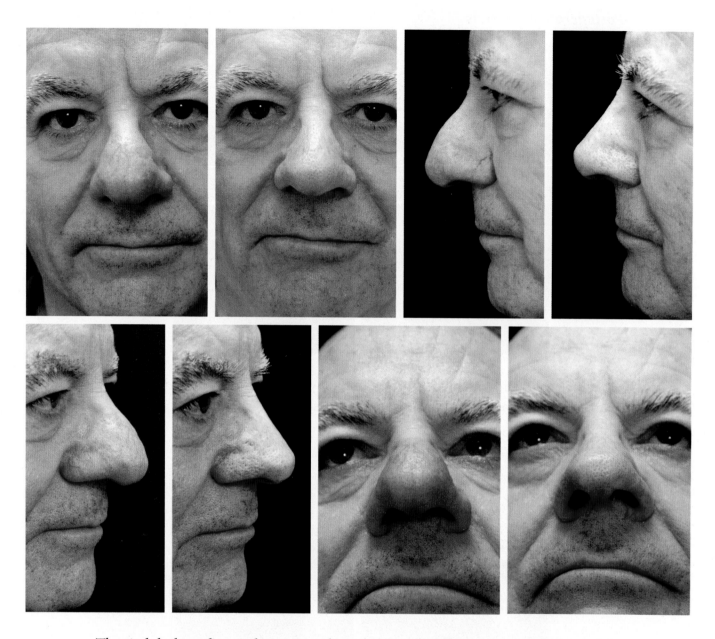

The tip lobule and nostrils are now shaped normally. Skin excision and the weight removed from the tip have rotated the base cephalad. Slight upper dorsal augmentation, direct shaving, supratip excision, nasal shortening, and columellar grafting have reduced the apparent nasal base size. Disease resection sufficient to create a straight dorsum was not performed; it would have produced a full-thickness defect. Scarring was reduced by the combination of skin reduction and skeletal augmentation.

Rhinophyma surgery matches the surgeon's right brain against disease.

BIBLIOGRAPHY

Anderson JR. Straightening the crooked nose. Trans Am Acad Ophthalmol Otolaryngol 76:938-945, 1972.

Baser B, Shahani R, Khanna S, et al. Calvarial bone grafts for augmentation rhinoplasty. J Laryngol Otol 105:1018-1020, 1991.

Bashour M. History and current concepts in the analysis of facial attractiveness. Plast Reconstr Surg 118:741-756, 2006.

Baum SJ. Nasal projection. Arch Otolaryngol 103:262-267, 1977.

Beheri GE. Rhinoplasty in Egyptians. Aesthetic Plast Surg 8:145-150, 1984.

Berry RL, Edwards RC, Paxton MC. Nasal augmentation using the mandibular coronoid as an autogenous graft: report of case. J Oral Maxillofac Surg 52:633-638, 1994.

Boccieri A, Pascali M. Septal crossbar graft for the correction of the crooked nose. Plast Reconstr Surg 111:629-638, 2003.

Boo-Chai K. The management of ala ptosis in Oriental rhinoplasty. Aesthetic Plast Surg 10:17-20, 1986.

Brain DJ. The management of the deviated nose. J Laryngol Otol 95:471-486, 1981.

Byrd HS, Solomon J, Flood J. Correction of the crooked nose. Plast Reconstr Surg 102:2148-2157, 1998.

Cannistrá CN, Guerrieri L, Iannetti G. Deviated nose: technical proposition for prevention of recurrences. Aesthetic Plast Surg 22:206-210, 1998.

Celik M, Tuncer S. Nasal reconstruction using both cranial bone and ear cartilage. Plast Reconstr Surg 105:1624-1627, 2000.

Cheney ML, Gliklich RE. The use of calvarial bone in nasal reconstruction. Arch Otolaryngol Head Neck Surg 121:643-648, 1995.

Clark DP, Hanke CW. Electrosurgical treatment of rhinophyma. J Am Acad Dermatol 22:831-837, 1990.

Colton JJ, Beekhuis GJ. Management of nasal fractures. Otolaryngol Clin North Am 19:73-85, 1986.

Constantian MB. An algorithm for correcting the asymmetrical nose. Plast Reconstr Surg 83:801-811, 1989.

Curnier A, Choudhary S. Rhinophyma: dispelling the myths. Plast Reconstr Surg 114:351-354, 2004.

Daniel RK. Hispanic rhinoplasty in the United States, with emphasis on the Mexican American nose. Plast Reconstr Surg 112:244-256; discussion 257-258, 2003.

Dingman RO, Natvig P. The deviated nose. Clin Plast Surg 4:145-152, 1977.

Ducut EG, Han SK, Kim SB, et al. Factors affecting nostril shape in Asian noses. Plast Reconstr Surg 118:1613-1621, 2006.

Ellis DA, Gilbert RW. Analysis and correction of the crooked nose. J Otolaryngol 20:14-18, 1991.

Farina R, Cury E, Ackel IA. Traumatic nasal deformities. Aesthetic Plast Surg 7:233-236, 1983.

Flowers RS. Nasal augmentation by the intraoral route. Plast Reconstr Surg 54:570-578, 1974.

Foda HM. The role of septal surgery in management of the deviated nose. Plast Reconstr Surg 115:406-415, 2005.

Gilbert JG. Treatment of posttraumatic nasal deformity. N Z Med J 100:713-715, 1987.

Gilbert SE. Overlay grafting for lateral nasal wall concavities. Otolaryngol Head Neck Surg 119:385-388, 1998.

González-Ulloa M. The fat nose. Aesthetic Plast Surg 8:135-140, 1984.

Grimes PE, Hunt SG. Considerations for cosmetic surgery in the black population. Clin Plast Surg 20:27-34, 1993.

Gruber R, Kuang A, Kahn D. Asian-American rhinoplasty. Aesthet Surg J 24:423-430, 2004.

Gruber RP, Weintraub J, Pomerantz J. Suture technique for the nasal tip. Aesthet Surg J 28:92-100, 2008.

Grymer LF, Fogstrup J, Stoksted P. The deflected nose—surgical correction. J Laryngol Otol 96:719-724, 1982.

Gurley JM, Pilgram T, Perlyn CA, et al. Long-term outcome of autogenous rib graft nasal reconstruction. Plast Reconstr Surg 108:1895-1905, 2001.

Guyuron B. The aging nose. Dermatol Clin 15:659-664, 1997.

Guyuron B, Griffin A, Hoefflin S, et al. African-American rhinoplasty. Aesthet Surg J 24:551-560, 2004.

Hallock GG. Cranial nasal bone grafts. Aesthetic Plast Surg 13:285-289, 1989.

Har-El G, Shapshay SM, Bohigian RK, et al. The treatment of rhinophyma. 'Cold' vs laser techniques. Arch Otolaryngol Head Neck Surg 119:628-631, 1993.

Hodgkinson DJ. The olecranon bone graft for nasal augmentation. Aesthetic Plast Surg 16:129-132, 1992.

Jeppesen F. Anterior wedge excision in correcting deflections of the nasal dorsum. Ear Nose Throat J 71:49-58, 1992.

Jeppesen F. Anterior wedge excision in deflected nasal dorsum. A pilot study. Rhinology 29:201-212, 1991.

Johnson CM Jr, Anderson JR. The deviated nose—its correction. Laryngoscope 87:1680-1684, 1977.

Kabaker SS. An adjunctive technique to rhinoplasty of the aging nose. Head Neck Surg 2:276-281, 1980.

Kabaker SS. An approach to aesthetic rhinoplasty in the non-Caucasian nose. Arch Otolaryngol 103:461-467, 1977.

Kane NP, Kane LA. Open reduction of nasal fractures. J Otolaryngol 7:183-186, 1978.

Kilic A. The nasal bone graft for nasal augmentation. Plast Reconstr Surg 108:274-275, 2001.

Kline RM Jr, Wolfe SA. Complications associated with the harvesting of cranial bone grafts. Plast Reconstr Surg 95:5-13, 1995.

Lawson VG. Management of the twisted nose. J Otolaryngol 7:56-66, 1978.

Levine B, Berman WE. Demineralized bone grafts in rhinoplasty. Ear Nose Throat J 74:222-223, 1995.

Maniglia AJ. Surgical correction of the traumatized nose. Otolaryngol Clin North Am 16:609-621, 1983.

Mann DG, Pillsbury HC III. Correction of the "right hooked" nose. Laryngoscope 91:1562-1564, 1981.

Maran AG. The deviated nose and the nasal airway. J R Soc Med 72:848-851, 1979.

Martin H. Surgery of the crooked nose. Arch Otolaryngol 92:583-587, 1970.

McCurdy JA Jr. Aesthetic rhinoplasty in the non-Caucasian. J Dermatol Surg Oncol 12:38-44, 1986.

McKinney P, Shively R. Straightening the twisted nose. Plast Reconstr Surg 64:176-179, 1979.

Megumi Y. Augmentation rhinoplasty with soft tissue and cartilage. Aesthetic Plast Surg 12:89-93, 1988.

Merkx CA. Treatment of pseudo-arthrosis of the mandibular body by a sliding bonegraft. Arch Chir Neerl 23:273-285, 1971.

Orak F, Senyuva C, Bayramicli M, et al. Reversed roof graft for the severely deviated nose. Aesthetic Plast Surg 19:31-36, 1995.

Ortiz-Monasterio F, Lopez-Mas J, Araico J. Rhinoplasty in the thick-skinned nose. Br J Plast Surg 27:19-24, 1974.

Ortiz-Monasterio F, Olmedo A. Rhinoplasty on the mestizo nose. Clin Plast Surg 4:89-102, 1977.

Parkes ML, Kamer FM. The mature nose. Laryngoscope 83:157-166, 1973.

Parkes ML, Kanodia R. Avulsion of the upper lateral cartilage: diagnosis, surgical anatomy and management. Laryngoscope 91:758-764, 1981.

Patterson CN. The aging nose: characteristics and correction. Otolaryngol Clin North Am 13:275-288, 1980.

Pirsig W. Wedge resection in rhinosurgery: a review of the literature and long-term results in a hundred cases. Rhinology 26:77-88, 1988.

Planas J. The twisted nose. Clin Plast Surg 4:55-67, 1977.

Porter JP, Olson KL. Analysis of the African American female nose. Plast Reconstr Surg 111:620-626, 2003.

Powell NB, Riley RW. Facial contouring with outer-table calvarial bone. A 4-year experience. Arch Otolaryngol Head Neck Surg 115:1454-1458, 1989.

Ramsay SC, Yeates MG, Ho LC. Bone scanning in the early assessment of nasal bone graft viability. J Nucl Med 32:33-36, 1991.

Robbins TH. The noselift procedure for rhinoplasty in the older patient. Br J Plast Surg 38:264-266, 1985.

Rohrich RJ, Adams WP Jr. Nasal fracture management: minimizing secondary nasal deformities. Plast Reconstr Surg 106:266-273, 2000.

Rohrich RJ, Hollier LH. Rhinoplasty with advancing age: characteristics and management. Clin Plast Surg 23:281-296, 1996.

Rohrich RJ, Muzaffar AR. Rhinoplasty in the African-American patient. Plast Reconstr Surg 111:1322-1339, 2003.

Rohrich RJ, Griffin JR, Adams WP Jr. Rhinophyma: review and update. Plast Reconstr Surg 110:860-869, 2002.

Rohrich RJ, Gunter JP, Deuber MA, et al. The deviated nose: optimizing results using a simplified classification and algorithmic approach. Plast Reconstr Surg 110:1509-1523, 2002.

Rohrich RJ, Hollier LH Jr, Janis JE, et al. Rhinoplasty with advancing age. Plast Reconstr Surg 114:1936-1944, 2004.

Romo T III, Jablonski RD. Nasal reconstruction using split calvarial grafts. Otolaryngol Head Neck Surg 107:622-630, 1992.

Sheen J, Sheen A. Aesthetic Rhinoplasty, 2nd ed. St Louis: CV Mosby, 1987.

Siemssen SO, Siemssen SJ. Sliding osteotomy of the nasal skeleton: a possible method of altering the length of the external nose. Brit J Plast Surg 34:247-248, 1981.

Smith HW. Autogenous nasal bone grafts. Ear Nose Throat J 64:122-126, 1985.

Staffel JG. Optimizing treatment of nasal fractures. Laryngoscope 112:1709-1719, 2002.

Stucker FJ. Non-Caucasian rhinoplasty. Trans Sect Otolaryngol Am Acad Ophthalmol Otolaryngol 82:417-422, 1976.

Thatte RL, Deshpande SN, Thatte MR. A radical approach in the treatment of the deviated nose. Br J Plast Surg 43:596-602, 1990.

Uchida M, Kojima T, Hirase Y. Secondary correction of the bilateral cleft lip nose by excision of the columellar forked flap and nasal remodeling with reverse-U flaps: a preliminary report. Brit J Plast Surg 47:490-494, 1994.

Vilar-Sancho B. Rhinoseptoplasty. Aesthetic Plast Surg 8:61-65, 1984.

Watanabe K. New ideas to improve the shape of the ala of the Oriental nose. Aesthetic Plast Surg 18:337-344, 1994.

Wexler MR. Reconstructive surgery of the injured nose. Otolaryngol Clin North Am 8:663-677, 1975.

Willemot J. The crooked or twisted nose. Eye Ear Nose Throat Mon 49:412-413, 1970.

Won Kim S, Pio Hong J, Kee Min W, et al. Accurate, firm stabilization using external pins: a proposal for closed reduction of unfavorable nasal bone fractures and their simple classification. Plast Reconstr Surg 110:1240-1246, 2002.

Wright WK. Surgery of the bony and cartilaginous dorsum. Otolaryngol Clin North Am 8:575-598, 1975.

PART V

Secondary Rhinoplasty

"What would you say is the earliest sign of civilization?" she asked. . . . "Here is what I believe to be evidence of the earliest true civilization." High above her head she held a human femur . . . and pointed to a grossly thickened area [of bony union]. "Such signs of healing," she went on, "are never found among the remains of the earliest, fiercest societies. In their skeletons we find clues of violence. . . . But this healed bone shows that someone must have cared for the injured person—hunted on his behalf, brought him food, served him at personal sacrifice."

MARGARET MEADE
Quoted by Paul Brand and Philip Yancey
Pain: The Gift Nobody Wants

Be well aware, quoth then that Ladie milde,
Least suddaine mischief ye too rash provoke.

EDMUND SPENSER
The Faerie Queene

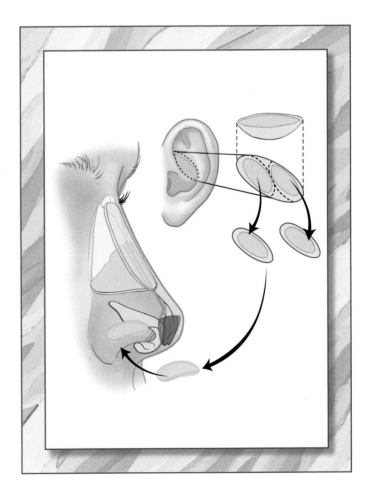

CHAPTER 17

Theory, Planning, and Technique

And there were gardens bright with sinuous rills,
Where blossomed many an incense-bearing tree. . . .
But Oh! That deep romantic chasm which slanted
Down the green hill athwart a cedern cover!
A savage place! As holy and enchanted
As e'er beneath a waning moon was haunted
By woman wailing for her demon-lover!

SAMUEL TAYLOR COLERIDGE
Kubla Khan

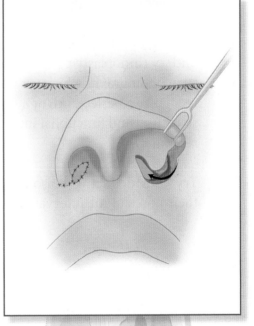

"I see nobody on the road," said Alice.
"I only wish I had such eyes," the King remarked
in a fretful tone. "To be able to see Nobody!
And at that distance too! Why, it's as much as
I can do to see real people, by this light!"

LEWIS CARROLL
Through the Looking Glass

Phenomenology and Diagnosis in Secondary Rhinoplasty

Successful primary rhinoplasty is the key to successful secondary rhinoplasty. Fundamental to both are familiarity with nasal phenomenology, soft tissue response to various skeletal alterations, and the effect of reducing support on the nasal airway. In practice, therefore, diagnosis is not necessarily more difficult in secondary patients than in primary ones if the surgeon understands normal anatomy and what happens as a result of the usual reduction maneuvers or the newer grafting or cartilage suturing techniques. In secondary patients, however, the approach is the reverse of primary rhinoplasty: instead of identifying anatomic traps and modifying the surgical plan accordingly, the surgeon observes the sequelae of failing to recognize those anatomic traps, and must correct the consequences.

Primary and secondary rhinoplasty are two sides of the same coin, which creates a unity between the operations. *If the surgeon removes or repositions deforming structures, maximizes function and equilibrium, uses incisions and dissection economically, and augments to create balance, contour, and structure, there is really no difference between primary and secondary rhinoplasty except the donor sites.*

Throughout this textbook, I have included the presurgical photographs of all secondary rhinoplasty patients for whom I have them. I encourage surgeons to obtain such photographs whenever possible. Like the musician who trains his or her ear to recognize a perfect fifth or a Lydian mode, the surgeon who can rapidly identify the structural and functional impact of previous surgery is already halfway toward correcting it.

Try your deductive reasoning on the following patients. What has happened to their noses in the interval between the photographs?

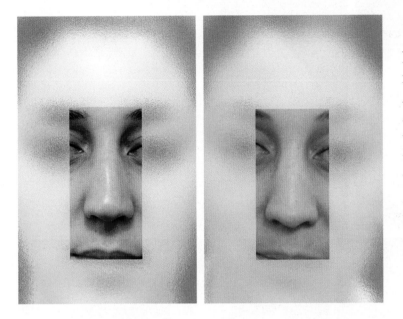

Notice that a dorsal reduction has been performed in this patient (her nose is wider). An inverted-V deformity has developed. The septal curvature has shifted from the left to the right. If the tip cartilages were reduced, the change was either minimal or the soft tissues were thick enough to resist change: nostril rim height is the same and there are no alar hollows. Upper lip plane and length appear unchanged; it is possible that no transfixing incision was made.

In contrast, what seems to have happened here? The dorsum and tip have obviously been reduced: the nose has shortened, the tip has narrowed, and a high septal deviation to the right has appeared. Lateral crural reduction has allowed the alar rims to retract, the right side more than the left. The nose has been shortened at the caudal septum, judging from increases in upper lip length and retrusion. The shadow over the bony vault indicates that a cartilage graft was placed.

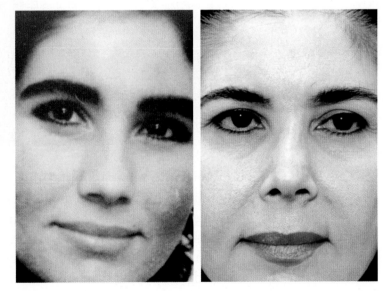

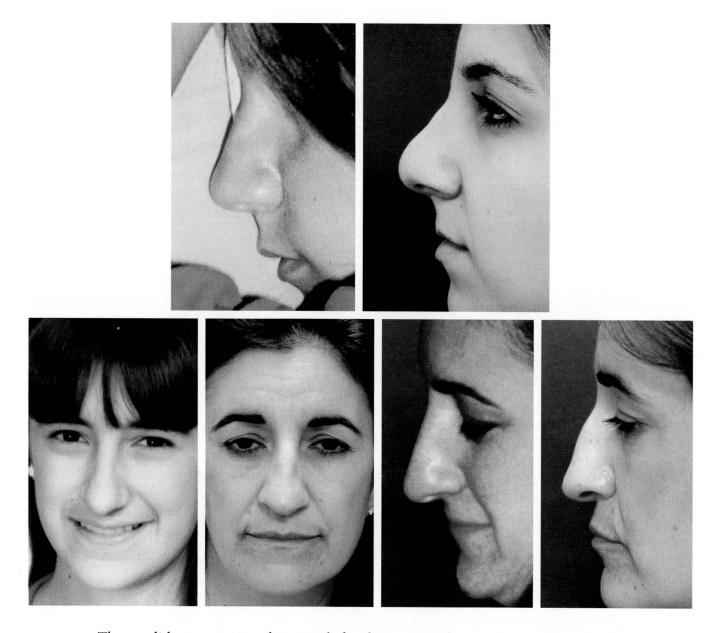

The candid preoperative photograph for this patient shows a low radix and a tip that is barely in line with the septal angle. Postoperatively, both dorsum and tip have evidently been reduced, enlarging apparent nasal base size, decreasing tip projection, and creating a supratip deformity. Although alar cartilage surface markings no longer remain (indicating a sizeable reduction), the patient's alar rim tissues have not retracted, confirming their substance.

This patient's nose seems to have lengthened since her yearbook picture, her upper lip has also become retrusive, and her middle vault is narrower. Because the bony dorsum appears no lower, it is reasonable to postulate a septal collapse even without examining the patient. Her lateral views confirm our observations.

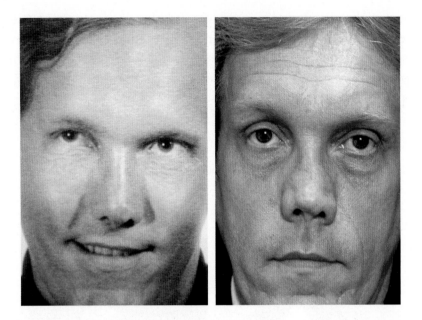

Here the effects of reduction are more obvious and devastating. Even without seeing the lateral view, the magnitude of the dorsal resection can be estimated by the relative increase in nasal width and loss of length. Caudal septal damage is signaled by the columellar retraction and increase in upper lip length, and the change in tip lobular shape and alar retraction mark the collapse caused by alar cartilage reduction.

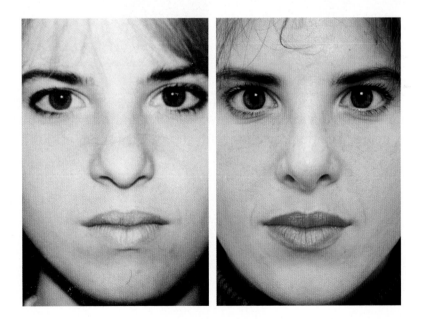

What has happened here? Although the dorsum is narrower, it seems lower. The malpositioned lateral crura have been reduced, allowing the alar rims to retract. The subnasale and superior upper lip seem to have dropped posteriorly, rotating the vermilion outward.

Because most malpositioned alar cartilages are also inadequately projecting, can you deduce the patient's profile appearance? In theory, the preoperative dorsum should be slightly higher, the tip inadequately projecting, and the lip more vertical. The postoperative dorsum should be lower, the tip still round, the alar rims higher, and the upper lip more retrusive.

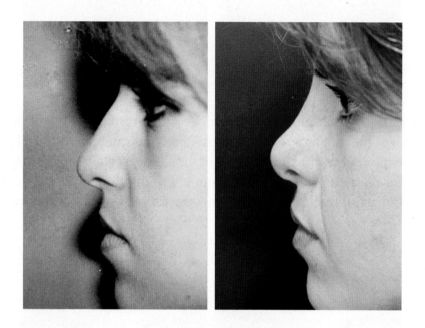

The patient's lateral view confirms an appearance that was almost completely predictable from the frontal view and a knowledge of common anatomic associations (in this case, inadequate tip projection with alar cartilage malposition).

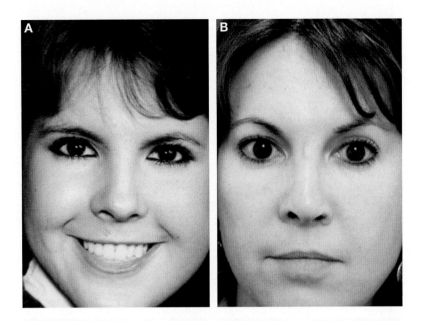

The most noticeable change in this patient is the nasal base. Dorsal height and middle vault width seem only slightly greater, yet the preoperative lateral crural convexities have disappeared and the alar rims have retracted. Although the patient is smiling in *A,* her upper lip still seems to have lengthened and become more retrusive in *B.* The airway has also diminished, indicated by the patient's involuntary nostril flare to support airflow.

Her oblique view therefore should show very little difference in dorsal height but a loss of tip projection, alar wall contour, and upper lip position.

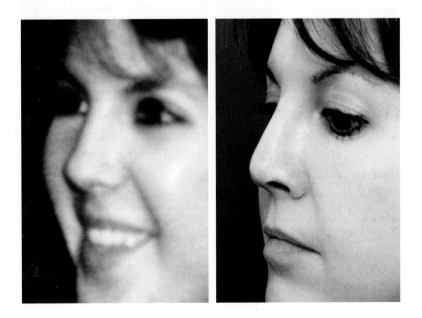

Our speculation matches the patient's appearance.

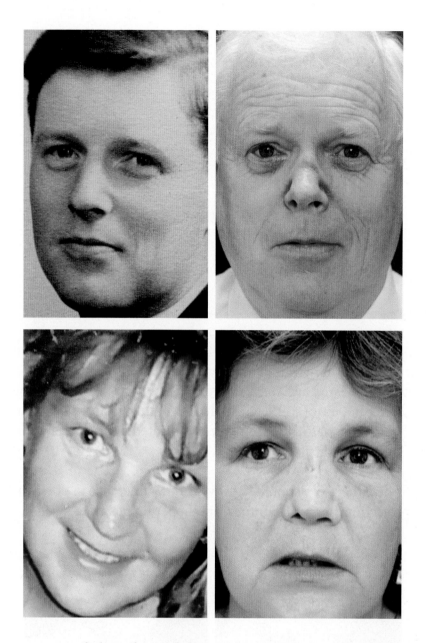

These patients reveal the effects of devastating panchondritis. Their premorbid frontal views show intact dorsa and normal nasal length and upper lip positions. But septal disease has changed everything. The noses have shortened, the middle vaults have collapsed, the columellae have retracted, and the upper lips have lengthened. Nasal width seems to have increased. The tip cartilages, largely sandwiched between the external and vestibular skin, have been affected less (though this is not always the case).

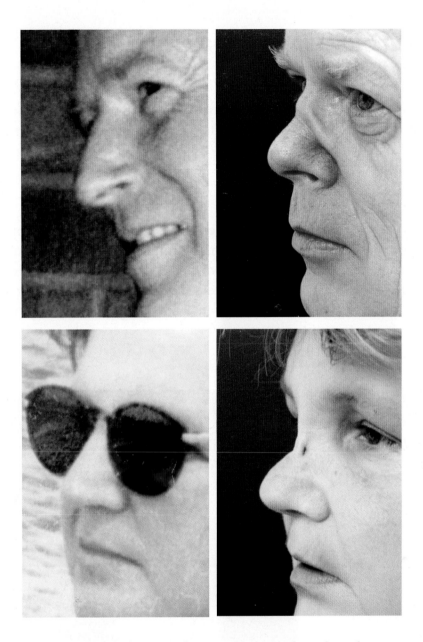

The oblique views support the speculations that were based on the patients' frontal appearances.

Surgeons discuss the lateral view more often than the frontal view, and they derive more information from it. The frontal view itself is foreshortened, and candid photographs limit detail. Nonetheless, notice how much information about surgical events, airway, remaining anatomy, and soft tissue response can be gathered from only the frontal view—often enough to predict important elements of other views without having seen them. As is true across the field of surgery, success in both primary and secondary rhinoplasty rests on correct diagnosis. Ultimately, it all comes down to anatomy.

Secondary Rhinoplasty Compared With Primary Rhinoplasty

Though primary and secondary rhinoplasty share common anatomy and phenomenology, three distinct differences separate the two: tissue tolerance, donor site depletion, and patient depletion.

TISSUE TOLERANCE

The tissues of secondary rhinoplasty patients have undergone irreversible changes; they will not tolerate extensive dissection, thinning procedures, and multiple incisions, and sometimes not even the columellar and tip exposure required for the open approach. Every prior operation alters soft tissue and skeletal characteristics. The skin becomes less pliable, less able to expand, and less tolerant of underlying pressure.

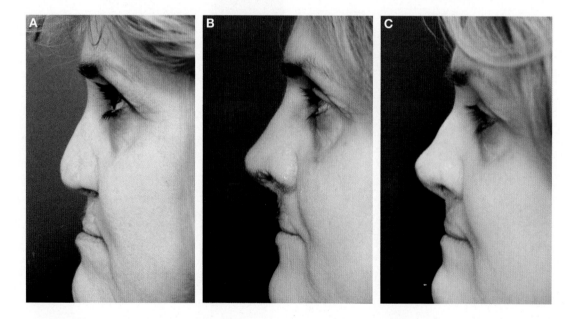

Unyielding soft tissues resist expansion and compress the grafts placed beneath them. A scarred, hypovascular bed increases the incidence of graft absorption, which is uncommon in primary rhinoplasty. Those elements are visible in this cleft patient, whose maxillary arch, dorsum, and tip were reconstructed with rib grafts; in addition, alar rim skin on the left (cleft) side was excised. Compare the result at 7 days *(B)* with the result at 1 year *(C)*. The patient's scarred tissues compressed the tip projection obtained, and a portion of the dorsal graft absorbed.

Surgical planning can be simplified somewhat by remembering that the only important deformities or anatomic variations are those that distort the surface or obstruct the airway. Anatomic facts that can be exposed only by an extensive dissection may be intellectual curiosities, but finding them is not relevant to treatment. Surgical objectives are based instead on internal septal and valvular examination and on inspection and palpation of the nasal surface.

Using the Open Approach for Secondary Rhinoplasty

Surgeons who use both the endonasal and open approaches often advocate a closed dissection for primary cases and reserve an open exposure for the most complicated, distorted, anatomically difficult cases. This strategy is exactly backward—in fact, established surgical teaching supports the opposite rationale for secondary surgery in almost all other body areas. The more difficult the case, the more limited the donor material, the more new support is required, the more scarred the soft tissue cover, the more important it is to avoid closure tension, and the more valuable it is to limit dissection, then the greater becomes the advantage of the endonasal approach. Surgeons who perform both open and endonasal rhinoplasty may therefore wish to rethink their strategy, and consider open access for well-vascularized, supple, primary cases and the endonasal approach for scarred and distorted secondary and tertiary patients. Columellar or nasal tip necrosis after secondary open rhinoplasty is almost never reported and rarely discussed, but it does occur, even in expert hands.

DONOR SITE DEPLETION

The population of secondary patients is changing. Thirty years ago, many surgeons would not attempt secondary rhinoplasty, and so most patients had undergone just a single endonasal operation and had intact septa. All that has changed, and today most secondary rhinoplasty patients have undergone two or more procedures by their original surgeon or by other surgeons; grafts and sutures have been tried, and donor sites have been exhausted and deformed. Surgeons who expect to perform secondary rhinoplasty must become facile with septal, ear, and rib cartilage, rib, and calvarial bone grafts. Each has its optimal uses.

PATIENT DEPLETION

Paralleling changes in soft tissue and donor sites, the patients themselves are depleted. Having undergone one or more unsuccessful procedures, secondary rhinoplasty patients have a lower tolerance for postoperative problems or disappointments. The surgeon electing to treat such patients must learn the specifics of the operation and perform a biologically sound surgical plan.

Often unspoken, but quite common, is a profound sense of guilt felt by the patient—guilt that he or she did not provide enough information to the surgeon, did not ask enough questions, did not do enough research into the surgeon's qualifications, or did not validate the correctness of the proposed procedure. This guilt, which seems deeper among rhinoplasty patients than others, increases patient anxiety and should be anticipated and recognized.

THE INTERVIEW

Secondary rhinoplasty patients are roundly considered to be a demanding and difficult group; but in their defense, there are virtually no other aesthetic operations in which a patient can lose ground after each procedure. Many patients whose rhinoplasties have worsened their external deformities and also created new airway obstructions could justifiably be more disagreeable than they are. It is therefore imperative that the surgeon construct a safe and biologically sound surgical plan, and also that both patient and surgeon have an accurate, explicit understanding of the aesthetic goals and the realities of the surgical problem—that is, what is possible and what is not. The patient must be guided to understand that every rhinoplasty is a compromise between the patient's aesthetic goals and the limitations that the operated skeleton and soft tissue configuration impose. Each patient's donor material varies in quantity and character, which determines its usefulness for a specific situation. What the secondary patient fears most and needs least is another unsuccessful result.

HISTORY

It is important to determine what the patient was originally trying to accomplish, whether that is still the goal, and whether it is attainable. Examine preoperative photographs. Try to untangle what the previous surgeon has done and what happened thereafter. In this regard, the secondary surgeon has an advantage that the primary surgeon did not: the ability to know preoperatively how this nose responds to surgery. Although most postoperative changes can be predicted, not all can: some soft tissue that appears able to contract will not, and some skeletal techniques work when they should not.

Inquire about previous trauma (which may alert you to unhealed septal fractures), sinus disease, epistaxis, and chronic rhinitis (which may indicate turbulent airflow or, much more commonly, excessive turbinate resection).

Patients are asked to supply previous operative reports if they can, but their value is limited. Surgeons struggling with the operation may not be able to report what they are seeing, and other surgeons exaggerate their functional work for the insurance company audience. I rely more heavily on my own examination.

NASAL EXAMINATION

I always examine the internal nose first to avoid being distracted in the discussion of aesthetics. Many patients know that they have bad airways, but in other patients, obstruction has developed more imperceptibly as edema from the first surgery resolved. I palpate the nasal septum to determine how much cartilage and bone can be harvested and, if a previous septoplasty has been performed, how much dorsal and caudal support remains. I examine the nose during quiet and forced inspiration to assess valvular competence, and I look for previously normal anatomy that has now become distorted (for example, malpositioned lateral crura buckled into the airway). I do examine the turbinates, but I am as conservative in treating them in secondary patients as in primary patients, because (1) most turbinate hypertrophy is reactive, not indicative of intrinsic disease, and (2) hypertrophy reflects cystic bony enlargement (not mucosal thickening), which can be treated in most cases by crushing and outfracture.

The external examination follows the same pattern as in primary patients. I identify deformities that can be seen or that obstruct the airway, areas of collapse or disequilibrium, soft tissues that require support for shape, and problems of proportion. As in primary patients, the surgical plan is founded on three criteria: (1) skin thickness and distribution, (2) tip lobular shape, and (3) the balance between nasal base size and dorsal height (see Chapter 7).

ASSESSING PATIENT ATTITUDE: THE ANGRY PATIENT

The way in which patients recall their previous surgeries forms a continuum, from patients who have poor results and seek any improvement but who like their previous surgeons, to patients with very good results who are desperately unhappy and furious with their previous surgeons.

The identity of the previous surgeon creates distinct management differences. The surgeon evaluating his or her own unhappy patient has the advantage of knowing the operative circumstances, the characteristics of the donor material, and the patient's personality, but has the disadvantage of having to manage both the patient's disappointment and his or her own. These are the circumstances that measure the surgeon's equanimity and test the degree to which informed consent has been obtained.

Alternatively, the surgeon evaluating someone else's unhappy patient need not overcome disappointment with the current result, but has less information about the original deformity, the patient's tissue idiosyncrasies and donor material, the procedures themselves, and the patient's personality. It is here that preoperative photographs and the surgeon's interviewing skills may have the greatest impact.

Patient anger can reflect hostility toward the previous surgeon or only disappointment with an unanticipated outcome. The distinction is an important one. Most surgeons want to help their patients, and most surgeons are doing their best—I try to diffuse patient anger by reminding them of those two facts. Often, a patient's attitude will then soften, allowing unhappiness with the previous surgeon to fade into the background so that our attention can turn to the rhinoplasty itself. But other patients remain fixed in their anger. Unless I can convert an angry patient's attitude from one of resentment and revenge to one of disappointment and understanding, I will not operate at that time.

Angry patients must also understand the margin of error inherent in human surgery. Some patients become convinced that seeing a surgical specialist or a rhinoplasty subspecialist inoculates them from another suboptimal outcome; Internet hyperbole and posturing have only intensified this belief. Whereas the discussion of functional and aesthetic problems and the techniques required to correct them may be similar in primary and secondary rhinoplasty, the donor sites and the chances of perfection differ.

The criteria for accepting a patient for surgery remain the same (see Chapter 20):
1. Can I see the deformity?
2. Can I fix it?
3. Can I manage the patient?
4. If there is a complication, will the patient remain controlled and cooperate with treatment?
5. Does the patient accept the margin of error inherent in surgery?

There are also secondary patients who should *not* have another operation, but it is hard for a surgeon to withhold care that he or she can provide. *Ultimately, the difficulty of the deformity (not necessarily its size) must be weighed against the patient's attitude toward it.* The patient must seem able to tolerate another imperfect result. For my part, I try to remember that I am not Lochinvar and I am too old to be a Boy Scout. When there is a danger of exceeding a patient's tissue or emotional tolerance, I have learned to step aside. Some patients return years later with new and more acceptable attitudes and tolerance for imperfect results. Some patients find other surgeons. The decision to operate is one of the most personal decisions that a surgeon can make, and it is an individual one that depends on the surgeon's own skill with a particular problem and his or her unique personality.

SUMMARY: PLANNING GUIDELINES SPECIFIC TO SECONDARY RHINOPLASTY

Identify the surgical conditions:
1. Which of the four critical anatomic variants are present and uncorrected?
2. What are the functional deficits?
3. What are the soft tissue conditions (stiffness, pliability, scarring, thickness) that will affect the surgical plan?
4. What are the *visible* deformities?
5. Imagine the correct balance: what areas need augmentation for shape, proportion, function, or stability?
6. Are the tissues sufficiently healed to permit the necessary dissection and augmentation?
7. What donor sites will be needed?
8. How can incisions and dissections be limited?

The skeletal and soft tissue deformities and the quality and availability of building materials have been predetermined and are unique to each patient. They are beyond the surgeon's control. Secondary rhinoplasty tests the surgeon's ability to overcome those obstacles, minimize mental errors, and apply complex surgical techniques. Secondary rhinoplasty is a test like no other.

Applicable Techniques
ALAR BASE FLAPS

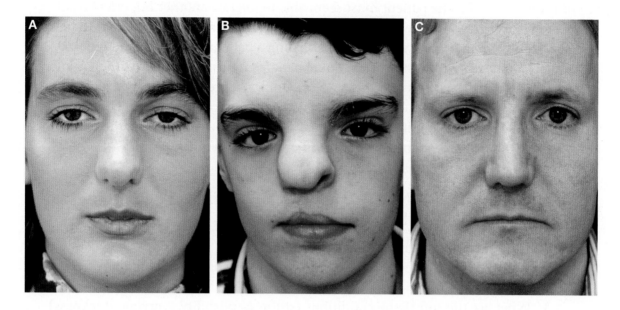

Though most patients and surgeons conceive alar base width as either normal or wide, the base can also be too narrow. Narrow bases occur less commonly in primary rhinoplasty *(A)*. Much more frequent is medial displacement of the base on the cleft side after lip repair *(B)* or after alar wedge resections in tertiary rhinoplasty *(C)*. Neoclassical aesthetic standards dictate that alar base width should equal intercanthal distance, an axiom that is true in only 40.8% of the Caucasian population, 3% of the African American population, and 35.4% of the Chinese population, according to the study by Bashour.

When the alar base is properly positioned, nostril or vestibular stenosis can be improved by composite grafts, using either the alar lobule or the ear as a donor site. In some circumstances, however, two simultaneous deformities exist: both nostril stenosis and malposition of the alar base. The alar base may be malpositioned in any direction. In these situations, composite grafting will enlarge the nostril but cannot correct the alar base displacement.

In 1931, Joseph described an inferiorly based flap that he transposed into the nasal floor to correct stenosis. Burget and Menick have employed the same flap elegantly in complex nasal reconstructions. Although my limited experience with the Joseph flap has been good, the transposition pivot point normally creates a dog-ear that may require secondary revision. The following is my modification of the flap, designed as a crescentic island on subcutaneous and musculocutaneous perforators.*

*While preparing my 1997 manuscript on this technique, I discovered that an identical flap had been described by Meyer in 1988.

PATIENT STUDY ONE

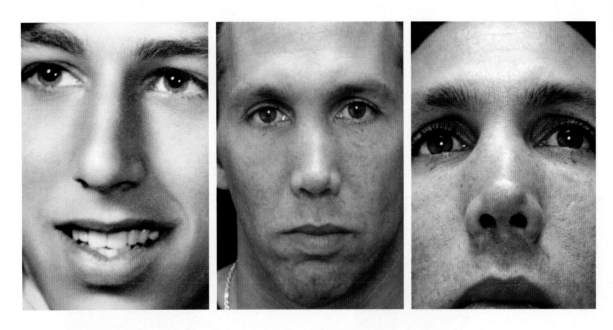

This tertiary rhinoplasty patient has an alar base that has been narrowed to bony vault width. Note also the difference in bony vault and upper cartilaginous vault widths that dorsal reduction has produced.

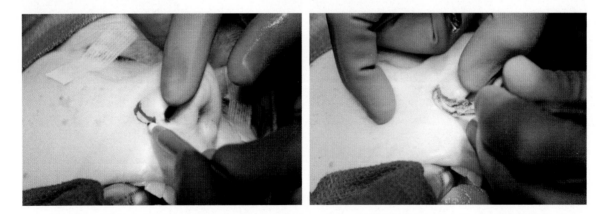

The flap should be designed as a crescent adjacent to the alar base (illustrated here in another patient). The medial flap edge must lie just lateral to the alar crease to avoid destroying this important landmark. The flap must be wide enough to correct the nostril stenosis, although 3 to 4 mm is all that is usually necessary. The lateral flap edge is incised at the appropriate position of the alar base on the cheek, or in cases of asymmetry, matches the lateral edge of the alar lobule on the normal side.

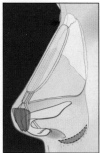

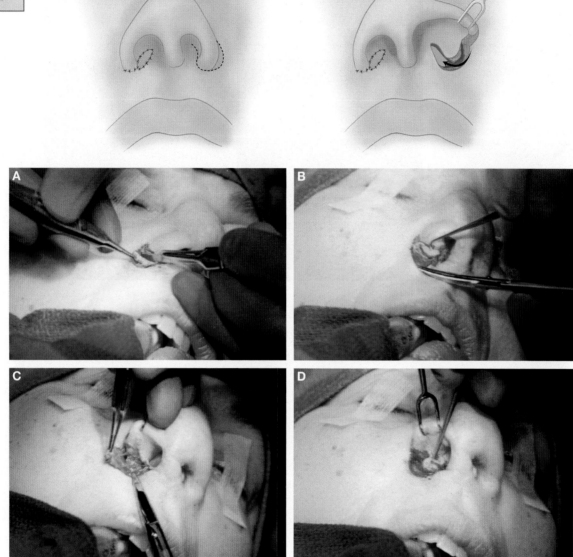

The flap is elevated as an island based on subcutaneous and musculocutaneous perforators (*A* and *B*) and on branches of the angular artery, which can be seen entering the flap base and should be protected if possible *(C: tip of scissors)*. Although it may at first seem more logical to transpose the flap so that its cephalic tip on the cheek becomes the posterior tip in the nasal floor, it is usually easier to rotate the flap into the defect *(D)*. Undermine the pedicle widely enough so that the flap transposition will not distort the donor site or cause tension on the repair, but be careful not to devascularize it. The flap normally rotates clockwise on the patient's left side and counterclockwise on the patient's right side.

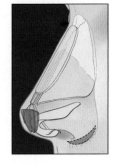

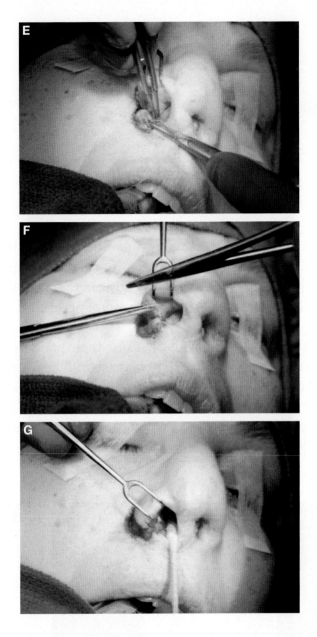

By reopening the nostril at the site of the previous alar resection (or the greatest tissue deficit) and freeing the displaced alar base, the surgeon can inset the flap into the nostril sill and floor (*E* and *F*). In *G*, the intranasal closure is complete. Closure of the donor site simultaneously corrects nostril stenosis and alar base malposition.

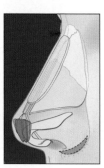

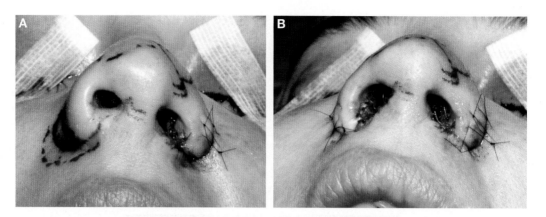

A surprisingly small flap can make a significant difference. In another patient, notice the nasal floor width created by this 3.5 mm wide flap. Flap length should be sufficient to span the length of the sagittal stenosis in the nasal floor, but must not extend beyond the alar crease. Overcorrection is not necessary.

Here are two other technical points. First, because these patients have a relative tissue deficit, the cheek flap inset at the alar crease should be as tension free as possible so that the alar base does not drift laterally later. The cheek area to be undermined is the outer line drawn on the patient's right side in *A*. Place deep sutures from the cheek flap to the muscle and subcutaneous tissue beneath the nasal floor so that the skin edges lie together gently before closure.

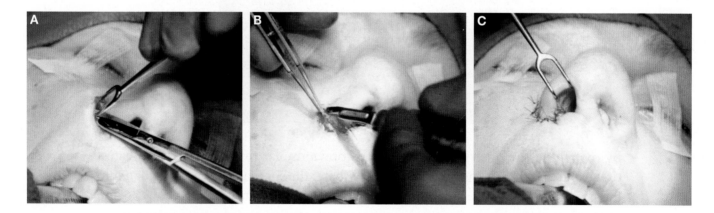

Second, it is important to create a declivity, not a flat surface, at the alar crease. Recall that the alar lobule curves posteromedially to meet the flatter cheek surface—the lobule does not meet the cheek surface edge-on. To help create this effect, it is often helpful to deepithelialize a 1 mm edge on the alar lobular side *(B)* and place inverting skin sutures to re-create this normal structure. Notice the magnitude of change produced on the patient's right side *(C)* from the 3 mm flap outlined at the beginning of the sequence. Preoperatively, the right nostril was smaller than the left.

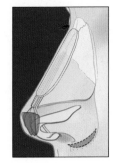

Postoperative Analysis

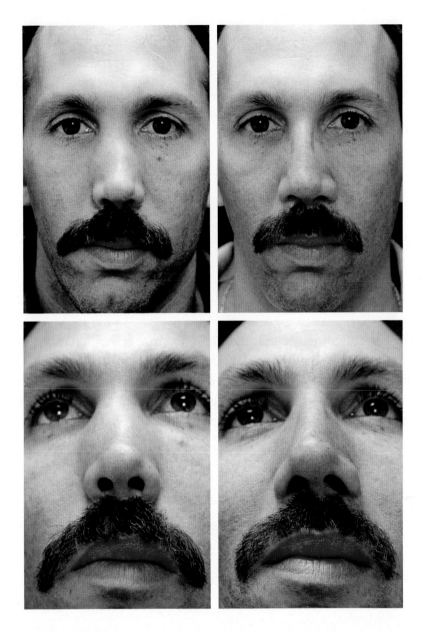

Eighteen months after the transposition flap, the nostril remains patent and the alar base width remains appropriate. A calvarial bone dorsal graft and conchal cartilage tip grafts were also performed in this patient.

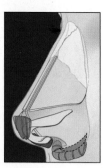

PATIENT STUDY TWO

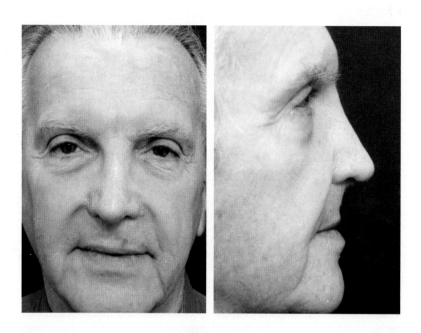

Although the patient's dorsum is straight and his nose is well balanced in the lateral view, three rhinoplasties have narrowed the base excessively. Note the hypertrophy of the alar base scars, signifying excessive closure tension. The patient's columella is thick and his Class III malocclusion exaggerates his upper lip position. His septum and both ears have been previously harvested.

SUMMARY OF THE SURGICAL PLAN

1. Harvest rib graft
2. Rib cartilage maxillary augmentation, greater in the perialar areas, less in the midline
3. Columellar grafts
4. Tip grafts
5. Bilateral alar base flaps

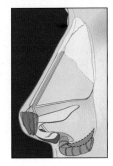

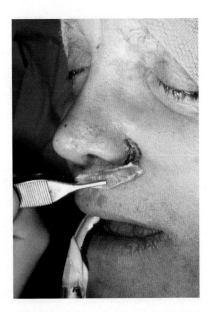

The patient's harvested rib shows the yellow, calcified appearance typical at this age. Notice the dimensions of the planned alar base flap, which will be set into the site of the previous alar base resection.

Postoperative Analysis

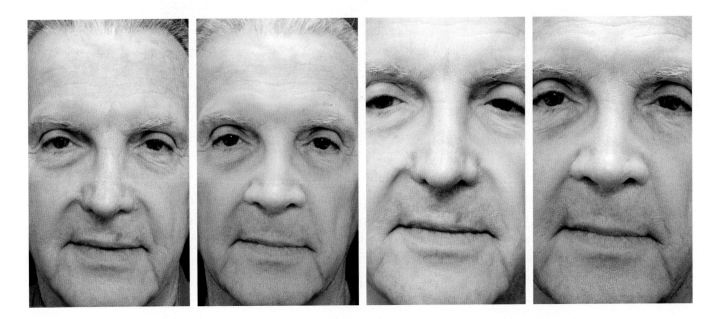

One year after surgery, the relatively small flaps have produced a significant change in alar base and nasolabial fold aesthetics. The scars have not hypertrophied, perialar maxillary augmentation has softened the upper lip depressions, and the repositioned bases have favorably altered alar rim contour.

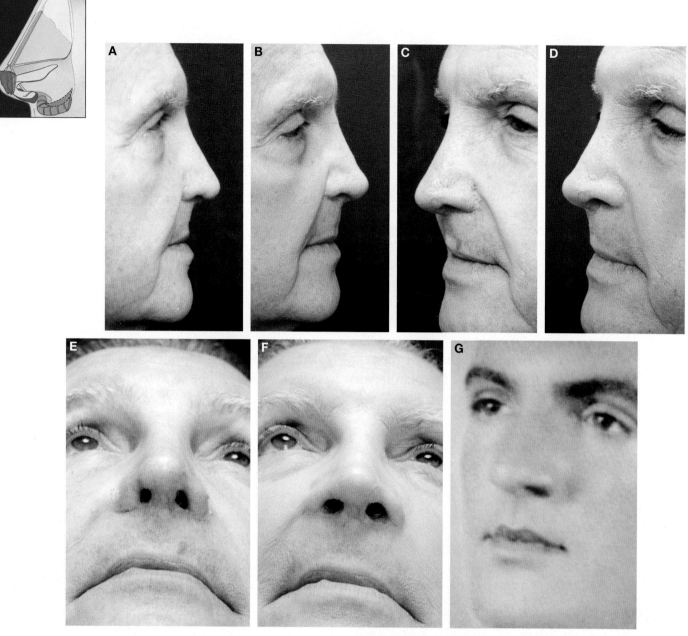

The alar base scars are not objectionable, and the columellar and tip grafts have helped rotate the nasal base and differentiate the tip lobule from the dorsum (*B* and *D*). However, the extraordinary tension on the closure has widened the base slightly and effaced the alar creases on inferior view (*F*). Comparing the postoperative appearance to the patient's midfacial contours as a young man (*G*), nostril length and nasal base contour have been partially restored.

The survival of alar base flaps has been uniformly complete in more than 70 patients. None of the flaps—whether unilateral or bilateral, performed as a separate procedure (Patient Study One) or simultaneous with other reconstructions (Patient Study Two)—have been lost. Even in patients whose donor tissue has been burned or scarred by previous procedures, survival has been uncomplicated.

However, remember that all these reconstructions were performed endonasally. *The safety of this procedure simultaneous with open rhinoplasty has not been established.* In this regard, the work of Rohrich et al (1995) that identified a dual blood supply to the nasal tip is germane. The lateral nasal vessels consistently appear 2 to 3 mm cephalad to the alar groove; the columellar artery (present in 68.2% of their dissections) can be divided during an open rhinoplasty, because the lateral nasal arteries (present in 100% of their specimens) adequately profuse the nasal tip. The authors of the work caution that previous alar base incisions or alar base excisions that extend more than 2 mm above the alar groove may damage the lateral nasal arteries. Because the alar base flaps described here are similarly perfused by the lateral nasal arteries, and because the flaps must be widely mobilized to rotate adequately, the surgeon who prefers open rhinoplasty should proceed with extreme caution; it may be unwise to perform an alar base flap simultaneously with open rhinoplasty. Even when using the endonasal approach, a surgeon should carefully limit the dissection in secondary and tertiary patients and make other access incisions precisely and only with specific indications. Further applications of the alar base flap can be found in the section on cleft rhinoplasty in Chapter 19.

CAUDAL SUPPORT GRAFT

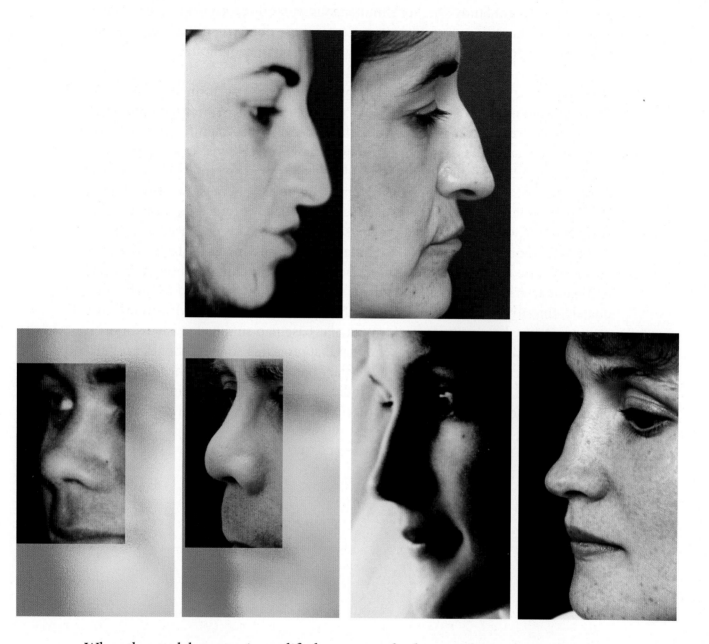

When the caudal septum is modified—even modestly, as we have seen in previous chapters—the subnasale can sharpen and the upper lip lengthens. When more of the septum is involved (for example, after septal collapse or surgical removal of the distal septum), the entire nasal base drops inferiorly and the nose lengthens. Maxillary arch retrusion alone can be corrected by maxillary augmentation. Loss of nasal base support, however, requires something more extensive that cannot easily be corrected by dorsal or tip modification alone. The most powerful solution is replacement of what is missing: the caudal septum and septal angle.

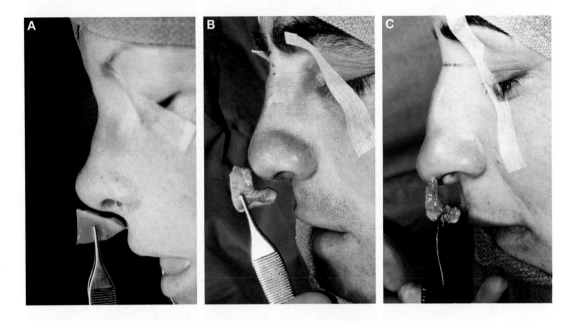

When rib cartilage is harvested for the rest of the reconstruction, a flat graft taken from the center of the rib works very well, provided it is large enough (A). However, when rib is not being harvested or if the rib is unusually calcified or distorted, the concha can be folded to create an excellent replacement for the distal septum (B and C). Here I use the method of Sheen and Sheen. The concha can be folded along either axis to suit the defect. Folding the graft and securing its shape with 5-0 nylon sutures increases its rigidity and therefore its strength. It is important that the portion being fitted into the columella be thin enough to avoid widening this delicate structure. The graft is placed through a short incision in the membranous septum on one side, just posterior to the columella, through which scissors dissection separates the membranous septal flaps (already empty from the septal collapse or resection). The portion of the graft that replaces the distal dorsal septum and septal angle slides in first, at which time the graft rotates either clockwise (for left-handed surgeons) or counterclockwise (for right-handed surgeons) until the tip of the caudal end can slip into place and slide into the posterior columella. It is important that the dissection not be too wide (particularly posteroinferiorly), because the graft would float in the pocket and not provide proper anterior projection.

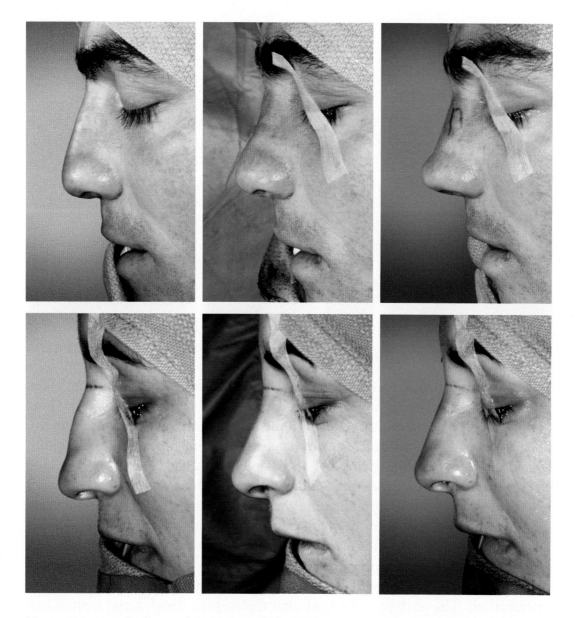

These patients illustrate the power of the technique and the importance of proper nasal base position. Each patient is shown at the beginning of the surgery *(left)* and after dorsal reduction, maxillary augmentation, and placement of the caudal support ear cartilage grafts shown on p. 1113 *(center)*. Notice the effects of maxillary augmentation and caudal support grafts: the upper lips have become vertical, the subnasales have become less sharp, the bases have rotated anterosuperiorly, and the columellae have become more evident. Dorsal and tip grafts were added to complete the reconstructions *(right)*.

Postoperative Analysis

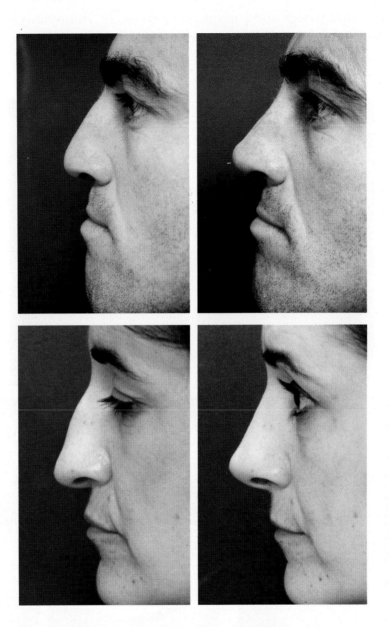

In these patients dorsal grafts were added as onlays and were not cantilevered. No columellar struts were used. Their upper lip positions were created by maxillary augmentation, and the nasal base rotations were achieved by replacing the missing caudal septa.

MAXILLARY AUGMENTATION

Because upper lip carriage and contour are affected by rhinoplasty, correction of any resulting deformities should be part of the reconstruction.

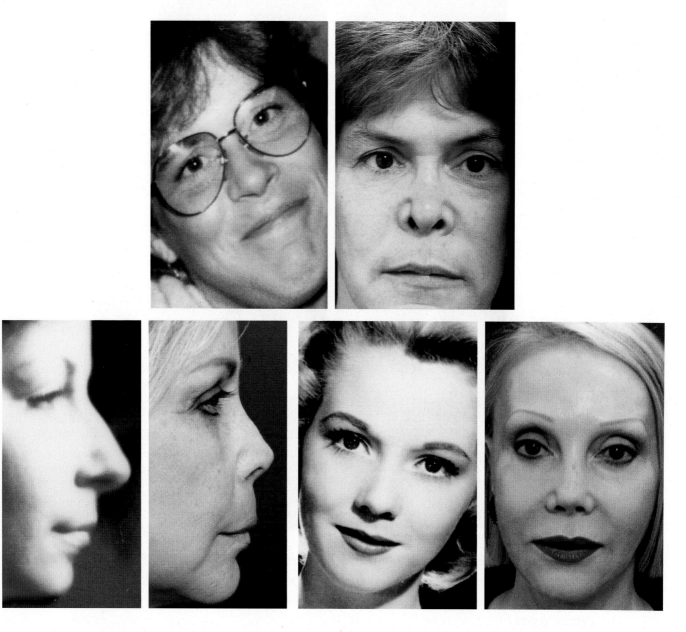

Not only facial clefts but trauma, cocaine, and especially rhinoplasty all affect upper lip position and contour. A retrusive upper lip occurs commonly with a long nose; in fact, it is uncommon to see a long nose with a full subnasale and strong upper jaw. The association of a lengthened upper lip and sharp subnasale after septal injury or chondritis should make the surgeon skeptical of the argument that only changes in the nasal spine, depressor septi muscle, or frenulum can alter surface contours. The common thread in each of these cases is the caudal septum.

Treatment of maxillary retrusion is most easily and effectively performed at the maxillary arch, not the caudal septum. In fact, caudal septal replacement alone does not move the lip forward very far. I make the decision to perform maxillary augmentation and/or caudal septal replacement independently, based on upper lip position and whether the columella is supported. Either area may be treated independently, or both may be treated together.

Technique: Autogenous Augmentation

Although donor cartilage from septum, ear, rib, or calvarium will augment the maxillary arch, rib is most commonly used in practice. Neither septum nor ear cartilage is available in sufficient quantity to justify their use where other donor sites will suffice. I have occasionally used ear cartilage to augment the maxillary arch in cleft patients (where alloplastics are always unwise), but rib cartilage is used much more often.

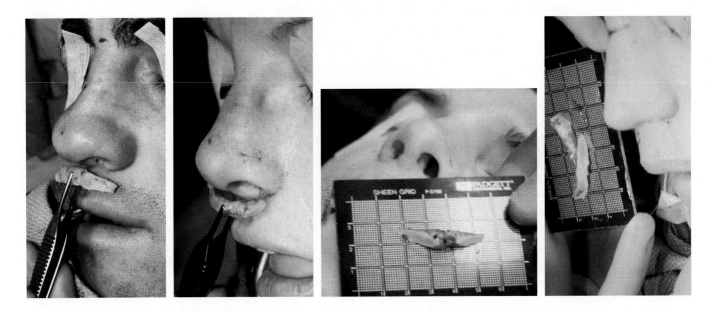

Although the tip of the tenth rib forms a very good single-unit maxillary augmentation, I more commonly augment the arch with a two-piece graft, for two reasons. First, in many patients, the perialar areas, not the midline, are the deepest, so the graft must be wider laterally. Second, a two-piece augmentation allows more normal lip movement and feels less like a rigid bar, which can annoy some patients.

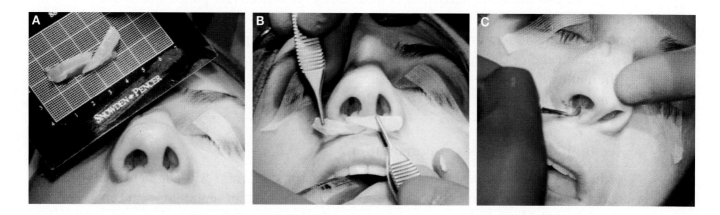

The donor rib is cut into sections of appropriate length, depending on the depth of the defect. Exact shape is not important, but the edges should be contoured to avoid palpability either laterally or in the midline. The lateral ends of the grafts determine the amount of perialar augmentation, and the degree of midline overlap controls the position of the central lip. In this patient, each segment measures approximately 2.5 cm *(A)*. Their approximate final position is shown in *B*. Grafts are placed through a 5 mm incision of the right nasal floor *(C)*.

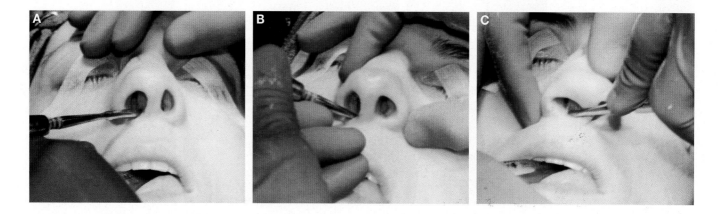

After incising down to the nasal spine, a Joseph elevator strips the periosteum in the desired area. Dissection must be kept high across the maxillary arch, and tight against the piriform aperture. Some caution is necessary here: there is less resistance to dissection toward the sulcus, and so it is easy to make the pocket too low, in which case the augmentation will be visible and palpable intraorally and annoy the patient. In *B*, my right thumb indicates the position of the elevator tip. After dissecting on one side, I use the elevator to strip the periosteum in the other direction *(C)*.

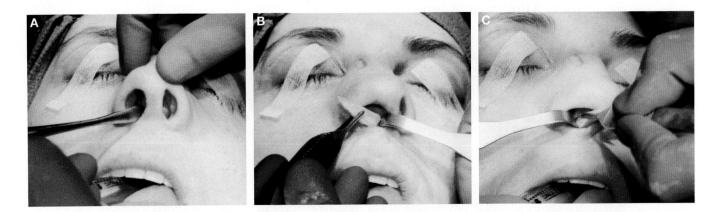

If necessary, I follow the Joseph elevator with a broad Cottle elevator, ensuring the proper pocket width *(A)*. Retracting the wound edge, the first graft is slipped into the pocket, widest and first *(B)*, followed by the opposite graft *(C)*.

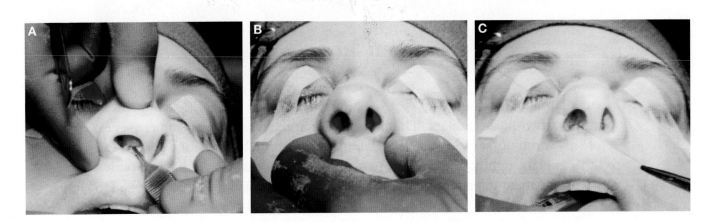

The tip of the second graft is folded over the nasal spine *(A)*. Graft position is checked by palpation and by noting the degree of midline overlap *(B)*. The correction is 1:1. If it seems excessive, the medial ends can be trimmed until there is little (or no) overlap, or additional slices of rib can be placed anterior to bring the midline forward. The wound is closed with fine, absorbable sutures *(C)*.

Technique: Alloplastic Augmentation

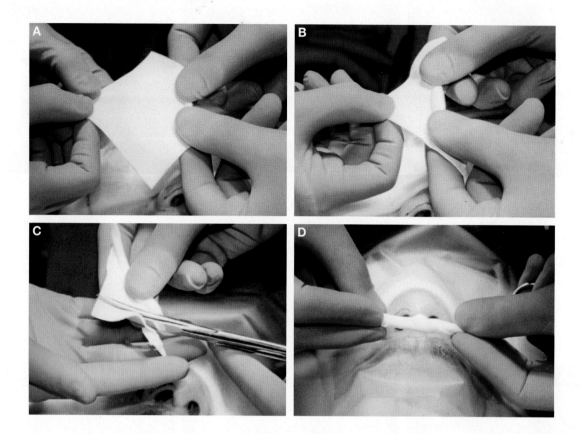

In a similar manner, 1 mm Gore-Tex sheeting can be rolled into a single implant or split into a two-piece implant. The material is supplied in 7.5 cm square pieces. While my scrub nurse holds the material under tension, I begin at one corner and roll the implant tightly until the proper central width has been achieved, which varies from patient to patient (*A* and *B*). The implant is then trimmed and rolled to the correct shape *(C)*. The implant must be wide enough to provide the proper surface effect, remembering that excessive width will distort upper lip movement or impinge on the labiogingival sulcus *(D)*.

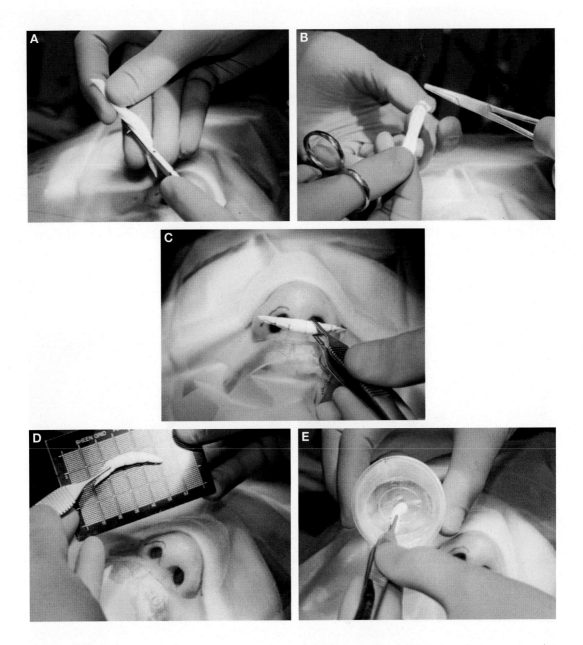

The implant is secured with penetrating and circumferential 6-0 nylon sutures (*A* and *B*), and is trimmed at each end. Sutures are added until it is bound snugly. The implant should extend just to the alar creases but not beyond them *(C),* and it can be curved to fit the maxillary arch *(D).* Notice also that a folded gauze pad protects the patient's eyes and that sterile adhesive drape isolates the nose. I perform the maxillary augmentation before any of the other rhinoplasty procedures, and without touching the skin with my gloved hand. While the bed is prepared, the implant is soaked in an antibiotic solution *(E).*

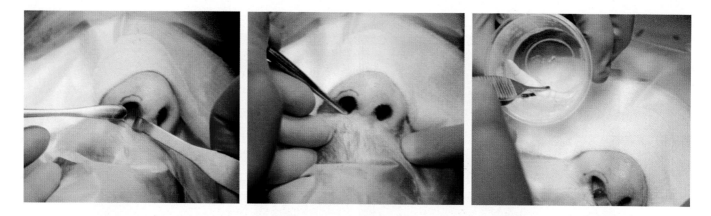

A Cottle elevator broadens the pocket, and the implant is retrieved from the antibiotic solution.

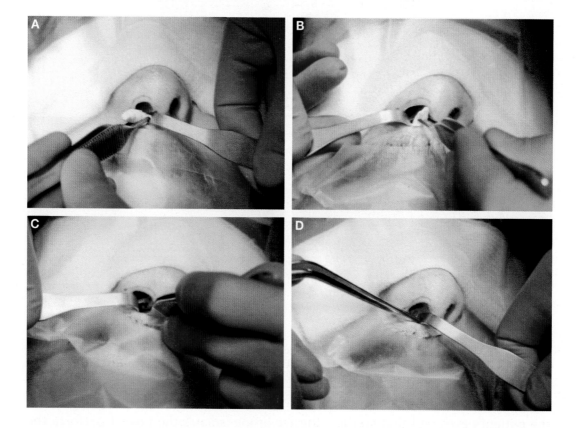

With a small curved retractor holding the pocket open, I slip the implant inside up to its midpoint *(A)*, after which the retractor picks up the other side and I tuck in the implant completely *(B)*. I can confirm symmetrical placement by palpation and by checking the position of the circumferential sutures *(C)*. I then slide over the implant with bayonet forceps to each of its ends to ensure that the tips have not folded over and that they lie flat *(D)*.

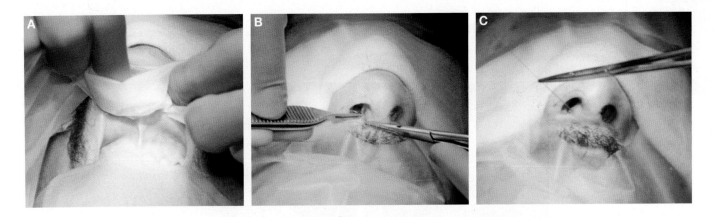

I check inside the sulcus to confirm that the implant is neither visible nor palpable *(A)*. The wound is then closed securely, with deep sutures opposing the entire depth of the wound on each side, including muscle *(B)*, and a second layer of skin closure of fine, absorbable sutures *(C)*.

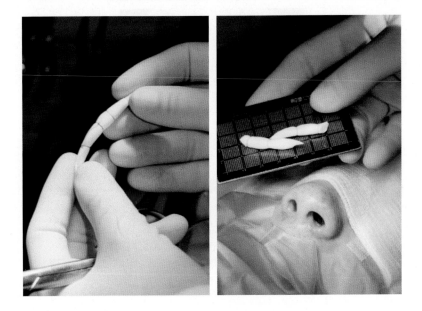

If the greater deficiency is in the perialar areas than in the midline, or if the maxillary arch is asymmetrical (which is often the case), the rolled implant can be split in the midline and the edges tapered, after which it can be placed as previously demonstrated for autogenous rib.

PATIENT STUDY ONE

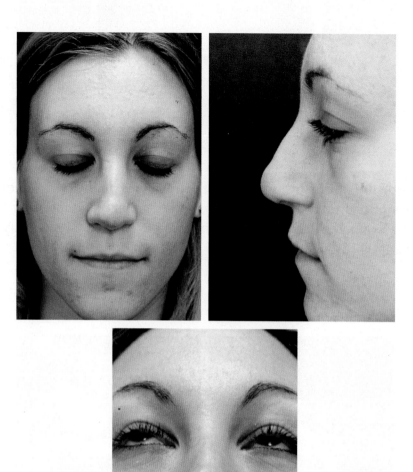

After two rhinoplasties, this patient's left high septal deviation remains. Her nose shows signs typical of a reduction disequilibrium: a low radix, a persistent dorsal hump, a blunt and poorly projecting asymmetrical tip, and a left nostril that is smaller than the right and displaced more medially. The caudal septum had been resected to the septal angle, producing a depression above the tip and a flaccid and unsupported columella.

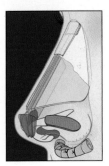

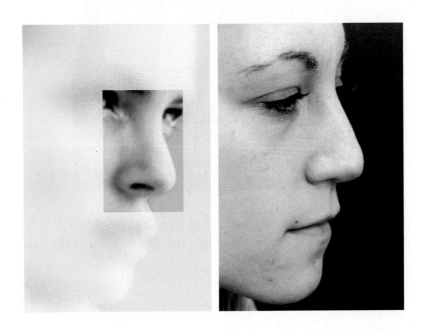

The patient's desired goal is impossible to achieve except at the metalevel. This is an opportunity to show the patient the differences in radix height and tip projection—the ingredients necessary for a straight profile and good nasal balance.

SUMMARY OF THE SURGICAL PLAN

1. Gore-Tex maxillary augmentation
2. Limited skeletonization over bony and upper cartilaginous vaults
3. Dorsal reduction, left greater than right (preoperative asymmetry)
4. Septoplasty
5. Harvest composite and caudal support grafts (then change gloves)
6. Asymmetrical spreader grafts, left greater than right
7. Caudal support graft
8. Radix graft
9. Multiple tip grafts with buttress
10. Bone grafts to external valves
11. Axially oriented composite graft along left alar rim and floor to correct vestibular stenosis

---

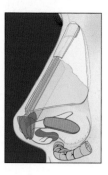

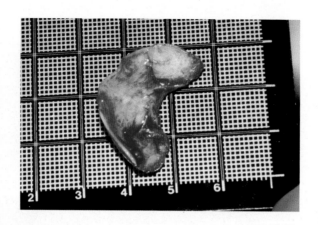

The right concha was harvested, preserving the skin on a portion of the cymba conchae (to be used for the composite graft); the rest will form the caudal support graft.

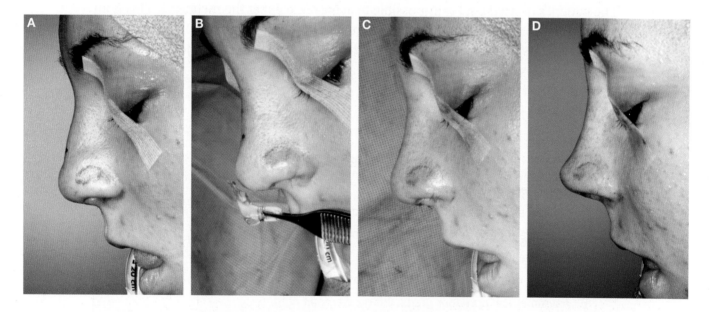

After maxillary augmentation and dorsal reduction, the boot-shaped caudal support graft was slipped into the caudal septum to replace the missing cartilage and correct the columellar retraction *(B)*. Compare the result after only these steps with the preoperative view *(C with A)*, and notice the change in upper lip position, columellar visibility, and nasal base projection. Dorsal, spreader, and tip grafts completed the reconstruction *(D)*.

Postoperative Analysis

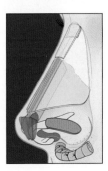

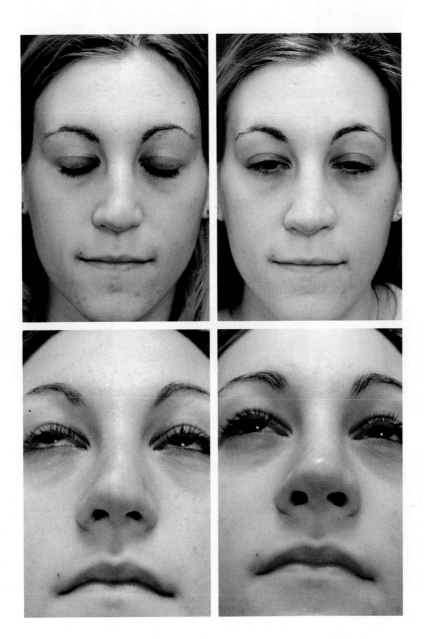

Fourteen months postoperatively, the nose is more symmetrical. Spreader grafts have aligned the high septal deviation, and radix and tip augmentation have supported the soft tissues and created tip contour. The left alar base has moved farther laterally. An axial composite graft, with its skin island in the vestibular floor and its cartilage ring running across the floor and around the left alar wall, has opened the smaller nostril on that side and supported the flatter left rim. Geometric mean nasal airflow increased 3.5 times over preoperative values.

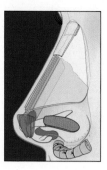

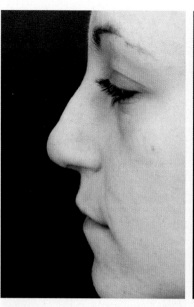 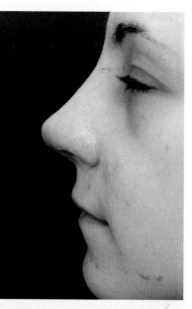

Preoperative   1 week postoperatively

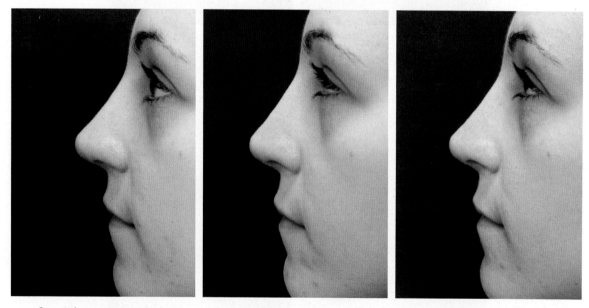

2 months postoperatively   6 months postoperatively   14 months postoperatively

Slight dorsal reduction, and radix and tip grafts have improved nasal balance, reduced apparent nasal base size, and created adequate tip projection. The maxillary augmentation has corrected the vertical position of the upper lip, and the caudal support graft has replaced the resected caudal septum and septal angle. As the postoperative months progress, the nose lengthens and edema reduces, but the dorsal, tip, and upper lip positions remain stable.

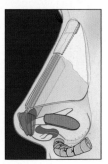

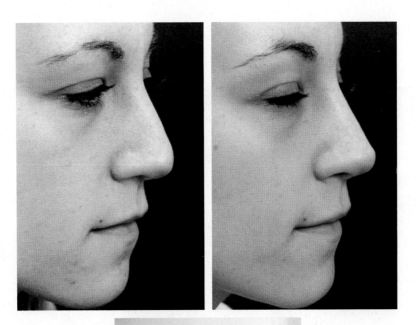

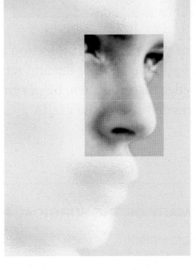

In the oblique views, many of the patient's preoperative goals have been realized. The dorsum is straight, the tip is adequately projecting, and the nose is more proportional. The tip is more angular, with a point of maximum projection and a flat supratip. The sharpness and retrusion of the subnasale have been softened.

To avoid creating excessive fullness, the surgeon must use caution in performing maxillary augmentation in patients with a lip configuration such as this. In this patient, a two-piece maxillary augmentation was placed, putting most of the correction in the perialar areas and less in the midline.

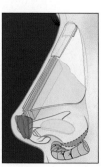

PATIENT STUDY TWO

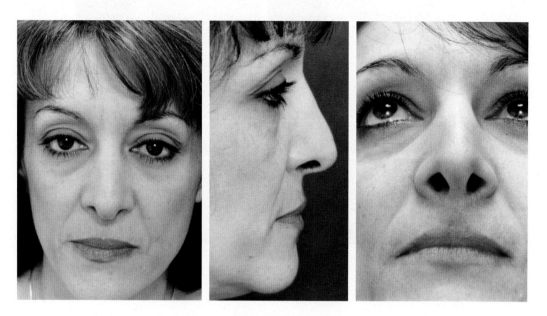

After three rhinoplasties, this patient lost tip projection and airway (notice the narrow middle vault), and her upper lip appears flat and retrusive. In addition to maxillary augmentation, alar wedge resections will be performed, recycling the excised lobular skin as coronally oriented composite grafts.

SUMMARY OF THE SURGICAL PLAN

1. Gore-Tex maxillary augmentation
2. Minimal skeletonization
3. Rasp bony vault for graft adherence
4. Transfix, shortening membranous septum 2 mm anteriorly
5. Septoplasty
6. Asymmetrical spreader grafts, thicker on right than left
7. Thin radix graft
8. Crushed cartilage tip grafts
9. Bilateral alar wedge resections, right greater than left
10. Alar rim to lobule transfers, right greater than left
11. Four-lid blepharoplasty with lateral retinacular canthopexy

---

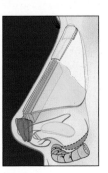

Postoperative Analysis

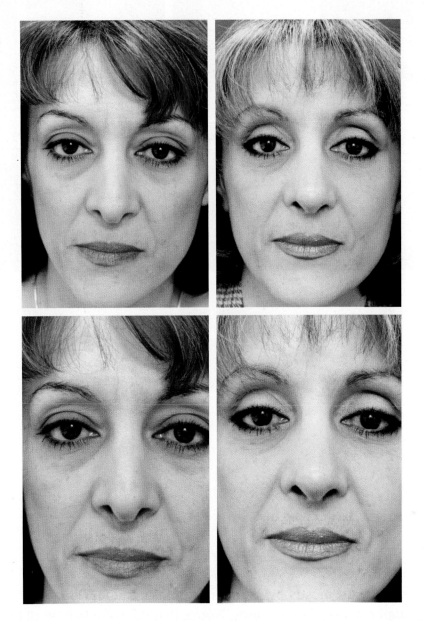

Two years later, the nose is slightly shorter on the frontal view, the middle vault is confluent with the bony vault instead of concave, and tip lobular support has appeared, with highlights demarcating the tip from the dorsum. The perialar creases have softened, and the upper lip appears less flat and retrusive. Alar wedge resections, removing both external and vestibular skin, have narrowed the base slightly, and the 3 mm wide grafts placed into short vestibular alar rim incisions have reduced the preoperative notches.

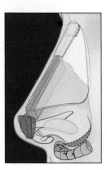

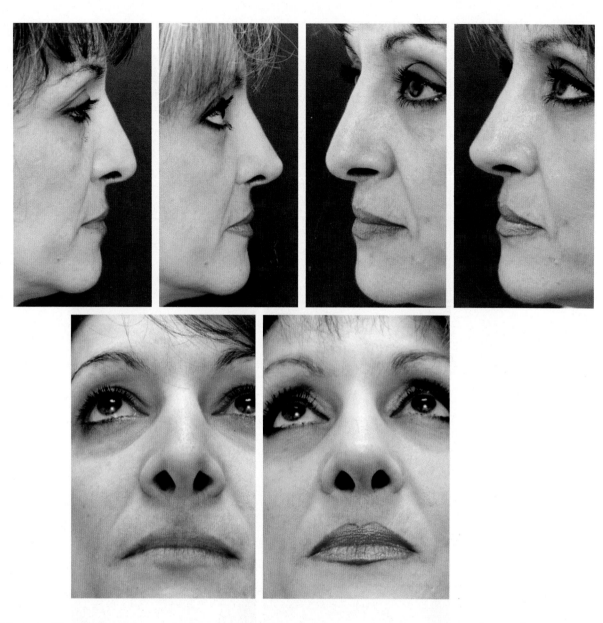

The profile is altered mostly by changes in nasal base position—the product of maxillary augmentation and tip grafts. Notice that the combination of tip grafting and small alar wedge resections has reduced apparent nostril size. The dorsum retains essentially all of its preoperative height, although radix and tip grafts have flattened the dorsal convexity. The columella remains narrow and unscarred, and although the alar wedge resection scars are visible on the inferior view, the floors remain smooth and unnotched. Geometric mean postoperative airflow increased 10 times over preoperative values.

CALVARIAL BONE GRAFT

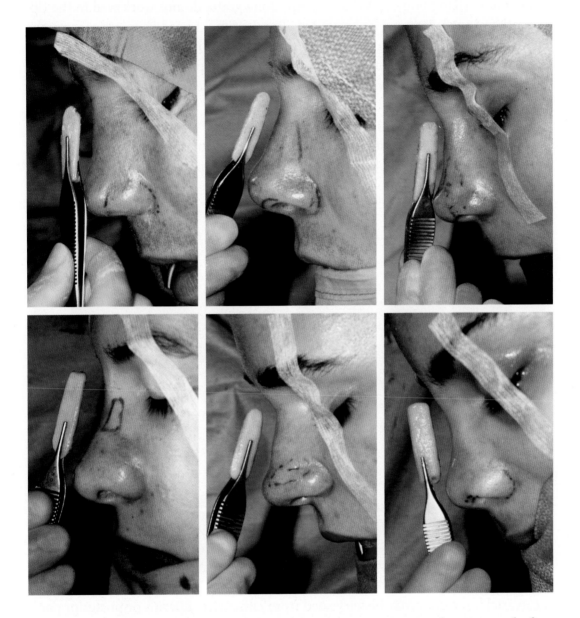

I used calvarial bone grafts for dorsal nasal reconstruction exactly 50 times before changing to rib cartilage for most cases. I never had a bad experience with calvarial bone except for the first one that I performed, which absorbed in the supratip. That one bad experience was a technical error: without the proper equipment, I used a high-speed, electric-driven drill designed for orthopedic surgery, which undoubtedly overheated the graft. After switching to an electric drill to harvest the graft at low speed under a constant, cooling water stream, absorption became negligible, even in patients followed for more than a decade.

Calvarial bone forms a smooth, straight, reliable dorsal graft. However, contouring calvarial bone for lateral wall grafts is tedious, and its survival when not in contact with an underlying bony bed is uncertain. Bone grafts do not work well in the tip, so another donor site must be harvested. To save time, I used alloplastics for maxillary augmentation, but that meant that three different materials were needed for a single reconstruction. It is for that reason that I now prefer rib graft reconstructions for most patients in whom septum is not available and conchal cartilage will not suffice.

Calvarial bone does have its place, particularly in adolescents and young adults whose white, elastic rib is likely to deform, or in other patients in whom their surgeons prefer calvarial bone.

Technique

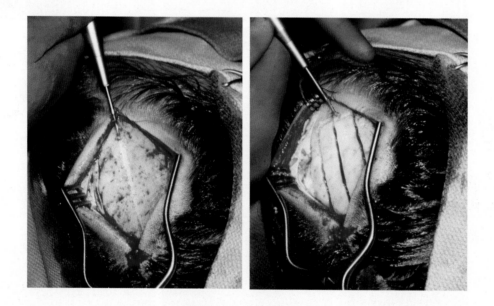

A calvarial bone graft may be harvested from either the superior or posterior parietal area, preferably on the patient's nondominant side. It is important to be far enough laterally to avoid the sagittal sinus. An incision is made perpendicular to the hair follicles and straight down through the pericranium to the bone. The surgeon then places the self-retaining retractor and tries to visualize the best location for graft harvesting.

A 2 mm cutting burr, running at low speed under a constant stream of water, outlines the graft, and then deepens the cuts through the outer table until bleeding indicates that the diploic space has been reached. As the surgeon cuts, holding the drill almost parallel to the surface of the parietal bone, he or she can gauge the substance of the bone and feel when resistance decreases, indicating the diploic space.

Using an angled chisel, the surgeon should begin harvesting laterally by taking a partial-thickness piece of bone and working toward the main graft. Removing a lateral piece allows the surgeon to angle the osteotome parallel to the diploic space, so that the main graft can be removed without fracturing it and without penetrating the inner table. It is extremely important that the surgeon maintain the angle of the chisel parallel to the surface plane of the skull, and remove the graft patiently and gently without twisting the osteotome, which might otherwise penetrate the inner table. In the patient shown here, the harvested grafts were unusually long.

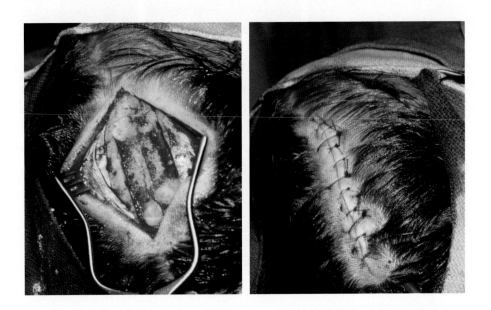

Once the main graft and the side graft have been removed, any bleeding points are controlled with bone wax. The lateral graft is placed in the deeper portion of the defect to minimize palpable irregularities in the skull, and the wound is closed with a few interrupted 2-0 chromic sutures, passing through all layers, and finished with 4-0 chromic sutures. The sutures should not be tied tightly to avoid postoperative alopecia, which has been very rare in my experience.

PATIENT STUDY ONE

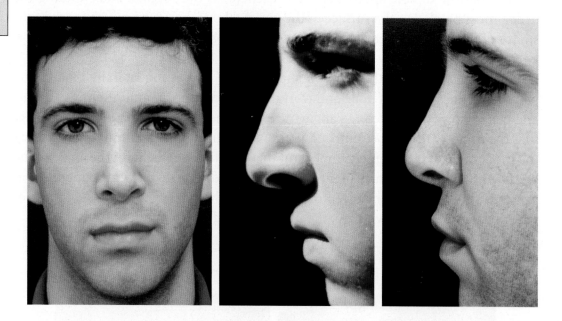

Two previous surgeries in this patient have created changes from his original preoperative nose that can be interpreted based on reduction and disequilibrium. Dorsal and tip reduction narrowed the middle nasal third, revealing a high septal deviation toward the right. Alar cartilage reduction allowed the tip lobule to contract posteriorly, producing a supratip deformity. The upper lip has lengthened and become retrusive. Septal cartilage was unavailable.

SUMMARY OF THE SURGICAL PLAN

1. Harvest calvarial bone and ear cartilage
2. Gore-Tex maxillary augmentation
3. Minimal skeletonization over dorsum
4. Rasp bony vault for graft adherence
5. Calvarial bone dorsal graft
6. Bilateral calvarial bone lateral wall grafts, thicker on left than right
7. Ear cartilage tip grafts

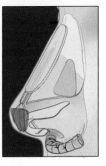

Postoperative Analysis

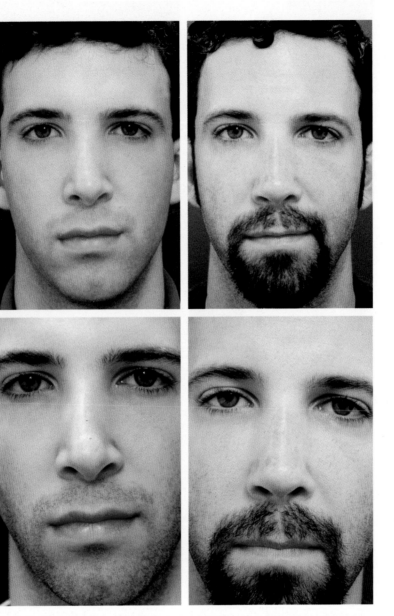

Seven-year postoperative views demonstrate what calvarial bone does so well: produce a straight, smooth dorsum in a patient who only needed a thin dorsal graft for a shallow defect. Maxillary augmentation has corrected the upper lip retrusion.

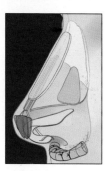

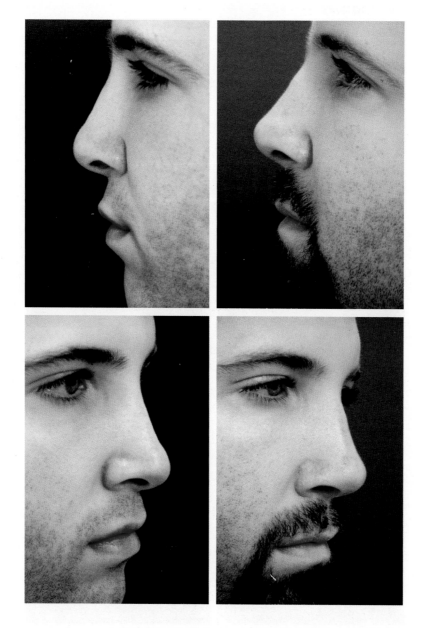

The dorsum remains straight, the upper lip is vertical, and the tip is adequately projecting. The dorsal graft edges are smooth and nonpalpable. Geometric mean nasal airflow increased 5.4 times over preoperative values.

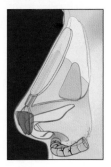

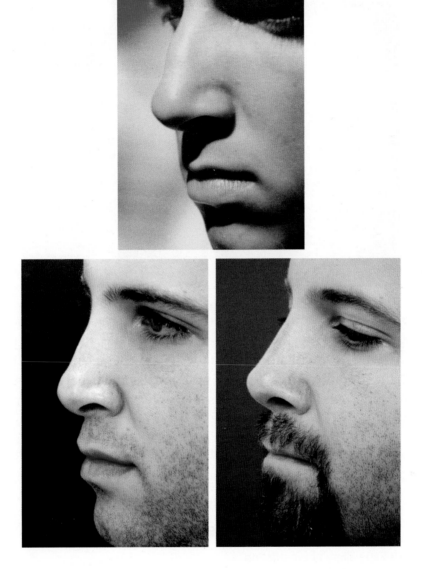

Comparing the patient's original appearance to his preoperative nose, the volume loss is evident. Tip reduction had allowed the alar creases to deepen, and the patient flared his nostrils to support his airway. Postoperatively, the dorsum is straighter and higher, and the alar walls remain supported by bone grafts. Nostril size seems smaller, partially because flare has diminished and because grafts have increased lobular size. No alar wedge resections were performed. The patient returned to ask for a further increase in dorsal height to restore his preoperative nasal volume; however, because the skin sleeve had permanently contracted, further augmentations were not possible.

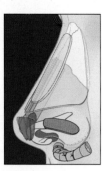

PATIENT STUDY TWO

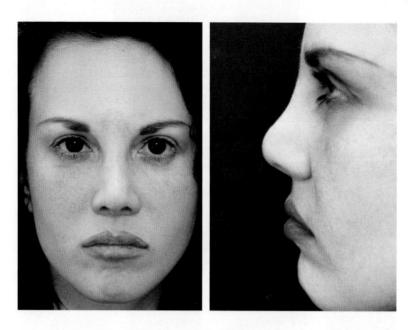

When nasal soft tissues are able to contract until they have nowhere else to go, the result is supratip deformity: the shape of unsupported nasal skin. This patient has a small, tight skin sleeve with no visible underlying skeletal landmarks: the middle vault is soft, the supratip is thick, the alar walls are flat and deeply grooved, the columella is unsupported, and the dorsum is low; only palpation of the bony vault offers any resistance.

SUMMARY OF THE SURGICAL PLAN

1. Gore-Tex maxillary augmentation
2. Harvest calvarial bone and ear cartilage
3. Minimal skeletonization over bony and upper cartilaginous vaults
4. Rasp bony vault for graft adherence, deepen radix
5. Calvarial bone dorsal graft
6. Ear cartilage tip grafts with calvarial bone buttress
7. Ear cartilage alar walls grafts
8. Ear cartilage columellar grafts

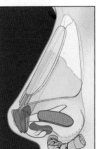

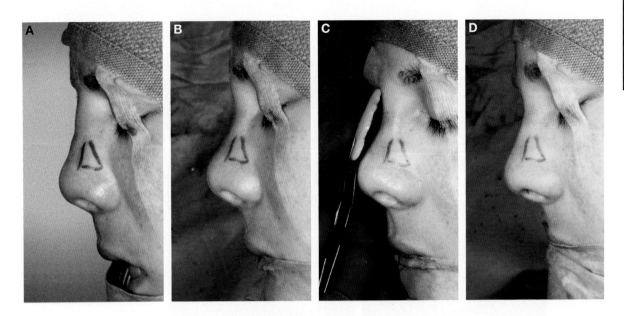

Compare the appearance at the beginning of the surgery with the appearance after maxillary augmentation alone (*A* and *B*). The nasal base has moved forward. After dorsal graft placement, the base rotates caudally *(D)*.

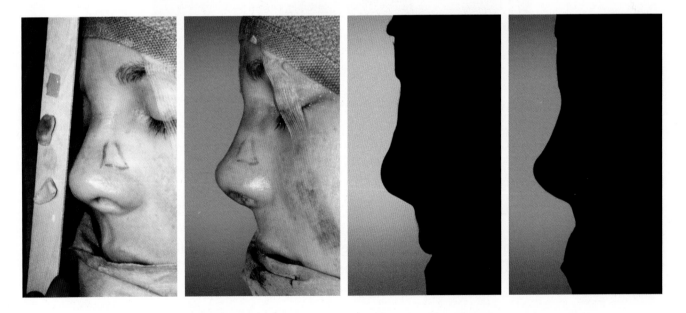

Solid ear cartilage tip grafts with a calvarial bone buttress (top of tongue blade) were used to complete the reconstruction. These tip grafts, which became visible, were revisited 2 years later (see Chapter 14). Silhouettes reveal the changes in nasal base size and dorsal contour that have taken place.

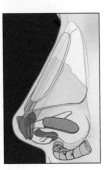

Postoperative Analysis

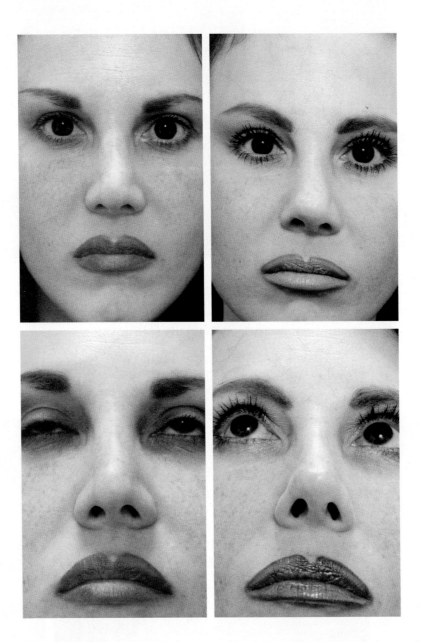

Ten years postoperatively, the dorsum remains smooth. Revised tip grafts are no longer visible. The upper lip retrusion has been corrected.

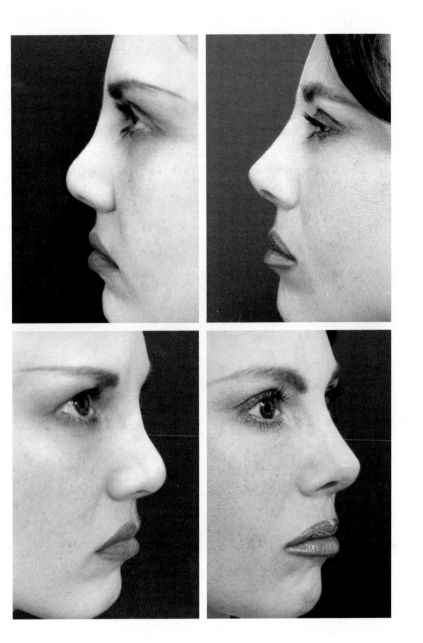

Alar wall grafts have filled the preoperative hollows and reconstructed the lateral crura. Each graft was placed in a separate pocket, combining incisions where possible: a cartilage-splitting incision was made on one side for access to the dorsum and placement of one alar wall graft; and short, vestibular skin incisions for the tip, opposite alar wall, and columella were also made. Dissection was kept to a minimum. *In tertiary patients whose skin is tight and heavily scarred, the surgeon should treat the tissues as he or she would treat irradiated skin. When exposure is wider than necessary, rough, or aggressive, tissue loss can occur.*

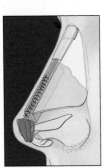

SKIN EXCISION

The caudal transverse excision and the cephalic transverse excision have both been discussed in Chapter 16. But there are times when a longitudinal excision is necessary, even though it is always a compromise. Although I have seen scars in Dr. Sheen's patients that I would not have known were there unless the patients told me, I have rarely attained a scar like that on one of my own patients. I avoid external excisions if I possibly can, and I spend a great deal of time discussing and illustrating the resulting scars with prospective patients.

PATIENT STUDY ONE

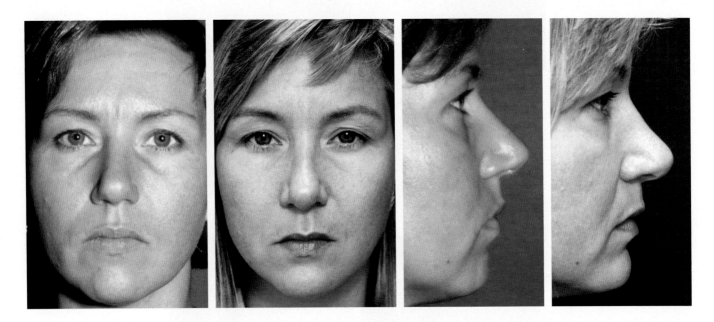

If all noses were shaped like this one, rhinoplasty as an operation would have disappeared long ago. This nose is virtually impossible to reduce successfully. The dorsum is straight, the tip is barely in line with the septal angle, and the tissues are moderately thick. Any disruption of this tenuous equilibrium should cause soft tissue distortion. Patients with such noses usually want the same shape in a smaller size; however, these patients must be guided to understand that such a goal is impossible. Even a conservative rhinoplasty changes each view for the worse. The middle vault becomes narrower, the alar walls collapse and groove, and the tip apparently increases in size and loses shape.

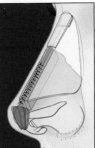

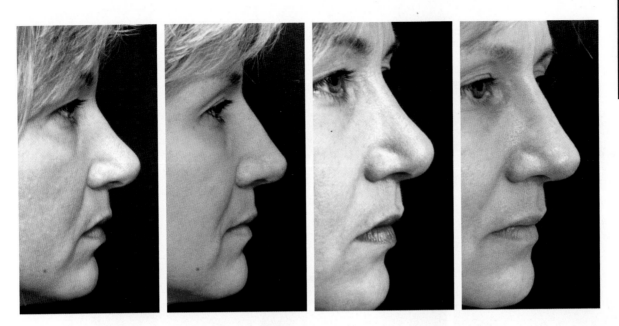

Dorsal and tip grafts, combined with a midline excision extending through the supratip to the point of greatest projection, have improved nasal balance and differentiated the dorsum from the supratip. The nasal base seems smaller because of direct excision and because of the dorsal grafts. The nose, however, remains large.

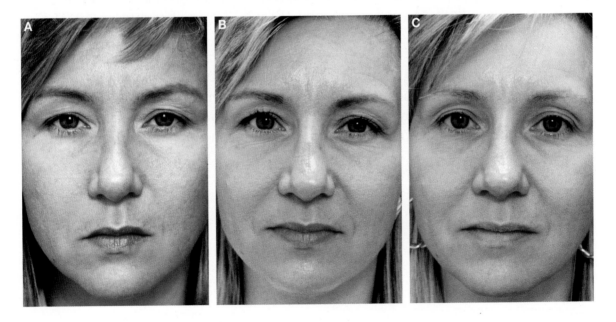

The patient is shown preoperatively *(A)*, and at 2 months *(B)* and 2 years after surgery *(C)*. The scar, although faint, is still visible.

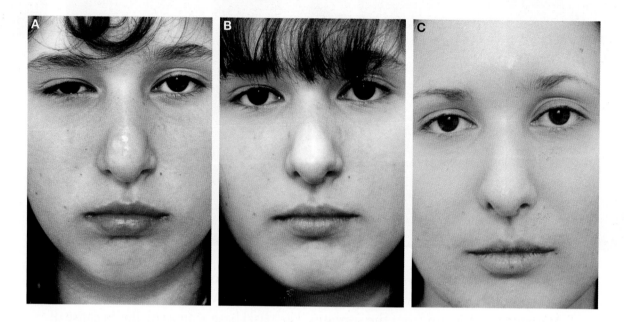

If skin excisions could always be performed on patients with fine, elastic skin, the scars would be much better, but most such patients do not require excision. This patient illustrates this principal. A midline excision was performed for excess soft tissue resulting from the involution of a cavernous hemangioma. The patient is shown preoperatively *(A)*, and at 7 months *(B)* and 13 years after surgery *(C)*. The scar is barely visible.

Coarser-skinned patients often have opportunistic bacteria in their large pores, producing maceration and epidermolysis if sutures remain too long. Dressings should be changed daily by the surgeon, the wounds should be cleansed and dried, and the sutures should be removed early. Even with such precautions, scars are frequently suboptimal.

PATIENT STUDY TWO

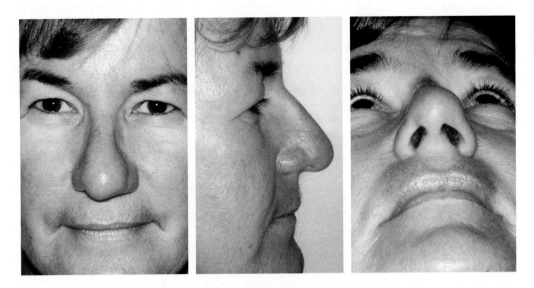

Paralleling the first patient in this subsection, this patient has a nose that is very difficult to reduce successfully. The tissues are thick and soft, the cartilages are bulky, and tip projection is barely adequate. The skin sleeve is long and loose, and the vertical plane of the lip inclines backward. Reduction will only increase apparent nasal bulk and length, and decrease the airway.

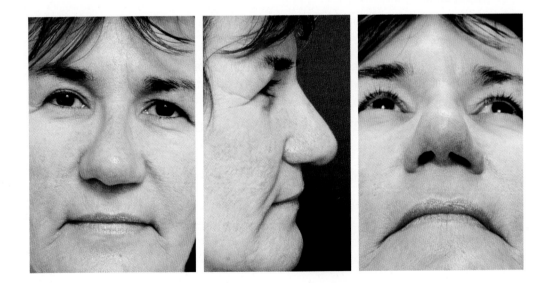

And that is exactly what happened. On the frontal view, the nose has lost what definition it had. The internal valves, not visible from the surface, have become incompetent. The columella has retracted and the upper lip has sunken posteriorly. On the lateral view, nasal length has increased and the subnasale has sharpened. From below, alar wedge resections have decreased nostril size and worsened the nostril-lobular ratio, accompanying a tip that has become rounder and less defined, although more symmetrical.

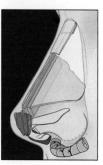

Restoring the airway involves two components: stabilizing the internal valves and increasing nostril size. The latter will also improve the nostril-lobular ratio and reduce apparent tip lobular volume. To shorten the nose, her surgeon must employ all of the strengthening mechanisms possible: maxillary augmentation, columellar augmentation (not as a strut but to increase soft tissue rigidity), and tip grafts. Because of the large skin sleeve volume, radix grafting would only improve nasal proportion modestly.

SUMMARY OF THE SURGICAL PLAN: FIRST STAGE

1. Gore-Tex maxillary augmentation, two pieces, right thicker than left (preoperative asymmetry)
2. Wide skeletonization over upper cartilaginous vault, limited over bony vault
3. Rasp bony vault for graft adherence
4. Shorten caudal ends, upper lateral cartilages, submucosally
5. Harvest composite grafts (change gloves afterward)
6. Septoplasty
7. Bilateral spreader grafts
8. Upper dorsal graft
9. Multiple tip grafts with buttress
10. Columellar grafts
11. Bilateral axial composite grafts, placing the skin islands in the nostril floors, with cartilage components augmenting the medial floors and alar walls

SUMMARY OF THE SURGICAL PLAN: SECOND STAGE (1 YEAR LATER)

1. Revise columellar scar, excise supratip skin
2. Excise left alar rim skin

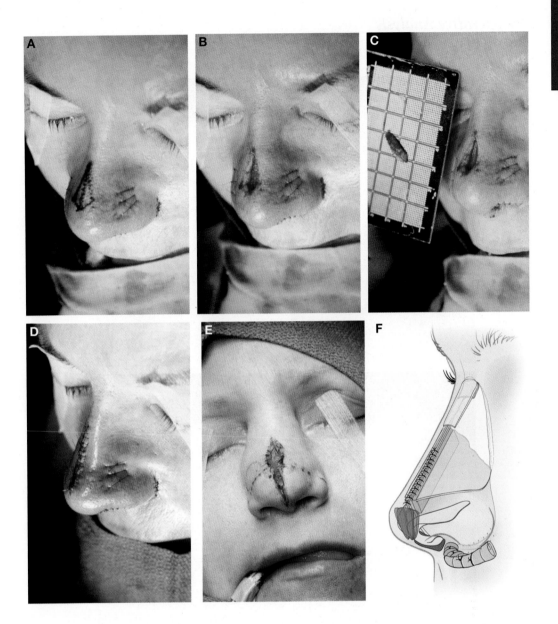

Mark the nasal midline and then the excision area, noting any soft tissue asymmetries. When the deformity is unilateral, place the scar along one of the dorsal reflections instead of the midline. It takes surprisingly little excision to affect the desired outcome, so the surgeon can decrease the chance of overcorrection by incising in the midline and confirming the amount of excision by overlapping the edges. In the patient in *A* through *D*, the excision measured only 4 mm at its widest point (which corresponded to the area of greatest supratip depression). When the tip lobule also must be narrowed, the excision design changes to two skewed diamonds lying end to end *(E)*. Their tips should meet at the point of maximum tip projection, which will be accentuated by wound closure.

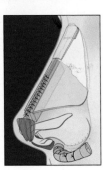

Postoperative Analysis

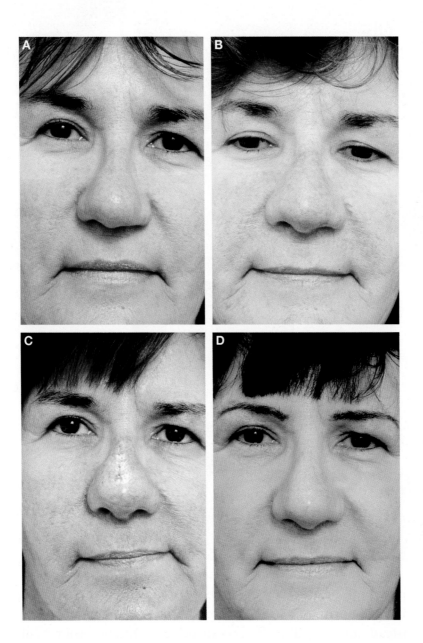

After the first surgery *(B),* the nose is shorter, the upper lip is more vertical, tip projection is adequate, and nasal balance is slightly improved. The supratip is still high and soft; it is not possible to augment this nose sufficiently to redrape all of the excess skin. At 1 week *(C)* and 1 year after the second stage *(D),* the nose has narrowed slightly on the frontal view, and the tip lobule is differentiated from the dorsum better.

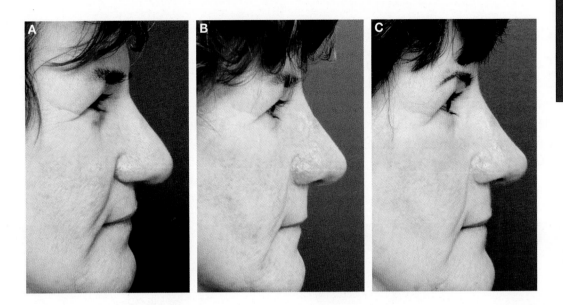

Excision of supratip skin has decreased bulk in the lower third of the nose (compare *B* and *C*). However, the degree of change between the patient's original appearance *(A)* and the finished product *(C)* is soberingly small, and this is still a large nose.

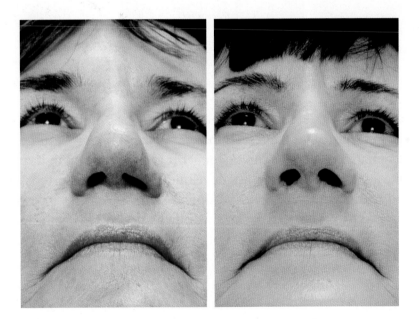

Geometric mean nasal airflow increased 13 times over preoperative values, which is unusually high, because the effects of both valvular and vestibular stenosis were treated. Axial composite grafts have recontoured the alar walls and widened the floors, improving the nostril-lobular ratio. The skin islands were inset exactly at the sites of the previous alar wedge resections.

COMPOSITE GRAFTS

Composite cartilage and skin grafts from the ear can supply lining in the coronal, axial, or sagittal planes, and they can restore alar rim height, increase external valvular support, and enlarge the airway. However, even more important than understanding how to use these grafts is recognizing the cause of the deformities, because we create most of them.

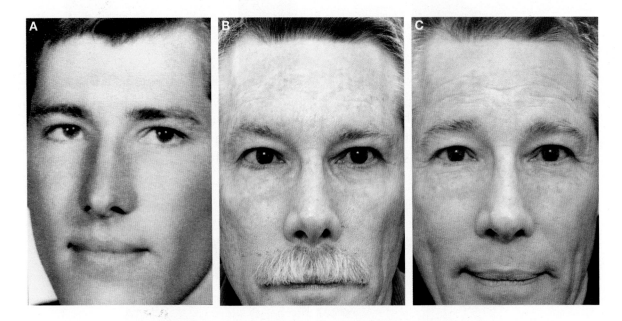

When the alar cartilages are reduced, the alar rims lose support *(B)*. Not all alar rims retract as a result, but if the resection is significant enough or if the soft tissues are thin, the remaining cartilage can no longer brace the alar rim in its preoperative position. Like a burn scar contracture developing, the lining shortens, pulling the rim cephalad with it. In the process, vestibular stenosis may occur. Even if lining has not been resected, external valvular incompetence reflects insufficient underlying support. Composite grafts correct both the lining and skeletal deficiencies *(C)*.

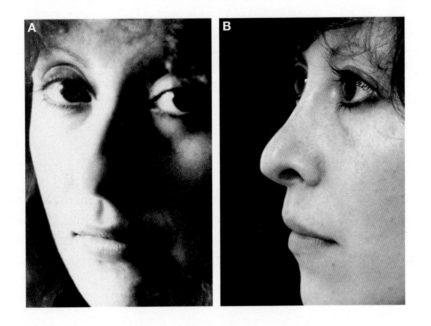

The pathophysiology worsens when the lateral crura are malpositioned. Malpositioned lateral crura are positioned so far from the rims that even unoperated patients may have arching nostril contours and external valvular incompetence *(A)*.* In a thin-skinned patient, lateral crural reduction sufficient to reduce a cosmetic deformity disrupts this fragile equilibrium and the rim retracts farther, producing a real lining deficit and valvular incompetence, in addition to the external deformity *(B)*. Therefore it is important to make the diagnosis of malposition preoperatively so that functional and aesthetic problems may be corrected together and so that a new obstruction does not develop.

*In my first review of external valvular incompetence, 61% of the primary patients had alar cartilage malposition.

Causes of Nostril Deformities in 100 Consecutive Secondary Rhinoplasty Patients Treated by Composite Graft Reconstruction

Cause	Number of Patients (%)
Previous rhinoplasty: Normal alar cartilage anatomy	50
Previous rhinoplasty: Alar cartilage malposition	33
Congenital deformity	7
Trauma	6
Tumor	4

A review of 100 consecutive patients on whom I had performed composite grafts indicated that the cause of the nostril deformity was a previous cosmetic rhinoplasty in 83%. Not surprisingly, 33 of the 83 patients (39.7%) had a previous alar cartilage malposition, based on their original preoperative photographs.

Composite Graft Use in 100 Consecutive Secondary Rhinoplasty Patients

Principal Indication	Number of Patients (%)
Alar notching or asymmetry in rim height	43
Insufficient nasal length	28
External valvular incompetence	14
Nostril/vestibular stenosis	11
Combined vestibular stenosis and lateral alar wall collapse	4

Composite grafts serve a variety of functions. The obvious function is reducing alar rim height and restoring a more normal nostril appearance, but the cartilaginous component not only prevents contraction of the skin island but also braces the external valve, correcting valvular incompetence. Used in addition to dorsally and caudally placed tip grafts, composite grafts can provide the illusion of greater nasal length. In addition, when oriented axially or sagittally, composite grafts will correct a nostril or vestibular stenosis.

Harvesting Technique

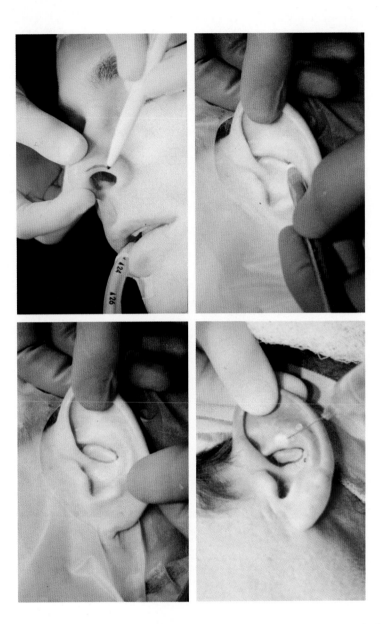

Before infiltration, the length of the defect is marked on the external skin, approximately opposite the site of the planned vestibular incision. The markings are then transferred to the ear. Any portion of the concha may be used, but the posterior wall should always be spared to avoid deforming the ear. I usually select the donor area based on the shape of the defect, previous scars or harvested areas, or locations that will be the least conspicuous. Local anesthesia is used to infiltrate the periphery of the graft, being careful not to separate the skin from the underlying cartilage.

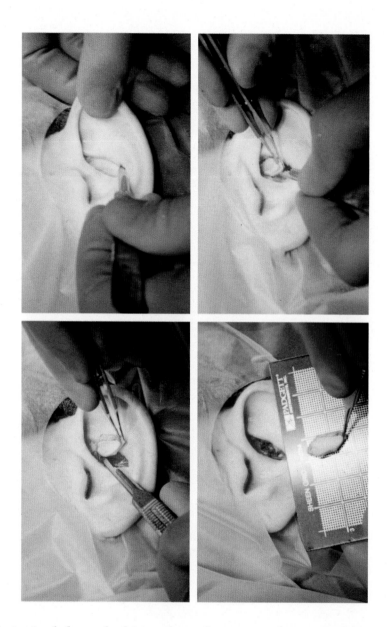

The graft is incised through skin and cartilage around its periphery and resected from the bed, protecting the underlying skin. In most patients, bilateral grafts are used, so the single piece will be split obliquely to provide two grafts of maximum width.

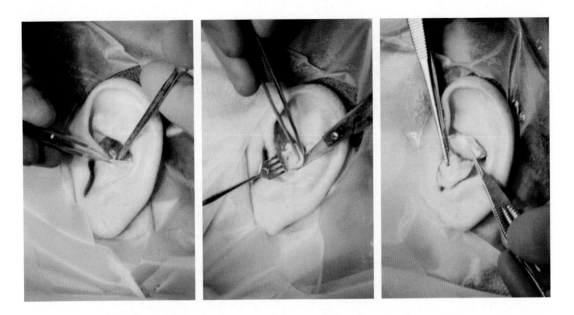

If additional cartilage is needed, a Cottle elevator or scissors can be used to dissect the rest of the concha through the same incision, still sparing the posterior wall. The entire harvest is shown.

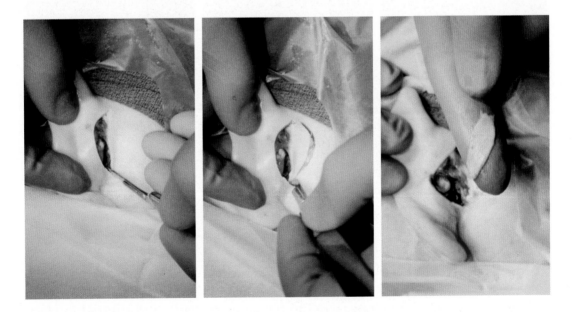

Visually marking the size of the defect or using a pattern, I cut and defat a full-thickness skin graft from the retroauricular skin.

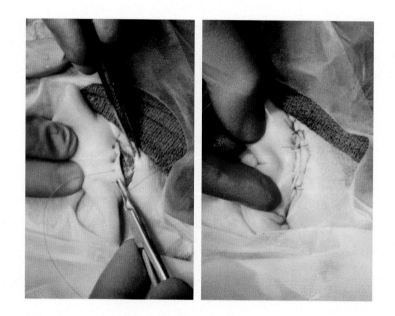

The donor site is closed in layers, using horizontal mattress sutures. The closure should lie exactly in the postauricular sulcus.

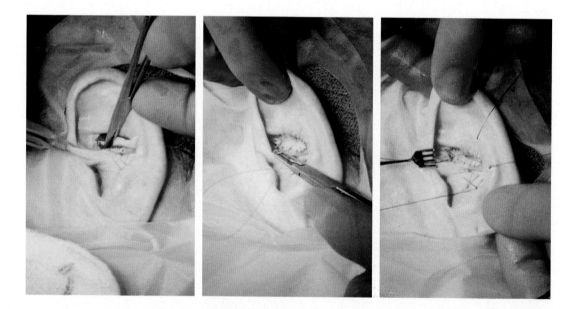

The full-thickness graft is transferred to the anterior defect and sutured in place with 6-0 chromic sutures. Basting sutures are added if necessary to coapt the anterior and posterior surfaces. I pass 3-0 nylon sutures through the ear and around a gauze bolster, which is placed in the sulcus to protect the postauricular and retroauricular skin.

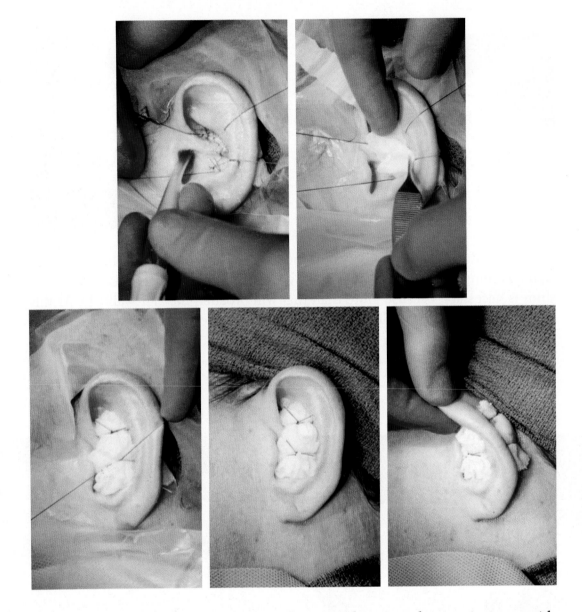

The external canal is filled with saline solution and suctioned, removing any residual preparation solution or blood to prevent external otitis. Half-inch petrolatum gauze is fed into the defect, and the sutures are tied over it. The sutures should be tied purposefully but not tight, because underlying skin necrosis is possible with excessive pressure. The dressing remains in place for 1 week.

Insetting Composite Grafts in a Coronal Orientation

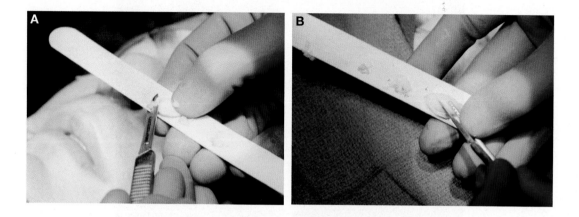

The composite graft as it comes from the ear is always too thick. Thin the cartilaginous component as much as possible without cutting through it. Usually only a shim is necessary, because more than that will broaden the alar wall *(A)*. At this point, the graft is split obliquely to provide two pieces of maximum width and length. If the degree of alar retraction is asymmetrical, the graft must be split accordingly *(B)*.

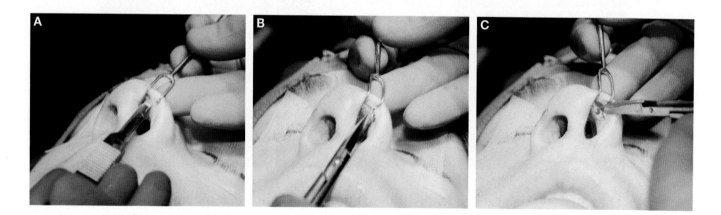

An incision is made opposite the external marking, 3 or more millimeters away from the alar rim. If the incision is made too close to the rim, the graft edge will be visible *(A)*. Dissect back toward the rim for approximately 2 mm to free the edge for attachment *(B)*; doing so allows the caudal suture line to lie flatter. The upper cephalic edge is dissected enough to free the tissues and release the contracture, but only as far as necessary *(C)*.

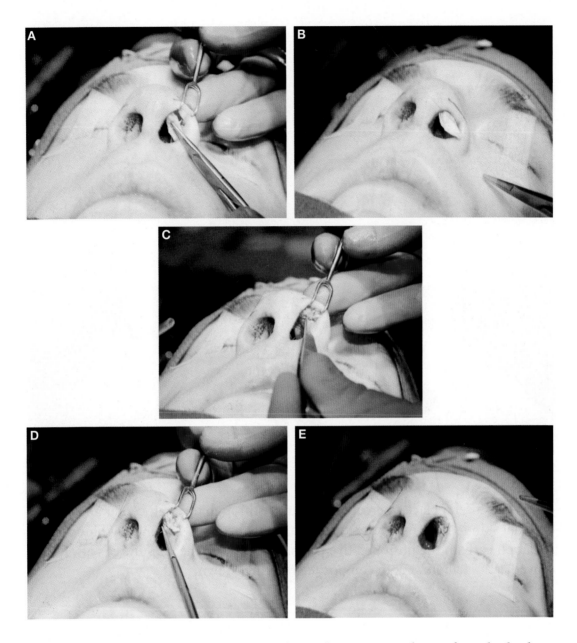

The caudal edge is inset first, suturing the widest point in the graft to the highest part of the defect (*A* and *B*). Then the rest of the caudal edge is inset. The surgeon uses a double hook to pull down on the alar rim until it reaches proper height, so that the required graft thickness can be assessed. It is important not to trim excess graft until this point, because, like releasing a burn scar contracture, more is often needed than might be anticipated (*C*). The cephalic edge is then inset (*D* and *E*). The right composite graft has already been placed in this series.

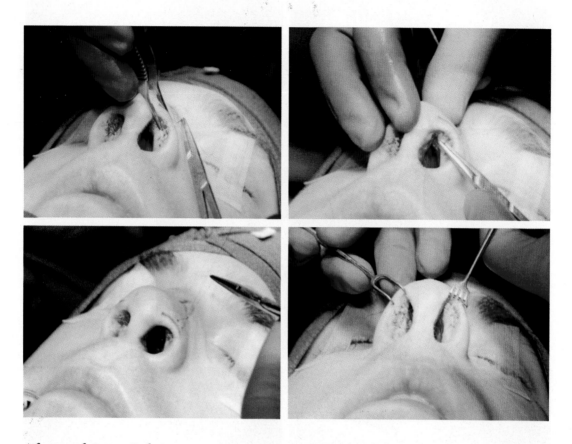

After graft inset, I place a percutaneous suture through the graft center and out the external skin to hold the graft snugly against its bed and prevent any blood accumulation early in the postoperative period. The percutaneous suture is always removed at 24-48 hours. Both composite grafts are shown.

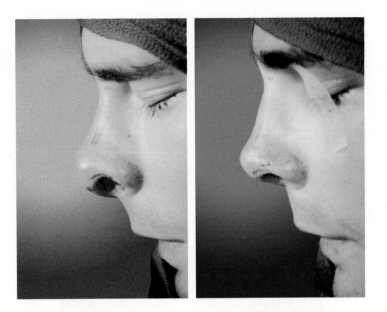

The composite graft correction is 1:1. In this patient, the dorsum and caudal septum were also reduced, and radix and tip grafts were added.

The Alar Lobule as a Donor Site

Occasionally, secondary patients require alar wedge resections, which can be recycled as composite grafts to correct alar retraction or vestibular stenosis.

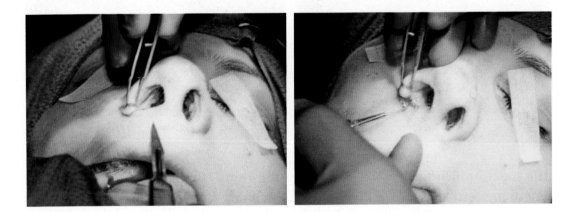

In this patient with asymmetrical alar bases, the right base will be used as a lobule for the left rim. Approximately 3 mm of external skin and 1 mm of vestibular skin will be removed. The inferior incision is made first, adjacent to the alar crease to avoid destroying this landmark. The No. 11 blade is rotated counterclockwise as it approaches and crosses the nasal floor to preserve a medial flap.

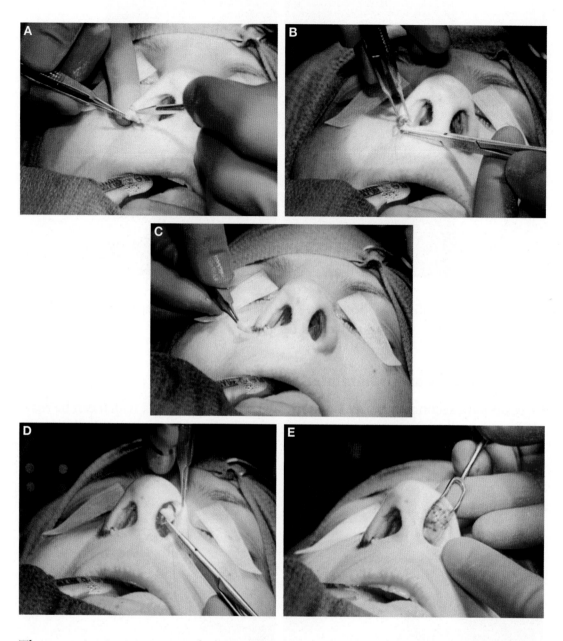

The superior incision is made, removing only a small wedge of tissue. Closure begins at the vestibular side of the rim and is completed. Inset of the caudal end graft is performed first *(D)*, and then along its superior surface *(E)*.

Donor Site Problems

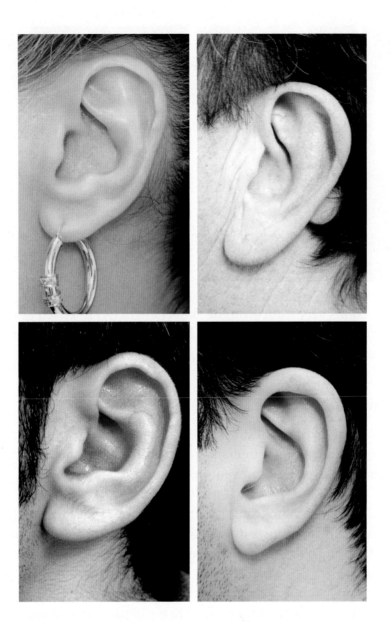

In a review of 100 of my own patients, donor site complications occurred in three patients, but with larger patient numbers, the complication rate is approximately 5%. Most patients with ear donor sites have imperceptible scars.

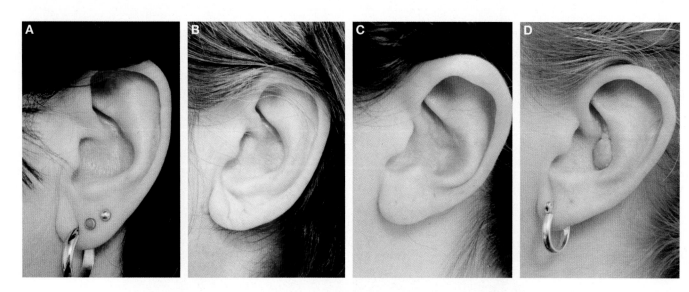

Graft imperfections vary from atrophic skin changes *(A)* to raised graft edges—the most common complication *(B* and *C)*. I have only seen one keloid in several hundred composite graft patients *(D)*.

Postoperative Care

I place routine rhinoplasty packs for 1 week. At that time, the skin islands should be obviously pink and healthy. Patients are instructed to apply petrolatum ointment twice daily for 1 more week to prevent desiccation.

When stenosis has been significant, I splint the airway with short sections of lubricated endotracheal tubing (usually 6 to 8 Fr), starting 2 to 3 days later, when the lining is not too fragile or tender to place them. The tubing only needs to be long enough to stay in place (less than 25 mm) but the diameter must be large enough to exert some pressure without being painful. Increasing sizes can be used as the sidewall softens. Tubes are worn at night for 2 to 6 months, depending on the severity of the preoperative condition. Tubes are routinely used when correcting stenosis—that is, when axial or sagittal grafts are used—but are less often needed for alar retraction, unless postoperative swelling has thickened the rims.

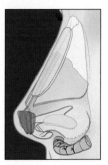

PATIENT STUDY ONE

COMPOSITE GRAFTS IN A CORONAL ORIENTATION

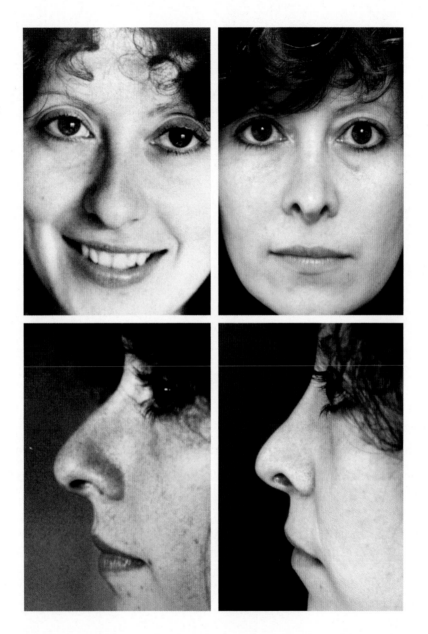

This patient's photographs appeared earlier in this section. Additional original pre-operative views confirm that the patient had all four critical anatomic variants: low radix, inadequate tip projection, narrow middle vault, and alar cartilage malposition (see Chapter 5). Despite the presence of a columellar strut (visible at the left side of the nasal tip), dorsal and alar cartilage reduction have created internal and external valvular incompetence and supratip deformity. No septal cartilage was available.

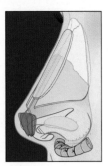

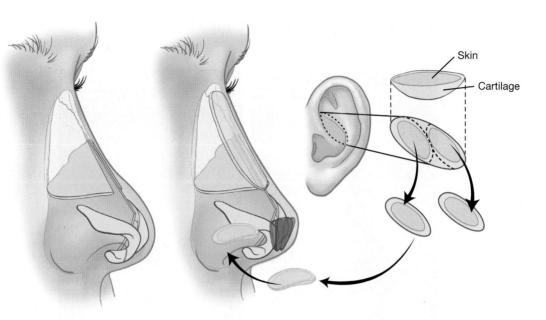

Skin

Cartilage

SUMMARY OF THE SURGICAL PLAN

1. Gore-Tex maxillary augmentation
2. Explore right tip, resect strut
3. Minimal skeletonization over dorsum, rasp bony vault for graft adherence
4. Transfixing incision, elevating caudal and membranous septa without shortening nose
5. Harvest calvarial bone
6. Harvest ear cartilage
7. Calvarial bone dorsal graft
8. Solid and crushed tip grafts
9. Bilateral composite grafts

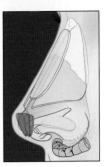

Postoperative Analysis

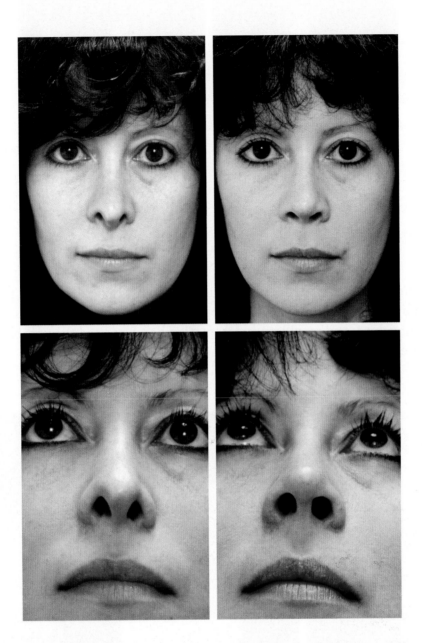

Fourteen months after surgery, the dorsal graft has expanded the middle vault and provided confluence between the upper and middle vaults. The alar rims remain stable, and the nasal base side walls are smooth, without notches.

1169

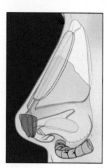

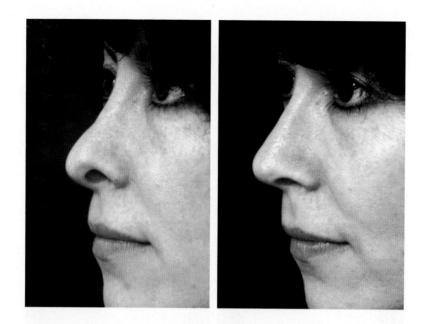

The dorsum is now straight, the supratip is flat, and the tip is adequately projecting. The combination of columellar elevation and alar rim reduction has improved basal relationships, and maxillary augmentation has corrected the vertical position of the upper lip.

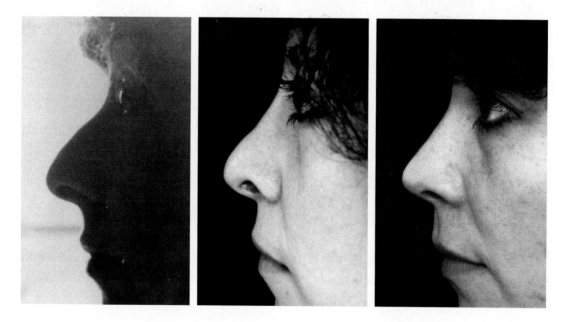

Comparing the patient's original preoperative nose with her nose after secondary rhinoplasty, an alternative original plan would have been slight caudal septal and dorsal reduction with radix, spreader, and tip grafts.

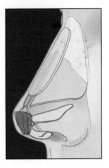

PATIENT STUDY TWO

COMPOSITE GRAFTS IN AN AXIAL ORIENTATION

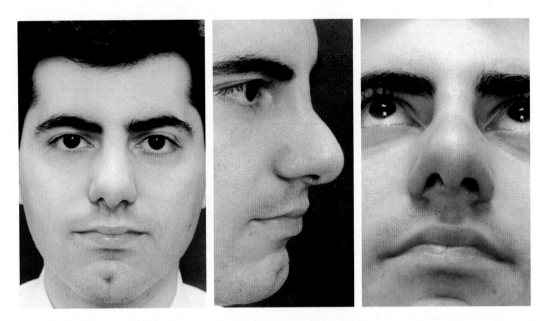

One rhinoplasty created a supratip deformity in this young man, but alar base resections had increased apparent tip lobular width. The nostrils were small and notched at the sites of the previous excisions. No septal cartilage was available.

SUMMARY OF THE SURGICAL PLAN

1. Harvest rib cartilage

2. Harvest composite grafts

3. Minimal skeletonization over bony and upper cartilaginous vaults

4. Rasp bony vault for graft adherence

5. Trim supratip

6. Dorsal graft of rib cartilage

7. Multiple tip grafts

8. Bilateral axial composite grafts

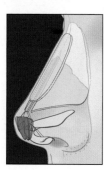

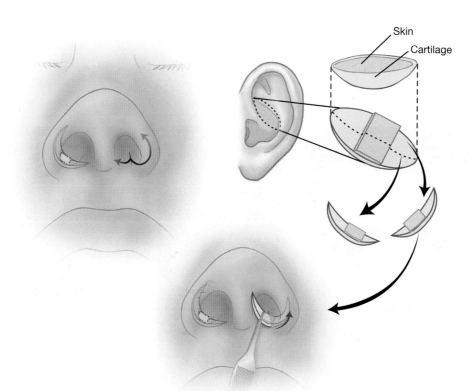

The graft is harvested in the same fashion as for coronal placement. Although less skin will be required for nostril correction, it is better to denude only the tips of the graft and leave a large central island until the size of the recipient defect can be established, because it may be larger than anticipated.

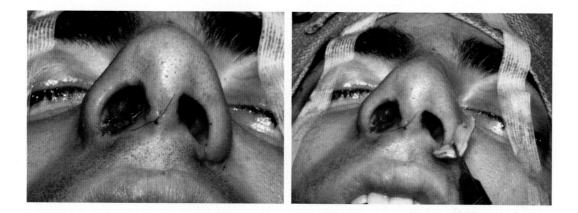

Here, the right side has already been corrected. The skin island required is often only 3 to 4 mm wide. Just as an extra millimeter of alar wedge resection can suddenly create a notch in the nostril floor, only a few millimeters of correction can relieve a notch.

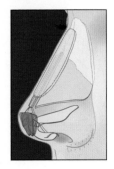

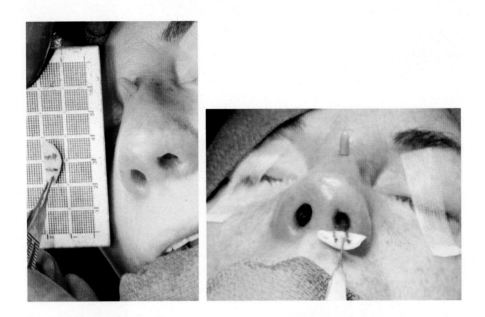

The complete technique is detailed here in a different patient with a unilateral deformity. A 2 cm graft has been harvested, and the skin island will measure 5 mm (as inked).

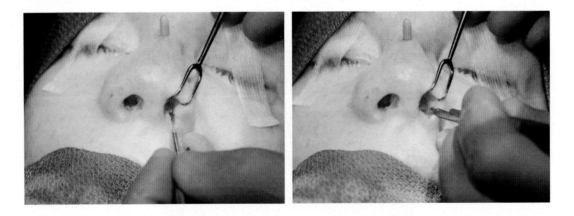

The floor is incised to re-create the defect at the point of greatest deficiency, which is usually the site of the previous scar.

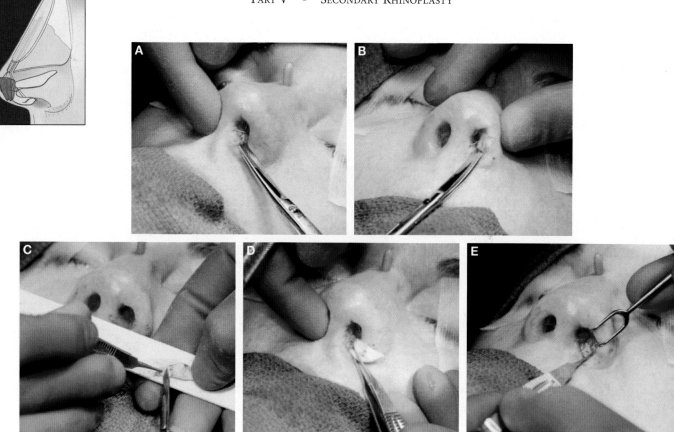

Scissors are used to separate the external and vestibular skin for a short distance medially along the floor *(A)*, and then laterally around the rim with counterpressure from the opposite hand *(B)*. Once the defect size has been established, the tips of the grafts are denuded of skin *(C)*. The graft first is slipped into the columella *(D)*, and the lateral end of the graft is slid into the alar wall *(E)*.

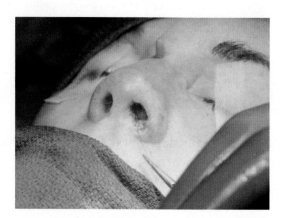

The skin island is fixed to the defect edges with 6-0 chromic sutures. If the tissues are particularly tight or a wider graft is needed, the floor can be split sagittally, with axial anterior and posterior extensions that form an H (rotated 90 degrees), into which the skin island will fit.

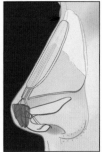

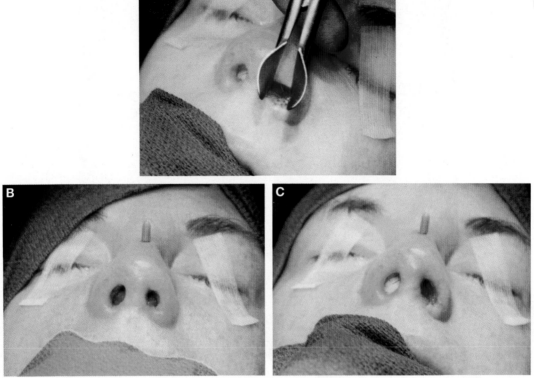

This technique corrects a vestibular stenosis when the alar base is properly positioned, and particularly when a flaccid or flat alar wall accompanies the floor deficiency (A). In this patient, a 5 mm skin island has increased internal nostril diameter by 30% (compare B and C). The blue cover marks the K-wire used to stabilize a rib graft used in this short nose. If the alar base is medially displaced, an alar base flap is preferable. The surgeon can determine the need for one technique or another preoperatively by pushing the alar wall laterally with an intranasal cotton-tipped applicator. If the alar wall and base move easily into the correct position, a composite graft will be sufficient; if not, the soft tissue deficit is more severe and an alar base flap will be necessary.

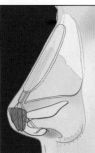

Postoperative Analysis

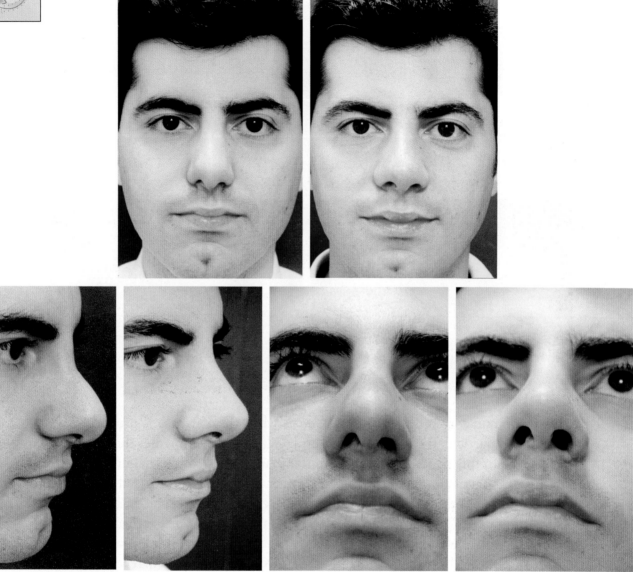

One year postoperatively, the nasal bases remain stable in their lateralized positions. The skin islands are not visible externally. The right alar wedge scar has remodeled after the decrease in skin tension, but the left side could still benefit from revision. Dorsal and tip grafts have redraped the soft tissues and corrected the supratip deformity.

Composite Grafts in a Sagittal Orientation

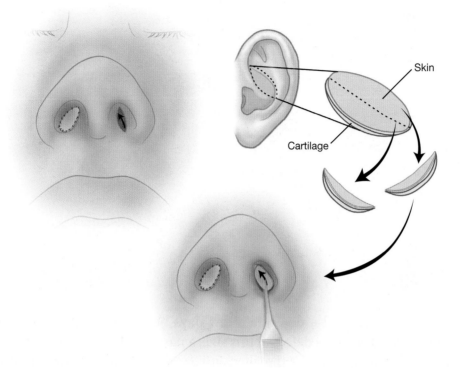

Less commonly, such as after trauma or in secondary cleft rhinoplasty, a soft tissue defect extends deeper into the airway. In these cases a sagittally oriented composite graft makes a significant improvement. Incise the nasal floor at the site of the previous alar resection, if there has been one, or at the point of greatest deficiency. Cut and gently spread only as deep as the thickness of the composite graft (usually about 3 mm), so that the defect will support the graft and the postoperative floor will be level.

After the size of the defect is certain, the graft is harvested in the same fashion as for coronal placement. For this orientation, the cartilaginous component should not be thinned: all of its heft will be needed to minimize the chance of recurrent stenosis. Inset the skin island with fine, absorbable sutures, and remember to use airway splints after removing the packing.

Composite Grafts Used Externally

Skin and composite grafts do not have the color and texture match advantages that local or regional flaps have, but neither do they create new facial scars. Though the color match is never perfect, composite grafts provide a good reconstructive alternative in selected cases.

PATIENT STUDY ONE

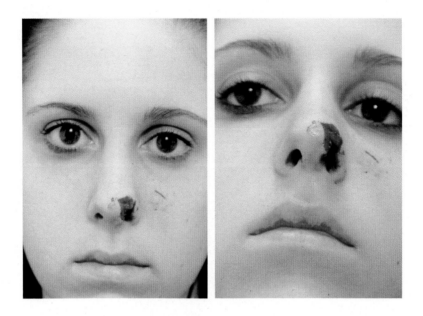

This teenage girl suffered a dog bite a few days before these photographs were taken. With a full-thickness defect of this size, a nasolabial flap is not large enough, and a forehead flap, the best of the alternatives, is a staged procedure that would add an additional facial scar. We agreed to try a composite graft and to use the forehead flap for definitive repair if a composite graft result proved unsatisfactory.

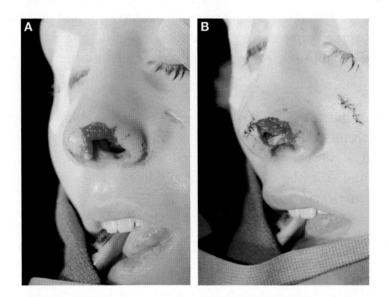

Intraoperatively, the wound edges were freshened, and the lining was advanced by freeing it from the undersurfaces of the upper and lower lateral cartilages *(A)*. The lining was then closed in a V-Y fashion, reducing the size of the defect to match the normal side, bracing the vestibular side along the alar rim with ear cartilage *(B)*.

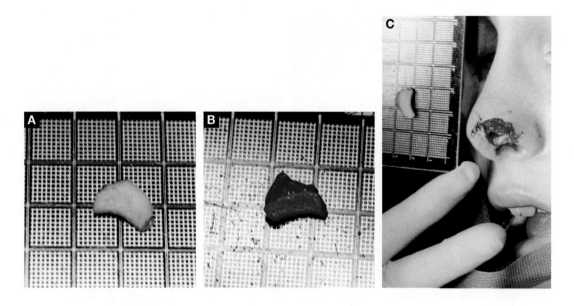

The composite graft was removed from the junction at the superior and transverse portions of the helix, removing retroauricular skin to fit the surface defect. The donor site was closed primarily along the back of the ear and by helical advancement flaps along the auricular edge. In *A* and *B,* the rim with its contained cartilage is inferior and the retroauricular skin is superior.

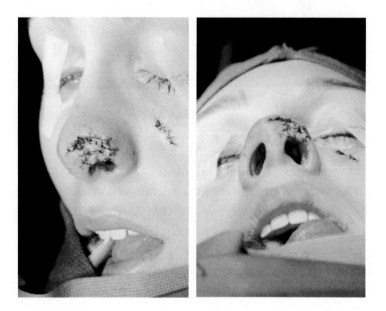

The graft was sutured into position along its intranasal side first and then externally, coapting the skin graft portion to its advancement flap bed with fine nylon sutures (removed at 48 hours). Graft take was complete.

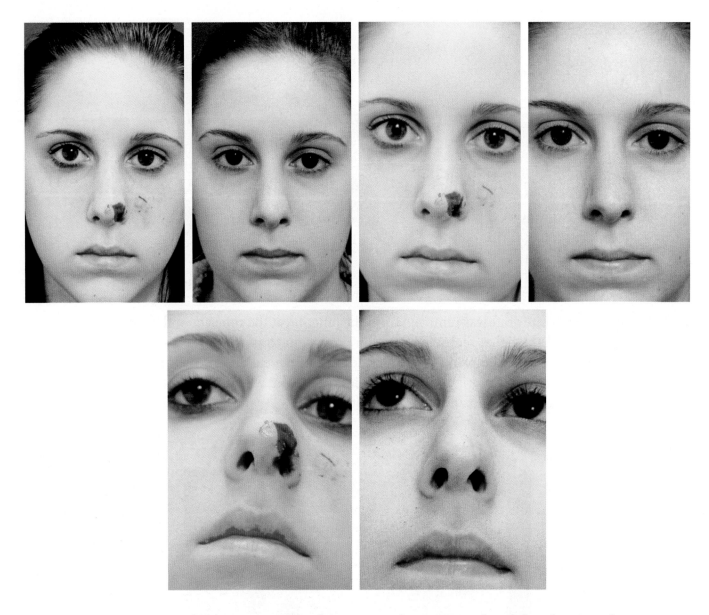

Fourteen months postoperatively, skin contour has improved and the alar rim, although not perfectly smooth, shows only minor imperfections. Fear has disappeared from the patient's eyes. Inferiorly, the tip lobule is symmetrical, and the nostril rim is continuous. The patient has no other visible donor scars.

Forehead flap donor scars are usually excellent, but in younger patients I prefer a one-stage correction that does not introduce new facial scars as long as the result will be sufficient.

PATIENT STUDY TWO

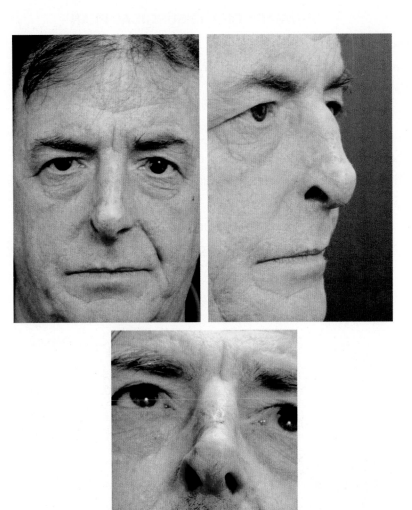

This man had undergone excision of a rhinophyma that resulted in a tight, contracted tip lobule and hypertrophic scarring. The middle vault was narrow and deviated toward the right, and airway obstruction was present.

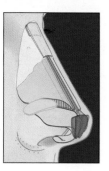

SUMMARY OF THE SURGICAL PLAN

1. Harvest composite graft
2. Limited skeletonization, narrow over bony vault
3. Rasp bony vault
4. Septoplasty
5. Spreader grafts—right thicker than left
6. Multiple tip grafts with buttress and crushed cartilage overlay
7. Release external contracture right alar wall
8. Composite graft right alar wall
9. Alar rim and sidewall bilateral osteotomies

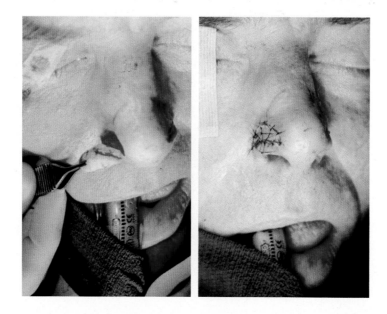

Based on the shape of the defect after release of the alar wall contracture, a composite graft was harvested and sutured into position, with its upper border aimed at simulating the cephalic margin of the normal lateral crus. Take was complete.

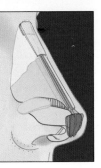

Postoperative Analysis

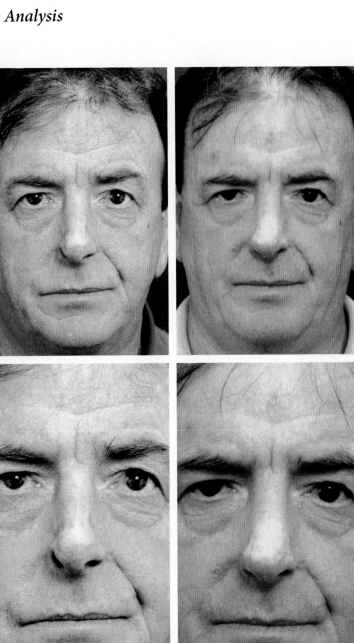

Two years postoperatively, alar base contours have improved. The right lower nose, although thicker than the left, no longer has a distracting asymmetry.

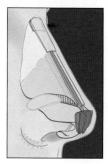

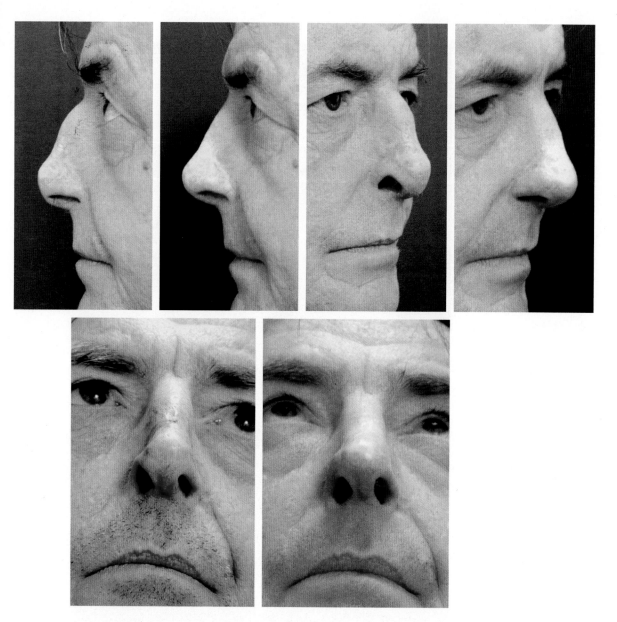

The dorsum is straighter, and the tip is more projecting. The right alar rim has returned to its normal height, and an appropriate lateral crural convexity contours the surface. From below, nostril size has returned to normal, although the alar wall is too thick. The patient declined revision.

Tip grafting in such patients is treacherous, particularly using an underlying buttress, because the tissues are scarred and unyielding. However, I needed the buttress to set the angle of tip rotation, which has improved; soft grafts placed anterior to the buttress formed the lobule itself. All grafts were placed without tension, and the wound was closed without tension. Despite that, the tip developed a worrisome blush on the evening of surgery, which resolved in 24 hours. Nasal circulation is never inviolable.

Donor Site Depletion

As more and more surgeons become familiar with varying autogenous donor sites, a group of secondary rhinoplasty patients is emerging with *donor site depletion,* a term that I coined in 1995. These patients have already had septoplasty or harvesting of one or more auricular, calvarial, iliac, or rib grafts. Some patients limit surgeons further by prohibiting donor sites that are painful (rib or iliac crest) or frightening (calvarium). Even primary rhinoplasty patients may have donor site depletion if the septum is bony and yields minimal useable cartilage (a circumstance that is more likely to occur in non-Caucasians or with posttraumatic noses). The surgeon faced with these patients must be familiar with techniques that allow acceptable functional and aesthetic results with suboptimal or minimal graft material.

It is here that the endonasal approach becomes especially helpful, because dissection can be limited and surface changes can be assessed accurately. Even scraps of leftover cartilage, none of which qualify as traditional tip grafts, can nevertheless reconstruct a lobule if pocket dissection is kept small and high so that even limited donor material can produce its maximal effect.

Another advantage of the endonasal approach is a decreased requirement for the grafts themselves. Because the columellar skin is never dissected from the medial crura, columellar struts are not necessary. Resection and replacement of alar cartilage lateral crura become an anatomic substitute for supporting alar or sidewall grafts. Crushed cartilage can be used in ways and places that would be difficult, if not impossible, through the open approach.

Technical Guidelines in Graft-Depleted Patients

1. Internal valvular reconstruction can be accomplished using either spreader grafts or dorsal grafts with equal functional effects. Geometric mean nasal airflow typically doubles with either graft type.
2. External valvular reconstruction can be accomplished by relocating malpositioned lateral crura, by using battens of cartilage or bone that span the area of rim collapse, or by composite skin/conchal cartilage grafts. Mean nasal airflow typically doubles with external valvular reconstruction alone by any of these methods.
3. Tip reconstruction may be accomplished by selective grafting of the skeletally deficient lobular parts using small, crushed grafts in limited pockets.
4. Thick skin limits the amount of reduction that can be performed successfully, because soft tissue contraction occurs only modestly, thickens the skin further, and creates increasingly blunt contours. The surgeon is wiser to plan a strategy that includes appropriate augmentation for balance, shape, or valvular support so that skeletal volume is redistributed rather than reduced.
5. Single-unit dorsal grafts are still needed for substantial bridge defects in thin-skinned patients. Not all patients can be treated with minimal donor material.
6. Multiple staggered grafts can form a smooth dorsum in patients with adequately thick soft tissue cover.

BIBLIOGRAPHY

Aiach G, Monaghan P. Treatment of over-reduction of the nose and subsequent deformities. Br J Oral Maxillofac Surg 33:250-261, 1995.

Bashour M. History and current concepts in the analysis of facial attractiveness. Plast Reconstr Surg 118:741-756, 2006.

Brand P, Yancey P. Pain: The Gift Nobody Wants. New York: Harper Collins, 1993, pp 274-275.

Brown JB, Cannon B. Composite free grafts of two surfaces of skin and cartilage from the ear. Ann Surg 124:1101-1107,1946.

Burget GC, Menick FJ. Aesthetic Reconstruction of the Nose, 2nd ed. St Louis: Mosby–Year Book, 1994.

Byrd HS, Salomon J, Flood J. Correction of the crooked nose. Plast Reconstr Surg 102:2148-2157, 1998.

Constantian MB. An alar base flap to correct nostril and vestibular stenosis and alar base malposition in rhinoplasty. Plast Reconstr Surg 101:1666-1674, 1998.

Constantian MB. Functional effects of alar cartilage malposition. Ann Plast Surg 30:487-499, 1993.

Constantian MB. Indications and use of composite grafts in 100 consecutive secondary and tertiary rhinoplasty patients: introduction of the axial orientation. Plast Reconstr Surg 110:1116-1133, 2002.

Constantian MB. Rhinoplasty in the graft-depleted patient. Oper Tech Plast Reconstr Surg 2:67-81, 1995.

Daniel RK. Rhinoplasty: a simplified, three-stitch open tip suture technique. Part II: secondary rhinoplasty. Plast Reconstr Surg 103:1503-1512, 1999.

Daniel RK. Secondary rhinoplasty following open rhinoplasty. Plast Reconstr Surg 96:1539-1546, 1995.

Erol OO. The Turkish delight: a pliable graft for rhinoplasty. Plast Reconstr Surg 105:2229-2241, 2000.

Gruber RP, Tabbal N, Sheen JH, et al. Panel discussion: treatment of complex nasal deformities. Aesthet Surg J 19:475-482, 1999.

Hilton L. Secondary rhinoplasty corrects bad "nose job." Cosmetic Surg Times 3(1), 2000.

Hodgkinson DJ. Cranial bone grafts for dorsal nasal augmentation. Plast Reconstr Surg 104:1570-1571, 1999.

Jackson IT. Long-term follow-up of cranial bone graft and dorsal nasal augmentation. Plast Reconstr Surg 104:882, 1999.

Jackson IT, Choi HY, Clay R, et al. Long-term follow-up of cranial bone graft in dorsal nasal augmentation. Plast Reconstr Surg 102:1869-1873, 1998.

Jackson LE, Koch RJ. Controversies in the management of inferior turbinate hypertrophy: a comprehensive review. Plast Reconstr Surg 103:300-312, 1999.

James SE, Kelly MH. Cartilage recycling in rhinoplasty: polydioxanone foil as an absorbable biomechanical scaffold. Plast Reconstr Surg 122:254-260, 2008.

Joseph J. Nasenplastik un Sontstige Gesichteplastik. Leipzig: Hertag von Curt Katbitzsch, 1931, p 205.

Juri J. Secondary rhinoplasties for men. Clin Plast Surg 18:763-773, 1991.

Kerth JD, Bytell DE. Revision in unsuccessful rhinoplasty. Otolaryngol Clin North Am 7:65-74, 1974.

Mazzola RF, Felisati G. Secondary rhinoplasty: analysis of the deformity and guidelines for management. Facial Plast Surg 13:163-177, 1997.

Meyer R. Secondary and Functional Rhinoplasty: The Difficult Nose. Orlando, FL: Grune and Stratton, 1988, p 297.

Millard DR. Secondary corrective rhinoplasty. Plast Reconstr Surg 44:545-557, 1969.

Muenker R. The bilateral conchal cartilage graft: a new technique in augmentation rhinoplasty. Aesthetic Plast Surg 8:37-42, 1984.

O'Connor GB, McGregor MW. Secondary rhinoplasties: their cause and prevention. Plast Reconstr Surg (1946) 15:404-410, 1955.

Pardina AJ, Vaca JF. Evaluation of the different methods used in the treatment of rhinoplastic sequelae. Aesthetic Plast Surg 7:237-239, 1983.

Peck GC Jr, Michelson LN, Peck GC. The external shaving technique in aesthetic rhinoplasty. Plast Reconstr Surg 97:33-39, 1996.

Peck GC, Michelson L, Segal J, et al. An 18-year experience with the umbrella graft in rhinoplasty. Plast Reconstr Surg 102:2158-2165, 1998.

Pensler J, McCarthy JG. The calvarial donor site: an anatomic study in cadavers. Plast Reconstr Surg 75:648-651, 1985.

Pitanguy I, Calixto CA, Caldeira AML. Analise critica e evolucao da rinoplastia secundaria. Revista Bras Cir 74:40-54, 1984.

Pollet J, Weikel AM. Revision rhinoplasty. Clin Plast Surg 4:47-53, 1977.

Rees TD. Current concepts of rhinoplasty. Clin Plast Surg 4:131-144, 1977.

Rees TD, Krupp S, Wood-Smith D. Secondary rhinoplasty. Plast Reconstr Surg 46:332-340, 1970.

Rohrich RJ, Gunter JP, Friedman RM. Nasal tip blood supply: an anatomic study validating the safety of the transcolumellar incision in rhinoplasty. Plast Reconstr Surg 95:795-799, 1995.

Rohrich RJ, Krueger JK, Adams WP Jr, et al. Rationale for submucous resection of hypertrophied inferior turbinates in rhinoplasty: an evolution. Plast Reconstr Surg 108:536-544, 2001.

Sheen JH. A change in the site for cranial bone harvesting. Prospect Plast Surg 4:48-57, 1990.

Sheen JH. A new look at supratip deformity. Ann Plast Surg 3:498-504, 1979.

Sheen JH. Rhinoplasty: personal evolution and milestones. Plast Reconstr Surg 105:1820-1852, 2000.

Sheen JH, Sheen A. Aesthetic Rhinoplasty, 2nd ed. St Louis: CV Mosby, 1987.

Stucker FJ, Smith TE Jr. The nasal bony dorsum and cartilaginous vault. Pitfalls in management. Arch Otolaryngol 102:695-698, 1976.

Szalay L. Early secondary corrections after septorhinoplasty. Aesthetic Plast Surg 20:429-432, 1996.

Thomas JR, Tardy ME Jr. Complications of rhinoplasty. Ear Nose Throat J 65:19-34, 1986.

Trussler AP. Revision rhinoplasty. Plast Reconstr Surg 122:309-310, 2008.

Webster RC. Revisional rhinoplasty. Otolaryngol Clin North Am 8:753-782, 1975.

CHAPTER 18

Regional Deformities

And there is a Catskill eagle in some souls
that can alike dive down into the blackest gorges,
and soar out of them again and become invisible
in the sunny spaces. . . . Even in his lowest swoop
the mountain eagle is still higher than the other
birds upon the plain, even though they soar.

HERMAN MELVILLE
Moby Dick

Our ignorance of the laws of variation is
profound. . . . But whenever we have the means
of instituting a comparison, the same laws
appear to have acted.

CHARLES DARWIN
On the Origin of Species by Means of Natural Selection

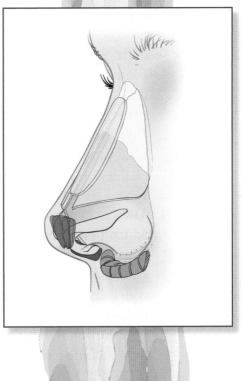

*P*rimary and secondary rhinoplasty both operate under the same natural laws. A surgeon seeing a primary deformity assesses the potential for reduction/disequilibrium, whereas a secondary surgeon sees the results of that disequilibrium. In concept and technique, therefore, there is very little difference between primary and secondary rhinoplasty except the donor sites.

But primary rhinoplasty and secondary rhinoplasty are not the same operations. In secondary rhinoplasty, the tissues have suffered and the patients have suffered. Decisions of dissection need to be planned carefully, placing safety first. Most patients have much more anxiety than they did before the primary surgery, because they now know that rhinoplasty is not always simple, and that a good result is not always guaranteed. Some patients are frantic for cosmetic improvement. Most have airway obstructions. Some are angry with their previous physicians, others have lost family support, and almost all have the spoken or unspoken fear that the next operation may also fail.

Some patients still seek the same unrealistic goals that they did before the primary surgery, others hope for less, and some only want to breathe well again. The surgeon must manage these goals and develop a plan with the patient that is corrective but not too bold, and enough but not too much. I follow Sheen and Sheen's tenets for secondary rhinoplasty:

1. *Establish realistic patient expectations.* Both patient and surgeon must understand why the original goals were not met. If they were never achievable, better goals must be set.
2. *Defer surgery until final resolution of tissues.* A surgeon must control all possible variables, and if augmentation will be performed, the tissues must be pliable enough to permit it.
3. *Have a well-defined aesthetic concept.*
4. *Make a proper diagnosis.* To this I would add that the surgeon must identify which of the anatomic variants were (and still are) present and what problems have been caused by failing to treat them.
5. *Limit the dissection.* This is critical, particularly for surgeons who like the wider dissection of open rhinoplasty. Treat tertiary skin as if it had been irradiated.
6. *Use only autogenous material.* Autografts provide the patient's best chance for a lifetime nasal reconstruction.

To Sheen and Sheen's six criteria, I would add two more, asking the following questions:

7. Can I see the deformity and can I personally fix it? These questions eliminate delusional patients and match the surgeon's individual experience and skill against the severity of the deformity and the patient's expectations.

8. Does the patient accept the margin of error inherent in surgery?

These last two criteria will have different answers among patients and surgeons, but if all criteria are satisfactorily met, the surgeon begins at a good place. These two criteria are discussed further in Chapters 17 and 20.

Dorsal Deformities

As I have emphasized from the beginning of this book, Nature's rhinoplasty rules are consistent, whether the operation is done open or closed, and whether the building material is rib cartilage, septum, ear cartilage, or calvarial bone. Unless we acknowledge that principle, the operation makes no sense. If the surgeon resects enough dorsum to open the cartilaginous roof, the middle third will always narrow. Dorsal resection affects nasal balance, apparent nasal base size, bony width, middle vault width, columellar position, and nostril contour. The degree of change, and how much it shows from the surface, depends on how aggressive the surgeon is and how capable the soft tissues are of responding. But the same things always happen. Therefore as you examine these patient examples, I hope that you are able to recognize patterns of nasal response and patterns of deformity, so that secondary nasal shapes become familiar, instantly triggering recognition of the surgical interventions that caused them. Taken backward one step, those secondary patterns teach the surgeon to see the predisposing deformities in the primary nose.

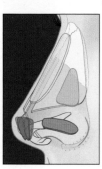

PATIENT STUDY ONE

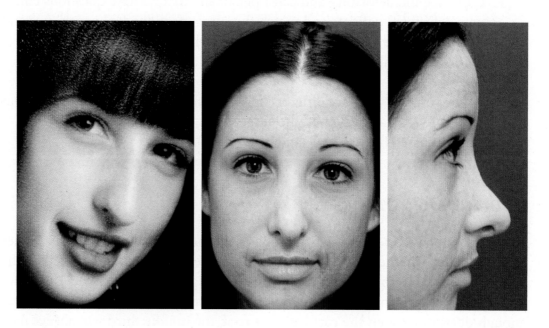

A single open rhinoplasty has converted a high dorsum and alar cartilage malposition to a nose with an obstructed airway. There is a high septal deviation to the right. Despite a distorting columellar strut, tip contour remains suboptimal.

SUMMARY OF THE SURGICAL PLAN

1. Minimal skeletonization to the radix through a single intercartilaginous incision
2. Transfix, resect columellar strut, trim caudal and membranous septa
3. Rasp dorsum for graft adherence
4. Harvest rib cartilage
5. Rib cartilage graft to nasal dorsum
6. Alar wall grafts
7. Left lateral wall graft
8. Tip graft

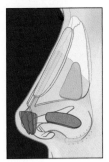

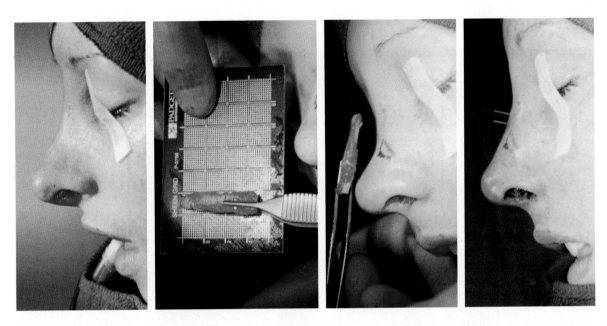

A 33 mm dorsal graft, covered with perichondrium on its anterior surface, was carved and placed, immediately correcting the dorsal defect and decreasing apparent nasal base size. The strut was resected, and the columella elevated. Smooth K-wires, to be removed at 7 days, immobilized the dorsal graft against an asymmetrical underlying platform.

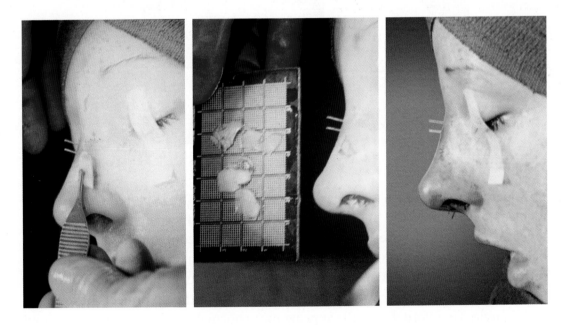

Slices of rib were used to cover the left lateral wall depression and contour the tip (two grafts were placed), which completed the reconstruction.

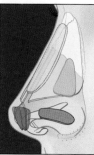

Postoperative Analysis

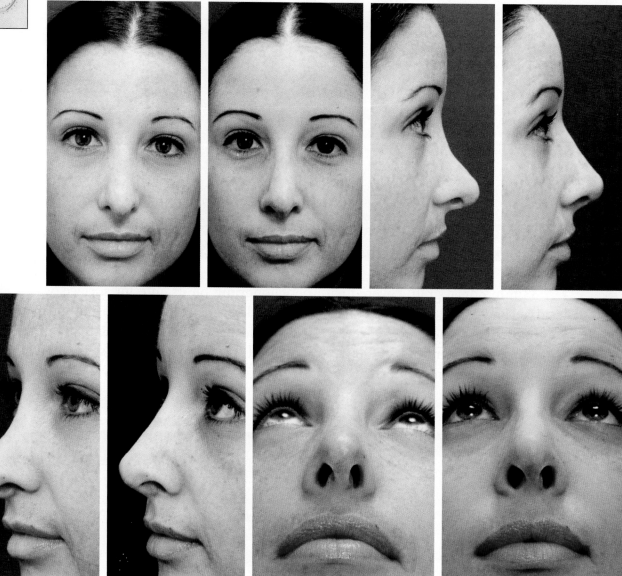

Postoperatively, the dorsal graft has narrowed the nose (no osteotomies were performed) but widened the middle third, correcting the internal valvular incompetence and ablating the inverted-V deformity. The major configurational change has been the conversion of a concave dorsal line to one that is straight. Notice that retroussé, which many patients identify as a desirable "curved" or "scooped" dorsal line, is not concave but straight; retroussé occurs when the tip projects beyond the septal angle. Therefore the profile appears more normal when it is straight, without a middorsal notch, and tip projection is adequate. As usual, a higher dorsum creates an apparently smaller nasal base, despite tip grafts. Columellar contour has improved after strut removal, and alar wall grafts have rounded the rims.

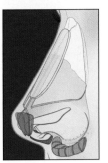

PATIENT STUDY TWO

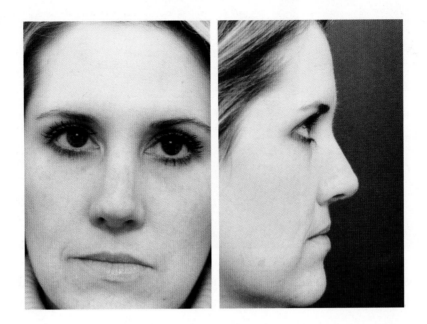

A single conservative rhinoplasty left this patient with a movable piece along the dorsum that she thought was a prosthesis. In addition, she had bilateral airway obstruction and a blunt tip. Her upper lip had fallen posteriorly, creating the appearance of Class III malocclusion, which she did not actually have. Her goals were a stable bridge, a vertical upper lip, an improved airway, and a more angular tip.

SUMMARY OF THE SURGICAL PLAN

1. Harvest rib cartilage

2. Remove dorsal implant

3. Two-piece maxillary augmentation, left thicker than right (preoperative asymmetry)

4. Rib cartilage dorsal graft

5. Multiple crushed cartilage tip grafts

6. Columellar grafts behind depressed scar

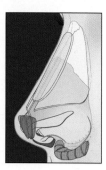

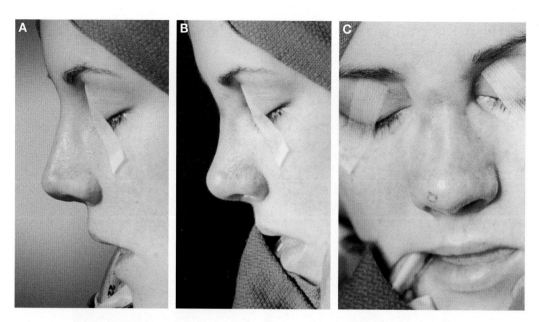

The supposed implant turned out to be the resected cartilaginous roof hiding a significant defect *(B)*, and covering a high septal deviation toward the patient's left *(C)*.

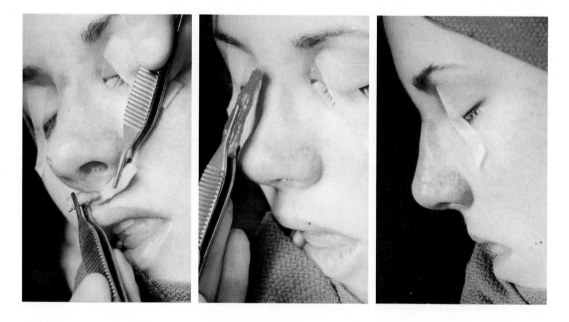

The tip of the ninth rib was trimmed and split to make a two-piece maxillary augmentation, thicker on the patient's left than right because of preoperative asymmetry. A more proximal section of the ninth rib was trimmed and beveled for a dorsal graft; sufficient calcifications remained to prevent it from curling, even though periosteum remained on the surface. Once in place, the dorsum became straight, and the nasal base seemed to diminish in size.

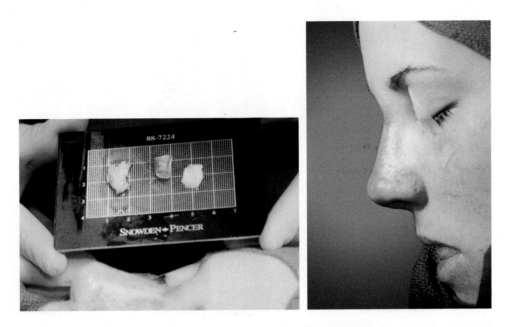

Slices of rib were crushed and used for the tip. Only two of the three slices shown were actually inserted, increasing projection and narrowing the tip slightly.

Postoperative Analysis

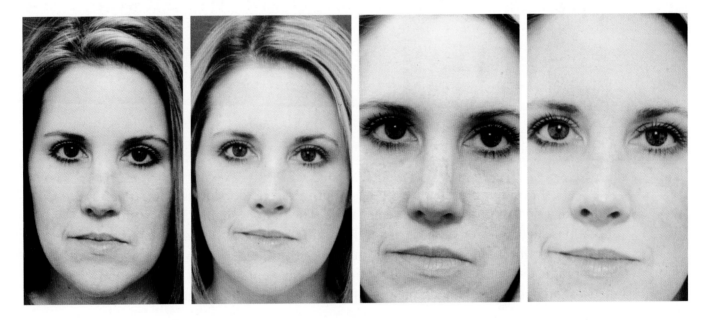

One year postoperatively, the dorsum is smooth and seems narrower, simply because it is slightly higher. No osteotomies were performed. Tip grafts have narrowed the tip lobule (no alar cartilage resection). Maxillary augmentation has improved upper lip position, correcting the retrusion in the subnasale and laterally.

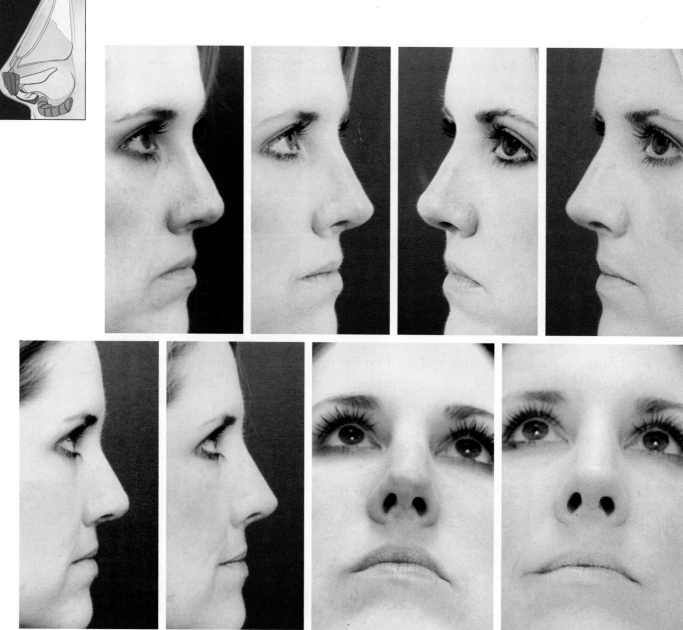

The vertical position of the upper lip has improved. The dorsum is now straight, ending in a tip that projects to the septal angle. The radix is slightly higher and the supratip is slightly lower, because of a redistribution of dorsal support. Notice that the dorsal graft placed was thickest in the upper third, tapering to a thin edge at the supratip. Despite a high septal deviation to the patient's left that created asymmetrical preoperative obliques, the postoperative obliques match more closely.

Tip augmentation has altered tip lobular shape slightly, and increased columellar support helps smooth the scar. Although I had planned to perform a linear scar revision as a secondary office procedure, the patient later decided against it.

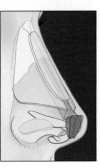

PATIENT STUDY THREE _____

A VARIATION ON RIB GRAFT DONOR SITE

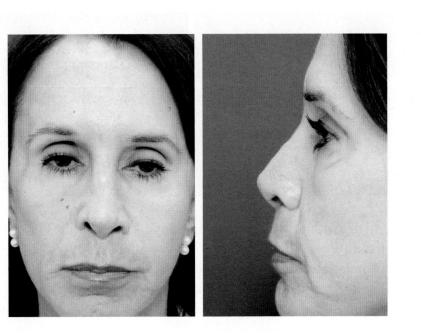

Four previous rhinoplasties created an irregular dorsum, a supratip deformity, alar retraction, and airway obstruction. One ear had already been harvested, and no septal cartilage remained. Simultaneously with the rhinoplasty and revision of a previous breast augmentation, a slice of sixth rib will be harvested for the patient's dorsum.

SUMMARY OF THE SURGICAL PLAN

1. Harvest composite graft
2. Harvest sixth rib graft through previous inframammary incision
3. Minimal skeletonization over dorsum
4. Rasp bony vault for graft adherence
5. Excise ellipse of membranous septum without shortening nose
6. Right spreader graft
7. Rib cartilage dorsal graft
8. Tip grafts
9. Bilateral composite grafts, right greater than left (preoperative asymmetry)

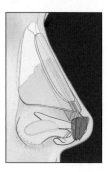

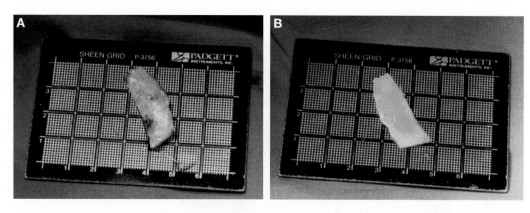

Taken tangentially with a No. 10 blade on a long knife handle, either the fifth or sixth rib (depending on patient anatomy) between the origins of the pectoralis major and minor muscles can supply an excellent dorsal graft that is 3 to 4 cm long. Perichondrium is always preserved to create a smooth surface cover *(A)*. In this patient, the yellowed undersurface indicates calcifications typical of her age *(B)*.

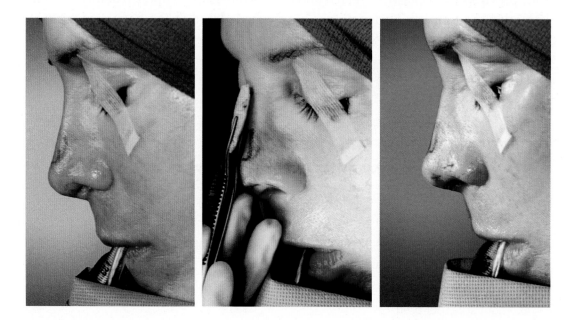

The graft was further thinned and scored on its surface to decrease perichondrial spring; the dorsum straightens once it is placed. A percutaneous suture marks the location of the left composite graft.

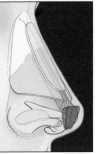

Postoperative Analysis

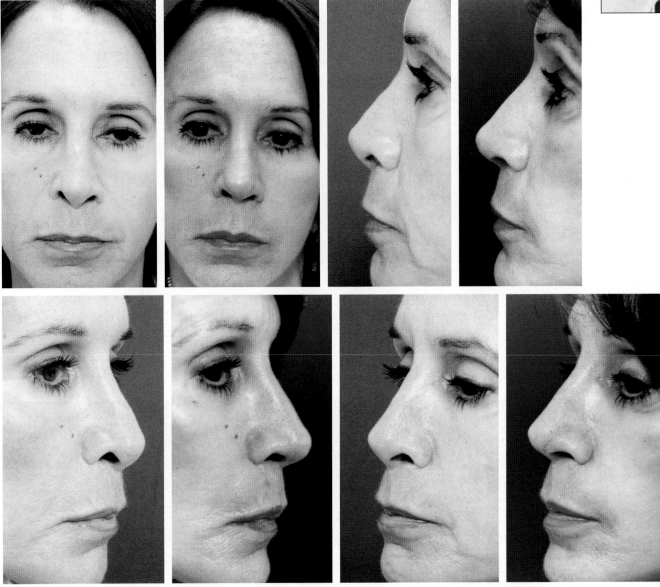

Two years postoperatively, the patient's dorsum remains straight, and nasal base aesthetics have been improved by columellar resection and composite grafts. Tip grafts have formed a better angle of rotation and created a columellar/lobular break. The oblique views match more closely, and the tip lobule now projects to the level of the septal angle.

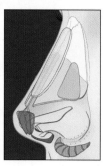

PATIENT STUDY FOUR

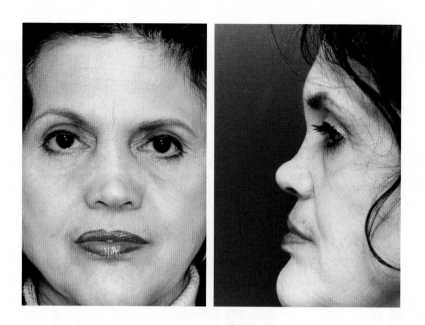

This patient underwent a primary rhinoplasty for airway obstruction that also involved a dorsal reduction. Some months later, noticing that the dorsum was so broad, her surgeon repeated his osteotomies. Most striking is the depth of the dorsal defect.

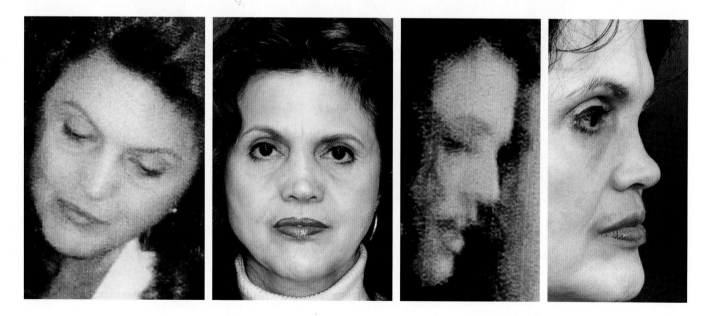

Comparison against the patient's original preoperative view illustrates the magnitude of the changes. Both the bony vault and the nasal base have widened, and the upper lip has become noticeably retrusive. The middle vault is narrower but flat. The nose has shortened and lost projection, and the entire midface seems to have become retrusive.

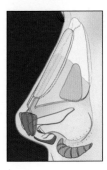

SUMMARY OF THE SURGICAL PLAN

1. Harvest eighth and ninth ribs
2. Moderate skeletonization over upper cartilaginous vault, limited skeletonization over bony vault
3. Rasp bony vault for adherence
4. Rib graft maxillary augmentation (single unit)
5. Rib cartilage dorsal graft
6. Rib cartilage lateral wall grafts
7. Columellar grafts
8. Multiple tip grafts

One goal for this patient is an increase in midfacial projection. A dorsal graft will improve dorsal and middle vault position, but cannot increase tip projection. Tip grafts improve tip projection but cannot correct maxillary retrusion. This patient is another example of the global effects of resecting only one nasal area (the dorsum), and illustrates how many secondary procedures are required to compensate for it.

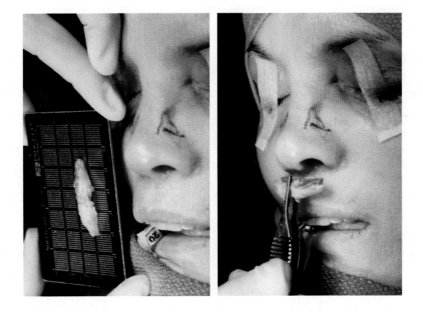

The ninth rib was carved to provide significant maxillary augmentation to reach from one alar base to the other. It was notched at its midpoint to fit over the nasal spine. The graft measured 35 by 8 mm at its midpoint. This is unusually large, but the supple, unscarred labiogingival sulcus would provide adequate cover in this patient. The graft was placed through a short incision in the right nasal floor to reposition the nasal base. Placing the maxillary graft first allowed the size of the dorsal graft to be more accurately assessed.

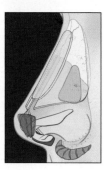

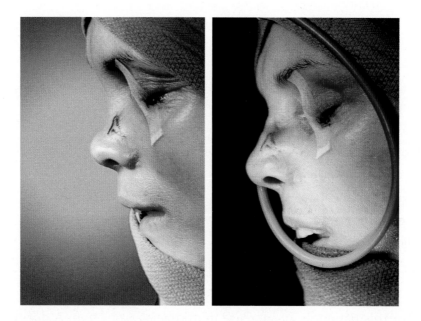

A Foley catheter was inserted into the skeletonized dorsum, and the balloon was gently inflated to expand the tight middle vault skin. Notice the difference in lip position created by the maxillary augmentation.

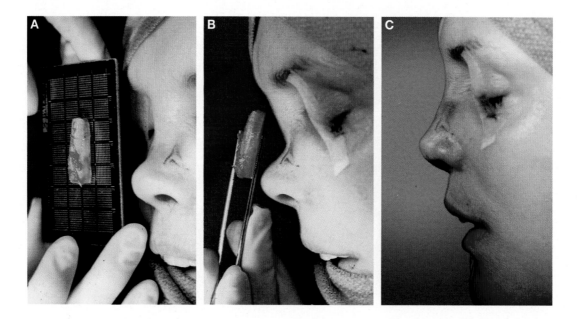

The dorsal graft was 3 cm long by almost 10 mm deep and heavily calcified *(A)*. After skeletonization, the soft tissues collapsed into the defect even further *(B)*. This is what the primary surgeon saw at the conclusion of his operation. The lateral skin markings indicate the location of rib cartilage slivers used to fill out the side-walls and camouflage the graft edges—such additional sidewall grafts are often necessary with large dorsal grafts.

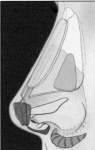

Postoperative Analysis

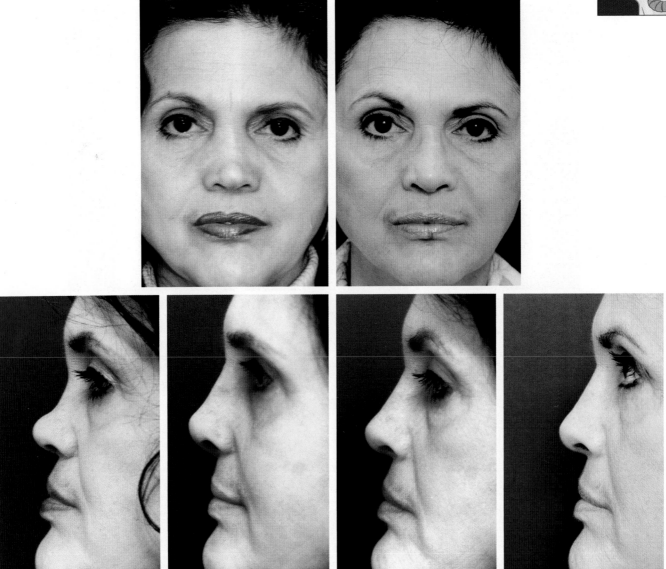

Preoperative   1 week postoperatively   6 months postoperatively   18 months postoperatively

All of the planned corrections are evident at 7 days after surgery. The nose lengthens slightly as edema resolves during the postoperative months, but the correction remains. At 18 months postoperatively, the dorsum remains straight, and the graft edges are not visible. Grafts must be large enough to provide the desired surface change; the soft tissues do not contract to reveal them.

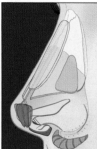

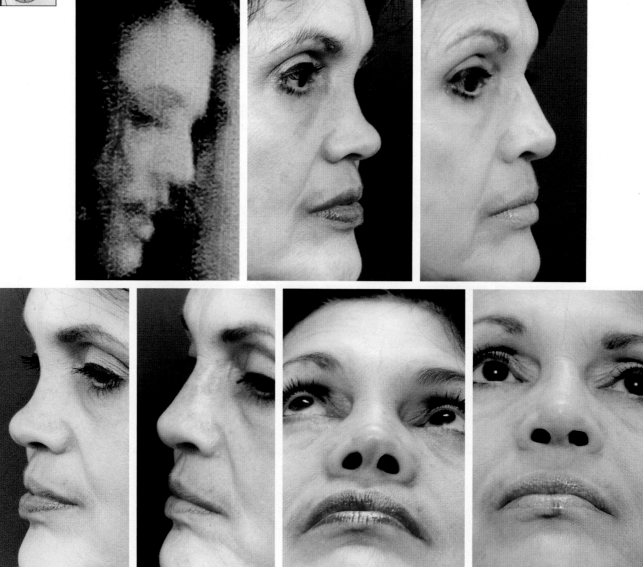

Comparing the postoperative views with the patient's original photo, many of the previous landmarks have reappeared. However, because the soft tissues have thickened irreversibly from contraction, not all nuances are recoverable. Mean postoperative airflow increased 4.2 times over preoperative values. The tip is symmetrical, and the nasal base is unscarred. Columellar grafts provide support and camouflage the intercrural groove.

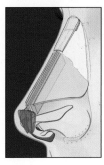

Middle Vault Problems

PATIENT STUDY ONE

If the surgeon plans only a reduction operation, the success of the entire procedure depends on the validity of two assumptions that we have already seen to be false (see Chapter 2): the reality is that soft tissues do not have an infinite ability to contract, and the nasal regions are functionally and structurally interdependent.

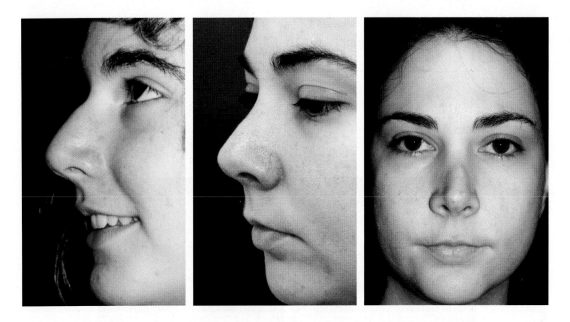

This young woman illustrates both of those principles. Before her first rhinoplasty, she had a low radix, a high dorsum, and inadequate tip projection. Dorsal and tip reduction have not only created a smaller version of her preoperative nose, but they also disrupted the continuity of the bony and upper cartilaginous vaults, creating an obvious inverted-V deformity and impairing her airway at the middle vault. Her reduced lateral crural remnants have buckled medially, creating alar hollows and obstructing the airways internally at the external valves. Based on our rhinomanometric data, her airflow is probably only 25% of what she originally had.

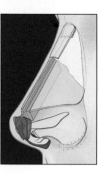

SUMMARY OF THE SURGICAL PLAN

1. Minimal skeletonization over middle vault, narrow over bony vault
2. Trim cartilaginous dorsum
3. Resect and relocate alar cartilage lateral crura
4. Elevate posterior membranous septum to lengthen nose
5. Septoplasty
6. Upper dorsal graft
7. Bilateral spreader grafts, right thicker than left
8. Tip grafts
9. Anterior columellar grafts
10. Posterior columellar graft

Postoperative Analysis

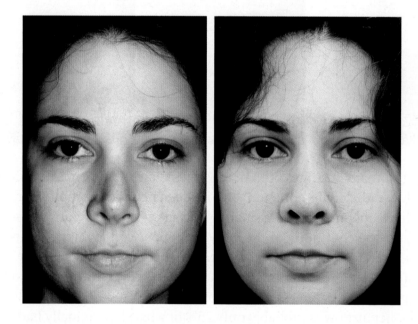

The resected and replaced lateral crura, reversed so that the convexities faced laterally, have ablated the alar hollows and created normal alar wall contours. Spreader grafts have opened the middle vault, and the radix graft combined with the dorsal resection has smoothed the dorsal plane.

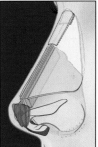

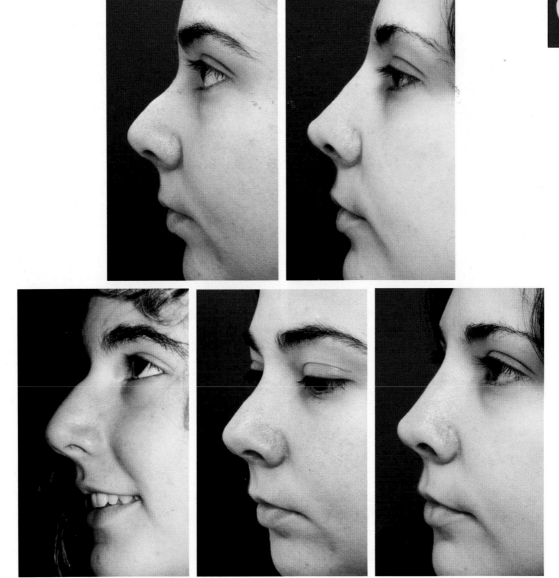

One-year oblique views show a reorganization of the dorsal line: the upper nose is larger and the lower nose is smaller, altering nasal balance and reducing apparent nasal base size. The posterior membranous septal resection has softened the sub-nasale, and multiple crushed tip grafts have increased projection to the level of the septal angle. The alar wall hollows have disappeared. Geometric mean nasal airflow increased 7 times over preoperative values.

PATIENT STUDY TWO

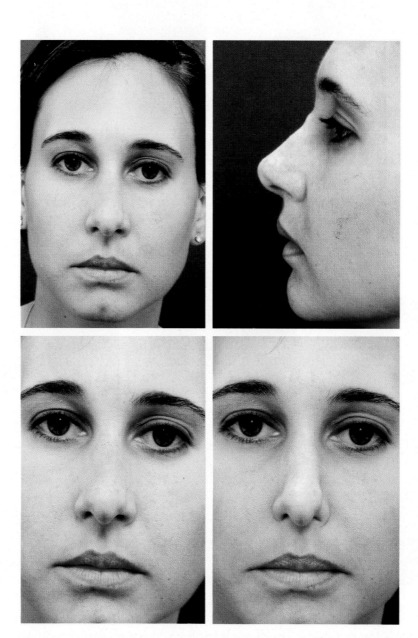

In this patient's first rhinoplasty, the surgeon recognized the low radix and grafted it correctly; but the graft was slightly short, and the substance of the graft proved too rigid for the thin radix soft tissues. Without spreader grafts, the middle vault narrowed. Only a small amount of septal cartilage remained. Inspiration collapsed the sidewalls caudal to the bony arch at the internal and external valves.

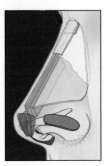

SUMMARY OF THE SURGICAL PLAN

1. Minimal skeletonization

2. Rasp radix, removing old graft

3. Harvest ear cartilage

4. Resect medial crural footplates through short membranous septal incisions; no transfixing incision

5. Septoplasty

6. Asymmetrical spreader grafts, thicker on right than left (preoperative high septal deviation toward the left)

7. Radix graft, longer than the original to blend with the dorsal resection, with a second short piece sutured to its posterosuperior surface

8. Bilateral alar wall grafts (crushed ear cartilage)

9. Multiple crushed tip grafts

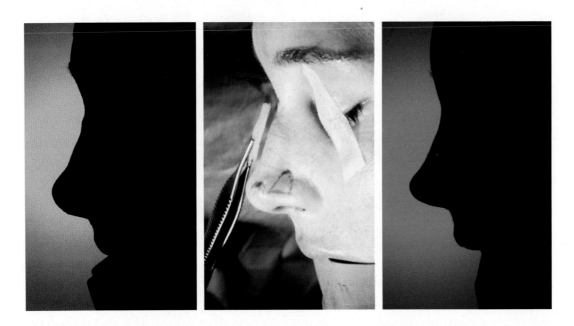

A new dorsal graft and tip grafts created subtle but real profile changes.

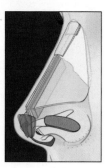

Postoperative Analysis

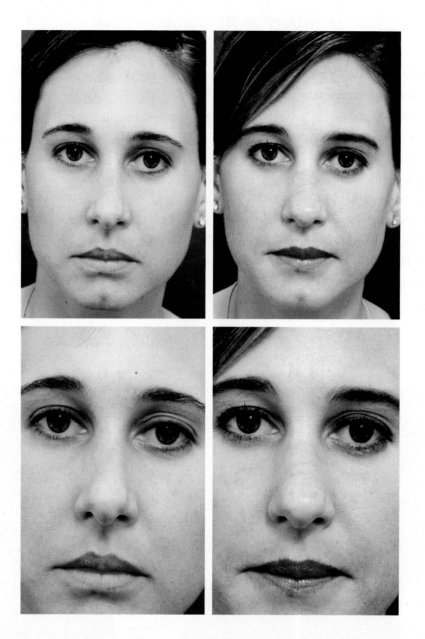

On the frontal view, the middle vault is slightly wider but symmetrical. The alar walls are normally convex, and the columella is narrow and unscarred. Mean postoperative airflow increased 8.4 times over preoperative values. The alar walls have become slightly more convex and support the airway. Multiple tip grafts have improved symmetry, but their distributed forces decrease the chance of visibility.

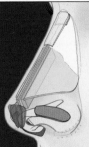

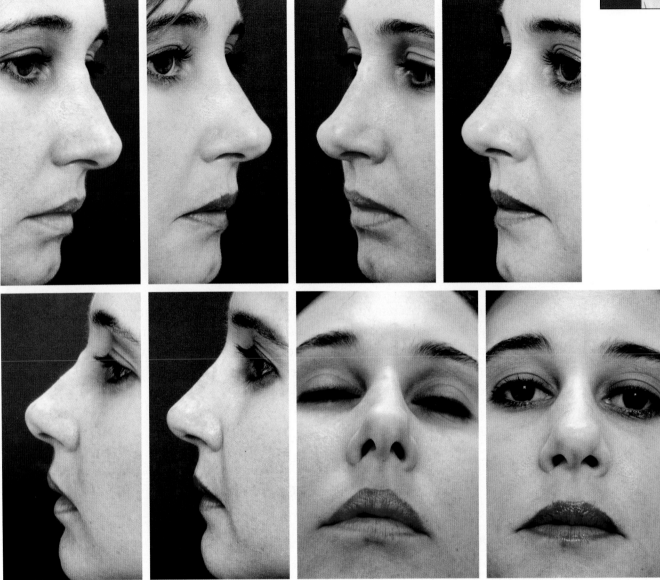

The dorsum is now straight, but the radix remains augmented, as the original surgeon had correctly intended.

The good news about grafting is that most problems are technical and under the surgeon's control and that imperfect results can be corrected—even in places as troublesome as the radix.

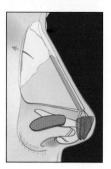

PATIENT STUDY THREE

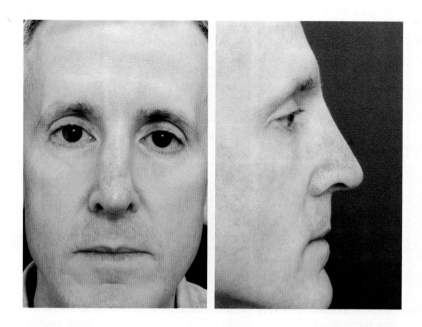

Three previous surgeries have created a straight dorsum, but the nasofacial angle is too vertical, the radix is too high, and the tip is inadequately projecting. The patient's thick soft tissues hide incompetence at the internal and external valves. Septal cartilage was unavailable, but because no dorsal graft was needed, the entire reconstruction could be performed with ear cartilage.

SUMMARY OF THE SURGICAL PLAN

1. Harvest conchal cartilage
2. Relocate lateral crural remnants
3. Moderate skeletonization over middle vault, narrow over bony vault
4. Rasp dorsum; reduce radix with angled chisel
5. Ear cartilage alar wall grafts
6. Right osteotomy
7. Spreader grafts (attempted but not possible)
8. Multiple crushed ear cartilage tip grafts

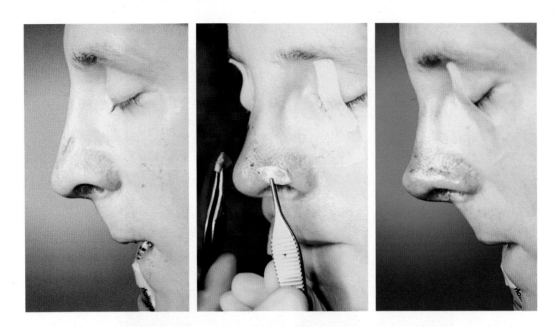

Ear cartilage was thinned and contoured to replace the missing lateral crura. A combination of dorsal reduction and tip grafting altered the nasofacial angle and differentiated the tip from the supratip and dorsum.

Postoperative Analysis

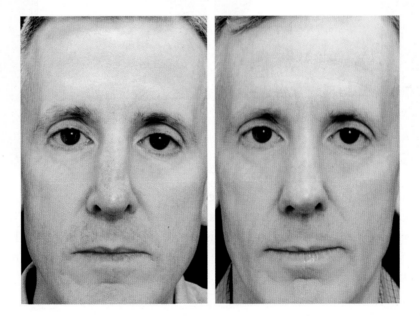

Four years postoperatively, the dorsum remains slightly wider because it is lower. The alar walls are better supported, and the patient no longer flares his nostrils, but some asymmetry persists. Geometric mean nasal airflow increased 5.3 times over preoperative values.

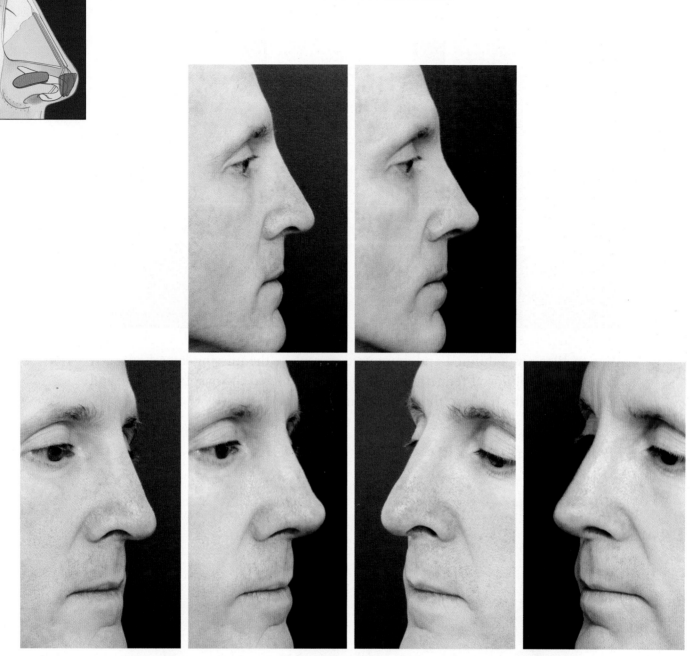

The nasofacial angle is less acute, and the tip projects beyond the septal angle. Repeatedly scarred soft tissues cannot always respond to augmentation; and in this case, the patient's flatter, more-scarred right tip did not expand as well as the left tip. The tip lobule remains twisted to the left; this is a soft tissue, not only a skeletal, difference.

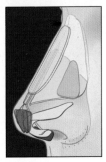

PATIENT STUDY FOUR

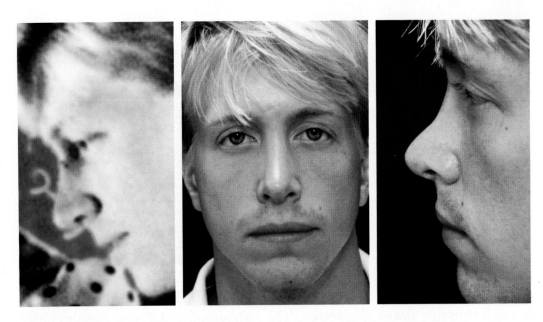

Reduction of this low, straight dorsum with inadequate tip projection has produced a more unbalanced version of the same nose: lower in its midpoint and collapsed in the middle third, with a high septal deviation twisting the tip toward the right. A mild supratip convexity has become a more significant supratip deformity. Only a small amount of septal cartilage was available. The patient's prior open rhinoplasty and columellar strut had failed to provide adequate tip projection, because the middle crus, deficient preoperatively, remained deficient. Only a small amount of septal cartilage remained.

SUMMARY OF THE SURGICAL PLAN

1. Harvest calvarial bone graft
2. Minimal skeletonization over bony vault and upper cartilaginous vaults; rasp bony vault for graft adherence
3. Remove columellar strut
4. Calvarial bone dorsal graft
5. Calvarial bone lateral wall graft, thicker on right than left
6. Limited septoplasty
7. Septal cartilage tip grafts
8. Septal cartilage graft to right columella

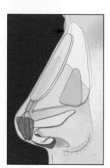

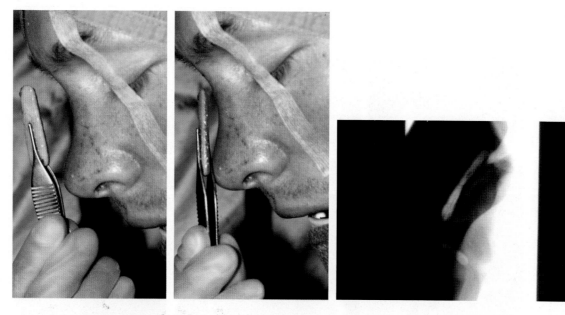

An outer-table calvarial graft was harvested and minimally beveled on its edges; too much thinning favors absorption. The radiograph is a 3-year postoperative view of another patient in whom a calvarial bone was used for the dorsum and the columella; both grafts are easily visible. (The patient had returned, because trauma had fractured the dorsal graft at its midpoint.)

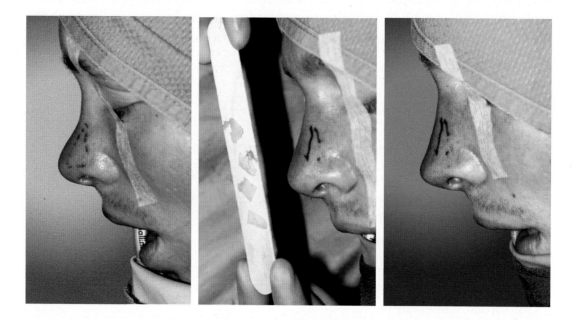

Compare the dorsal contour before and after placement of the dorsal graft alone. Solid and crushed tip grafts completed treatment of the supratip deformity.

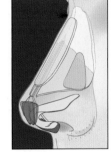

Postoperative Analysis

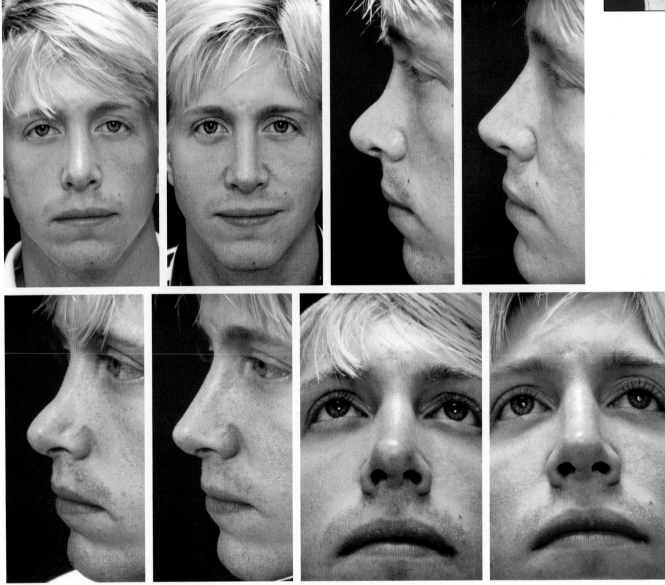

Two years postoperatively, the dorsal graft remains smooth, with its edges invisible. The middle vault has opened, pulled upward and laterally by the dorsal graft (exactly the reverse of what occurs with dorsal resection). The left-sided high septal deviation has been hidden. Inferior views confirm the new middle vault symmetry. The right-sided columellar graft has smoothed columellar contour. Geometric mean nasal airflow increased 4.3 times over preoperative values.

Nasal Base Problems

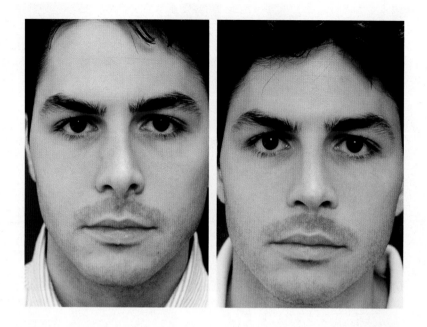

In some patients, the entire nasal base is disorganized: the tip is asymmetrical, the columella is lower on one side than the other, the alar rims are different heights, and the alar bases are asymmetrically positioned. Each component must be addressed separately. In this patient, spreader grafts align the middle third, tip grafts create symmetry and projection, and columellar resection and an alar base flap reduce notching from a previous wedge resection and reposition the alar base laterally. But, most problems are not so complex.

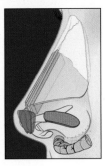

PATIENT STUDY ONE

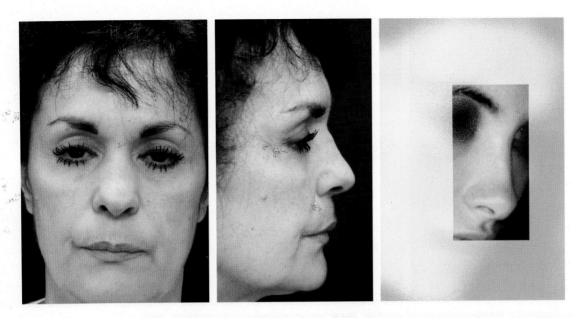

Although this patient was happy with her dorsal height and overall nasal configuration, she believed that her previous rhinoplasty had lengthened her upper lip and distorted her tip, leaving convex, malpositioned lateral crura that were too prominent. She preferred more angular tip projection. However, her medium-thickness soft tissues would not permit significant nasal base reductions, and her soft tissues could not be expected to contract significantly; thus only conservative changes were possible.

SUMMARY OF THE SURGICAL PLAN

1. Two-piece Gore-Tex maxillary augmentation

2. Resect and replace alar cartilage lateral crura

3. Minimal rasping of bony vault

4. Harvest ear cartilage (available septum previously resected)

5. Thin spreader grafts, right greater than left

6. Multiple tip grafts with buttress

7. Alar wall graft

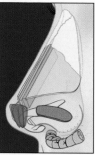

Postoperative Analysis

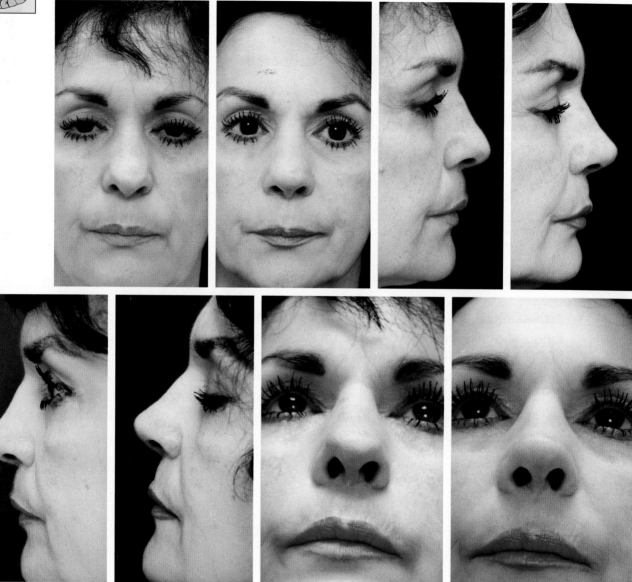

Resection and replacement of the alar cartilage lateral crura have softened the knuckles left by the previous reduction, which had allowed the cartilages to kink at the lateral genua. Because the patient was satisfied with her dorsal height, the dorsum was not reduced, but spreader grafts have rendered the middle vault more symmetrical. Maxillary augmentation has softened the subnasale. Tip grafts demarcate the tip lobule from the dorsum. Dorsal height is essentially unchanged, but the supratip is now flat, ending in a tip that projects beyond the septal angle. Even though no transfixing incision was made, the nose seems slightly shorter because of the change in tip lobular configuration. Geometric mean nasal airflow increased 6.4 times over preoperative values.

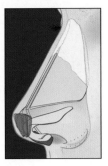

PATIENT STUDY TWO

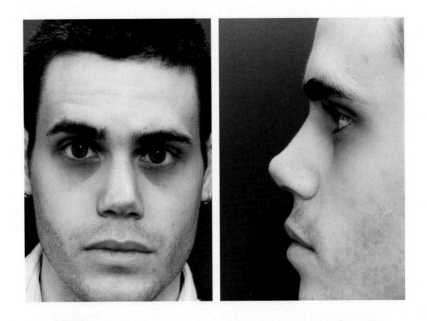

After three rhinoplasties, this man liked everything about his nose except the flatness of his nasal base. Septum was unavailable, but one ear remained unharvested.

This is not a difficult correction if performed endonasally. The surgeon makes the usual infracartilaginous access incision for the tip lobule, but fills only its caudal side, watching surface changes as the augmentation proceeds. Then, through an incision on the vestibular side of the columella, a separate pocket can be developed anterior to the medial crura and filled with softened cartilage, once again watching surface changes as successive grafts are added.

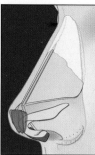
Postoperative Analysis

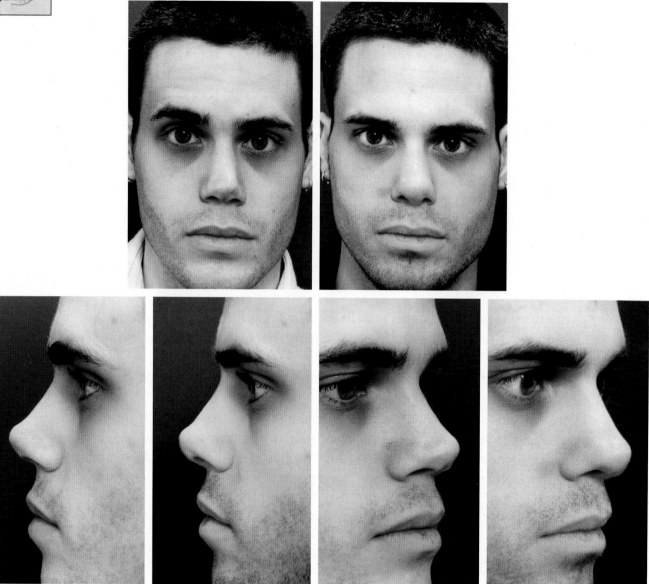

Four years postoperatively, the dorsum remains unchanged, but the patient's tip lobule and columella have been filled with autogenous grafts. The base is now proportionate to the upper nose, because new middle and medial alar cartilage segments have been simulated using only multiple softened grafts in limited pockets. This much expansion cannot always be undertaken in one procedure. The surgeon must be mindful of tip circulation and skin tension. In this patient's case, I was greatly aided because no other procedures, which may have altered nasal circulation, were simultaneously required.

PATIENT STUDY THREE

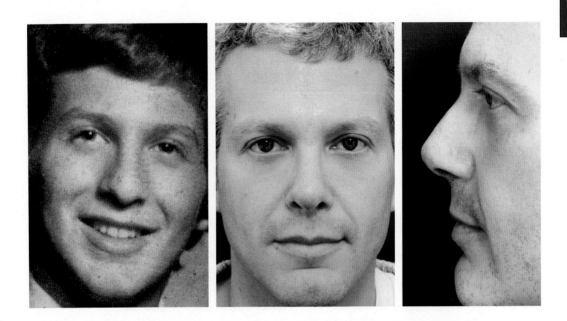

This man's interesting psychological history is more fully described in Chapter 20. He came to me many years after a successful secondary rhinoplasty by another surgeon to inquire about nasal base changes. He thought that his nostrils were too visible, and he wondered if his nose could be lengthened further and whether the inadequate tip projection of his original nose could be better re-created.

SUMMARY OF THE SURGICAL PLAN

1. Harvest composite grafts and ear cartilage for tip grafts

2. Bilateral composite grafts, coronal orientation, right greater than left

3. Multiple crushed cartilage tip grafts, placed caudally

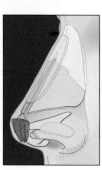

Postoperative Analysis

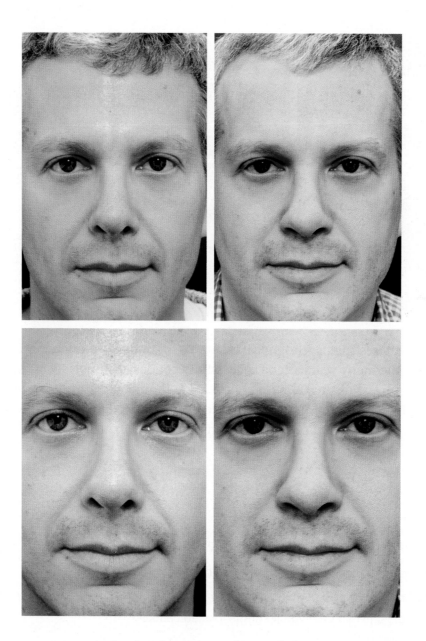

Three years postoperatively, the alar rims are lower and more symmetrical. The tip lobule is slightly broader and fuller inferiorly. Grafts that were deliberately placed caudally in the tip lobule and anterior columella have increased both real and apparent nasal length.

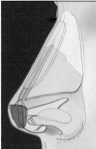

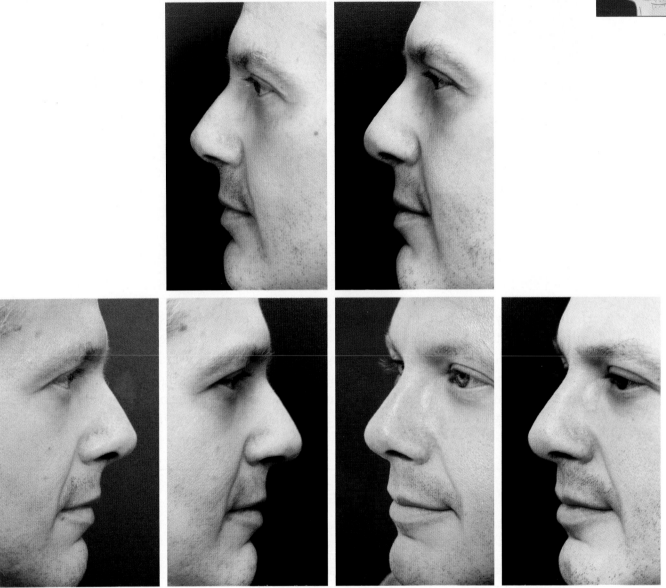

By further distributing the forces created by the prior tip grafts, the tip has become more blunt and apparently less projecting. Tip and nasal base contours more closely resemble the patient's original preoperative nose.

PATIENT STUDY FOUR

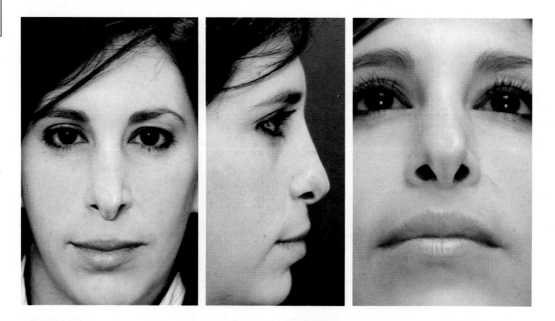

Highlighted by thin skin, this patient's tip is distorted by malpositioned lateral crural remnants and by a long middle crural segment, worse on her left than her right. The middle vault is narrow and asymmetrical, shifted toward her right; the dorsum is straight, but the nasofacial angle is too vertical. Although I considered maxillary augmentation to help increase nasal base projection, the patient's overjet and bimaxillary protrusion did not favor additional augmentation in that area.

SUMMARY OF THE SURGICAL PLAN

1. Resect lateral crural remnants; replace if possible
2. Moderate skeletonization over upper cartilaginous vault
3. Transfixing incision, shorten caudal septum
4. Resect middle crura through infracartilaginous incision
5. Slight rasping of bony vault shoulders
6. Septoplasty
7. Asymmetrical spreader grafts, thicker on right than left
8. Harvest ear cartilage
9. Alar wall grafts of ear cartilage
10. Multiple tip grafts
11. Columellar grafts
12. Bilateral osteotomies

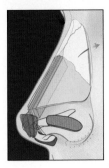

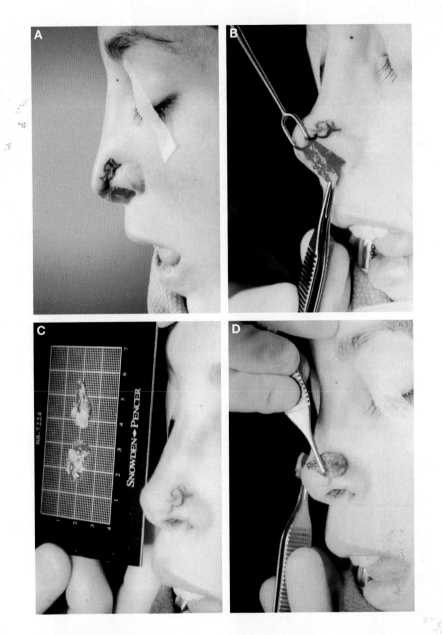

The malpositioned lateral crural remnants were first dissected free with the intent of repositioning them (B), but they were so distorted that they were removed and set aside to be used for the tip (C). Conchal cartilage grafts were shaped into lateral crura, thinning the cartilage and beveling the edges to avoid thickening the alar sidewalls (D).

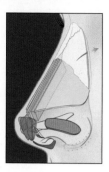

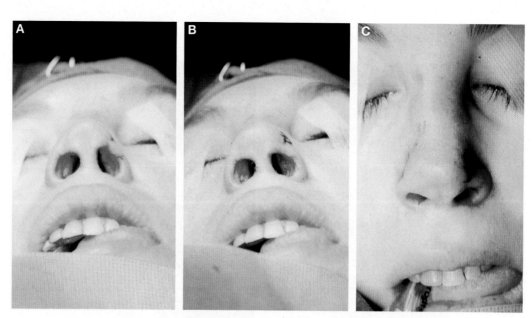

After the right lateral crus was replaced, notice the normalization of lateral nostril contour *(A)*. After placement of both alar wall grafts, the nostrils became oval and more symmetrical *(B)*. Frontal appearance improved after bilateral resection of the distorted middle and lateral crura and after ear cartilage alar wall grafts *(C)*.

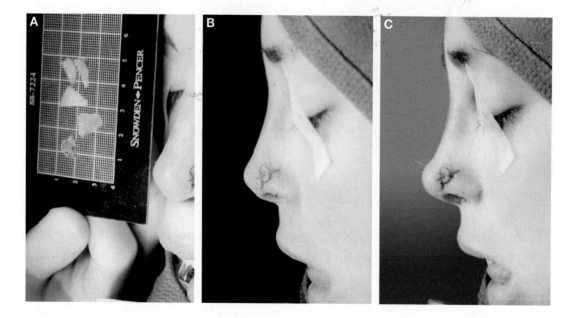

Multiple solid and crushed grafts have been prepared. A solid tip graft is placed first to establish the angle of rotation *(B)*. After crushed grafts are placed anterior to the buttress to reform the lobule and after additional grafts contour the columella, the nasal base has been re-created *(C)*.

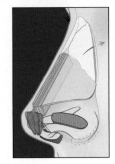

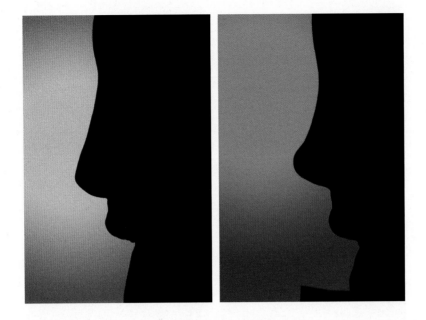

Silhouettes indicate the changes produced by a slight dorsal reduction and by rotation and projection of the nasal base.

Postoperative Analysis

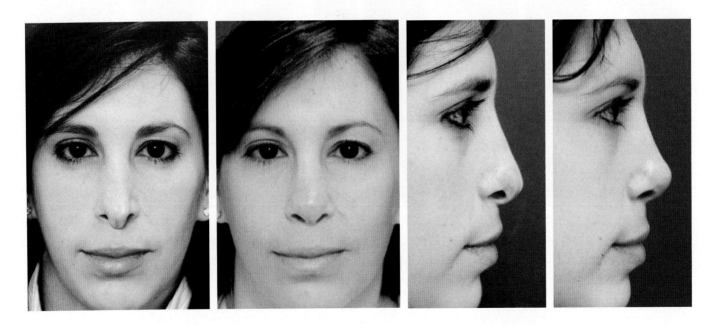

Eighteen months after surgery, the patient's nasal base distortion has improved, but is not perfect. Her middle vault is more symmetrical, and her alar cartilage deformity has been reduced by resecting the deforming parts and placing tip and alar wall grafts.

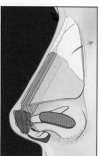

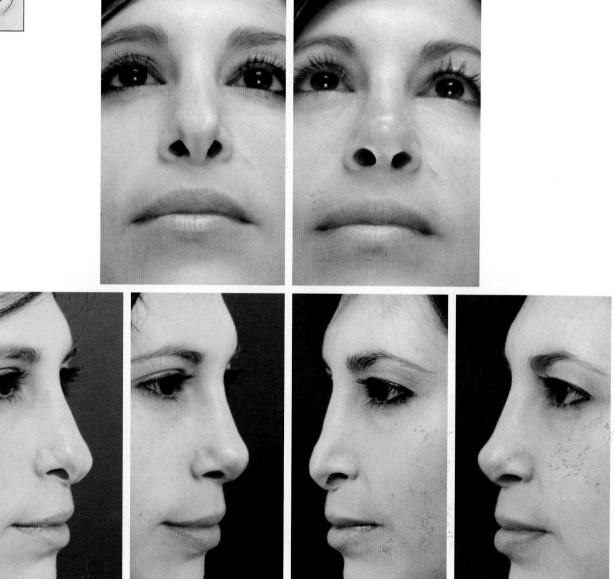

The nasal base shows better projection, and the tip no longer hangs from the septal angle. But some asymmetries remain, and the flat, tight tip lobule continues to insist on an angle of rotation that is too vertical.

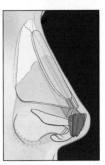

PATIENT STUDY FIVE

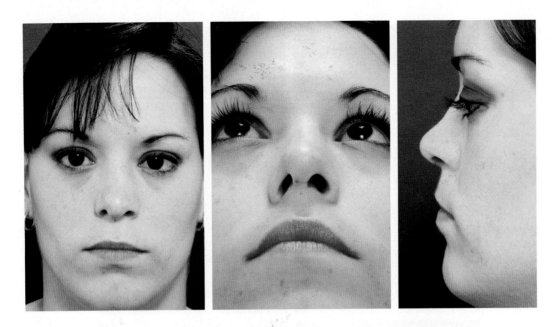

Although this woman has a high septal deviation toward her right, her primary deformities reside in the nasal base. The lateral crura are malpositioned: the left side is orthotopic, whereas the right side is malpositioned, carrying with it the right alar rim. Alar cartilage reduction in a previous rhinoplasty has flattened the malpositioned sidewall and decreased nostril size. The tip is adequately projecting, but the dorsum is slightly low relative to nasal base size, and the tip lobule itself is blunt.

SUMMARY OF THE SURGICAL PLAN

1. Harvest composite graft
2. Resect and relocate right lateral crus
3. Minimal skeletonization over dorsum
4. Rasp bony vault for graft adherence
5. Septoplasty
6. Right spreader graft
7. Thin dorsal graft
8. Crushed cartilage tip grafts
9. Axially oriented composite graft to open the right vestibular stenosis

---

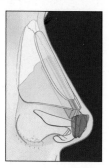

Postoperative Analysis

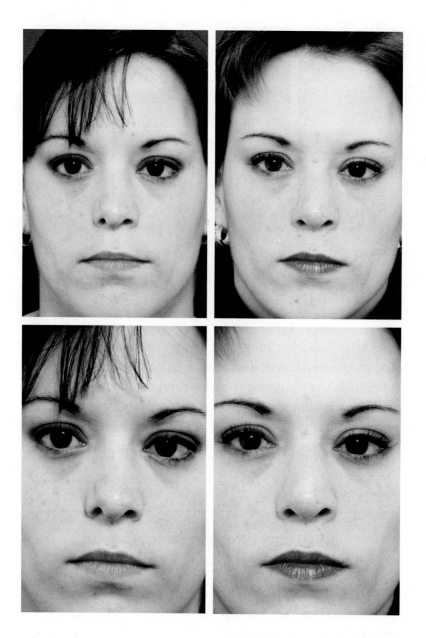

Sixteen months postoperatively, the nose is straighter, the alar walls are evenly supported, and nostril height is therefore equal.

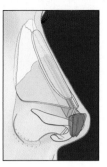

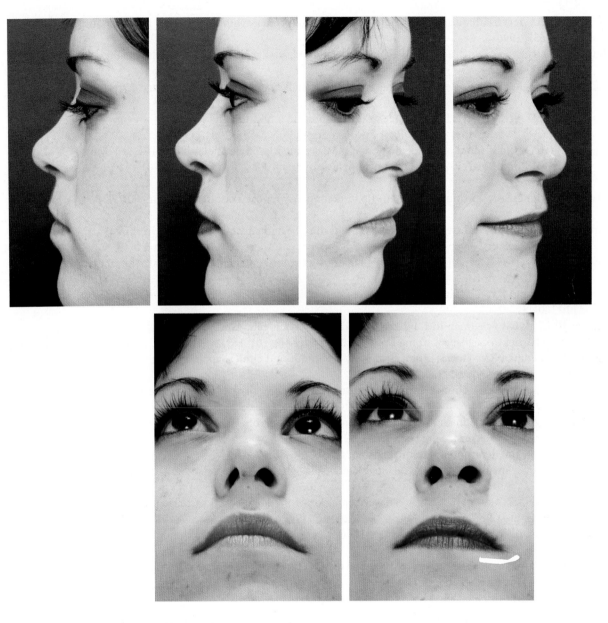

The axially oriented composite graft on the right, in which the skin island replaces the nasal floor deficiency, and the cartilaginous ring supports the sidewall and extends toward the columella, has opened the right nostril. The dorsum is slightly higher, the tip is better contoured, and the right alar wall is no longer hollow. Tip grafts have created a defined point of maximum projection. Multiple grafts distribute tip forces and decrease the chances of postoperative visibility. Geometric mean nasal airflow increased 10 times over preoperative measurements.

BIBLIOGRAPHY

Adham MN. A new technique for nasal tip cartilage graft in primary rhinoplasty. Plast Reconstr Surg 97:649-655, 1996.

Burget GC. Aesthetic reconstruction of the nose. In Mathes SJ, ed. Plastic Surgery, 2nd ed. Philadelphia: Elsevier, 2006.

Calvert JW, Brenner K, DaCosta-Iyer M, et al. Histological analysis of human diced cartilage grafts. Plast Reconstr Surg 118:230-236, 2006.

Camirand A, Doucet J, Harris J. Nose surgery: how to prevent a middle vault collapse—a review of 50 patients 3 to 21 years after surgery. Plast Reconstr Surg 114:527-534, 2004.

Clark MP, Greenfield B, Hunt N, et al. Function of the nasal muscles in normal subjects assessed by dynamic MRI and EMG: its relevance to rhinoplasty surgery. Plast Reconstr Surg 101:1945-1955, 1998.

Daniel RK. Rhinoplasty: creating an aesthetic tip. A preliminary report. Plast Reconstr Surg 80:775-783, 1987.

Gruber RP, Friedman RM. Lateral crural strut graft: technique and clinical applications in rhinoplasty. Plast Reconstr Surg 99:943-952, 1997.

Gruber RP, Kryger G, Chang D. The intercartilaginous graft for actual and potential alar retraction. Plast Reconstr Surg 121:288e-296e, 2008.

Gruber RP, Pardun J, Wall S. Grafting the nasal dorsum with tandem ear cartilage. Plast Reconstr Surg 112:1120-1122, 2003.

Gunter JP, Clark CP, Friedman RM. Internal stabilization of autogenous rib cartilage grafts in rhinoplasty: a barrier to cartilage warping. Plast Reconstr Surg 100:161-169, 1997.

Gunter JP, Friedman RM. Lateral crural strut graft: technique and clinical applications in rhinoplasty. Plast Reconstr Surg 99:943-952, 1997.

Gunter JP, Landecker A, Cochran CS. Frequently used grafts in rhinoplasty: nomenclature and analysis. Plast Reconstr Surg 118:14e-29e, 2006.

Gunter JP, Rohrich RJ, Friedman RM. Classification and correction of alar-columellar discrepancies in rhinoplasty. Plast Reconstr Surg 97:643-648, 1996.

Guyuron B. Alar rim deformities. Plast Reconstr Surg 107:856-863, 2001.

Guyuron B, Michelow BJ, Englebardt C. Upper lateral splay graft. Plast Reconstr Surg 102:2169-2177, 1998.

Jung DH, Choi SH, Moon HJ, et al. A cadaveric analysis of the ideal costal cartilage graft for Asian rhinoplasty. Plast Reconstr Surg 114:545-550, 2004.

Marin VP, Landecker A, Gunter JP. Harvesting rib cartilage grafts for secondary rhinoplasty. Plast Reconstr Surg 121:1442-1448, 2008.

Mowlavi A, Masouem S, Kalkanis J, et al. Septal cartilage defined: implications for nasal dynamics and rhinoplasty. Plast Reconstr Surg 117:2171-2174, 2006.

Neu BR. A problem-oriented and segmental open approach to alar cartilage losses and alar length discrepancies. Plast Reconstr Surg 109:768-779, 2002.

Peck GC Jr, Michelson L, Segal J, et al. An 18-year experience with the umbrella graft in rhinoplasty. Plast Reconstr Surg 102:2158-2165, 1998.

Rohrich R. An 18-year experience with the umbrella graft in rhinoplasty: discussion. Plast Reconstr Surg 102:2166-2168, 1998.

Rohrich R, Hollier LH Jr, Janis JE, et al. Rhinoplasty with advancing age. Plast Reconstr Surg 114:1936-1944, 2004.

Rohrich RJ, Muzaffar AR, Janis JE. Component dorsal hump reduction: the importance of maintaining dorsal aesthetic lines in rhinoplasty. Plast Reconstr Surg 114:1298-1308, 2004.

Sen C, Iscen D. Use of the spring graft for prevention of midvault complications in rhinoplasty. Plast Reconstr Surg 119:332-336, 2007.

Seyhan A. Method for middle vault reconstruction in primary rhinoplasty: upper lateral cartilage bending. Plast Reconstr Surg 100:1941-1943, 1997.

Sheen JH. Rhinoplasty: personal evolution and milestones. Plast Reconstr Surg 105:1820-1852, 2000.

Smith RA, Smith ET. A new technique in nasal-tip reduction surgery. Plast Reconstr Surg 108:1798-1804, 2001.

CHAPTER 19

Generalized Deformities

As natural selection acts solely by accumulating slight, successive, variable variations, it can produce no great or sudden modification, it can act by very short and slow steps. Hence the canon of "Natura non facit saltum" [Nature does not jump].

CHARLES DARWIN,
On the Origin of Species by Means of Natural Selection

. . . In your next breath, you are taking in 3×10^{19} [inert argon atoms]. . . . By the end of the year, the 3×10^{19} argon atoms [in that single breath] . . . will be smoothly distributed throughout all the free air of the earth. . . . The first little gasp of every baby born on earth a year ago contained argon atoms that you have since breathed. . . . Argon atoms are here from the conversations at the Last Supper . . . from the recitations of the classic poets . . . from the battle cries at Waterloo. . . . This story of argon . . . associates us intimately with the past and the future.

HARLOW SHAPLEY
Beyond the Observatory

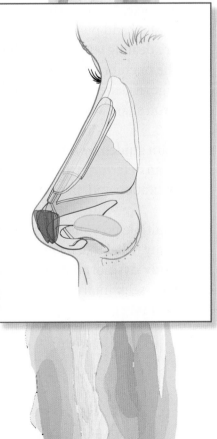

1237

*A*ny division of deformities into regional or generalized is naturally somewhat arbitrary, but since the beginning of this text I have pressed the argument that *different nasal areas are functionally and structurally interdependent,* not independent. It is partly the failure to recognize such interdependence that has made rhinoplasty difficult for so many surgeons. Most secondary rhinoplasty patients are understandably upset, in varying degrees, that they even need additional operations. In previous years, before the appearance of Internet chat rooms that allow patients to exchange their unhappy stories, many secondary patients believed that imperfect rhinoplasty results were uncommon, and that they had been almost uniquely unlucky.

I believe it is important that every patient, before consenting to surgery, understand the pathophysiology of his or her surgical problem and the logic of the proposed plan and to prefer it to alternatives that he or she may have heard or read. The most difficult problems are created by patients whose original goals were unrealistic, but who cannot be convinced of that even in the face of repeated disappointments.

A surgeon should never perform an operation that he or she does not personally endorse. "I didn't think that another reduction was going to work, but the patient pushed and pushed and so I went ahead…" creates an impossible predicament. We are dealing with Nature's laws, not the surgeon's. The outcome does not depend on the open or closed approach, or whether the surgeon uses septal, rib, or ear cartilage; it depends on biologic behavior. Success only occurs when patient and surgeon share a common goal and have a realistic way of achieving it.

I am guided by the patient's history, by what the previous surgeons did and why (if I can determine that), and by the patient's behavior and ability to withstand another operation and, in particular, to tolerate an imperfect result.

Multiple previous operations do not necessarily signify a psychological disorder. It is my belief that *a person who has self-esteem cannot have body dysmorphic disorder.* Body dysmorphic disorder is largely an affliction of patients without self esteem who seek internal acceptance by external means (such as through improved appearance).

What is more common, and much more gratifying, is the boost in self confidence and self acceptance that most patients achieve through successful plastic surgery of any kind, including rhinoplasty. You can observe this fact throughout this book simply by looking at the patients' eyes. Rhinoplasty is indeed brain surgery.

Supratip Deformity

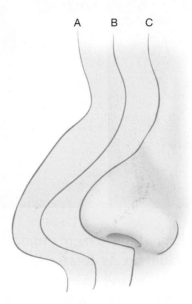

Supratip deformity describes the shape of an end-stage nose. When the nasal skeleton has been reduced by trauma, injury, congenital anomaly, or surgical resection beyond the capacity of the soft tissues to adapt, the skin sleeve assumes a characteristic shape containing some or all of the following features *(C):* low and narrow dorsum, collapsed middle vault, mid-dorsal notch, disproportionately large nasal base, round and shapeless tip lobule, retracted columella, arched alar rims, sharp subnasale, and retrusive upper lip. Depending on the patient's skin characteristics and the degree of skeletal change, some deformities may not occur. For example, patients with thin skin develop retracted alar rims more commonly than those with thicker skin, which can retain its position even without skeletal support.

Because supratip deformity only occurs when the soft tissues have reached their contractile limits, patients and surgeons must accept the fact that the postoperative nose cannot be made smaller unless skin is resected. This reality may present a conceptual problem for patients who believe that their noses have only become larger after every operation. Augmentation can correct the deformity but will not produce a smaller nose—it can only redistribute and support the skin sleeve. But augmentation is better than more reduction, which will accomplish nothing at all.

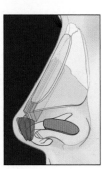

PATIENT STUDY ONE

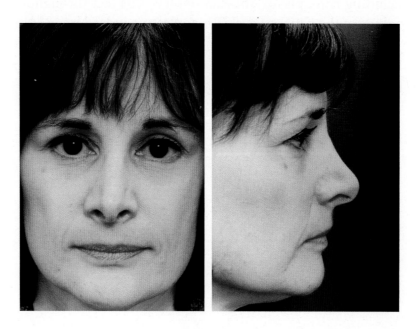

Two previous operations collapsed this patient's middle vault, hollowed her alar walls, and produced a round, blunt tip. As dorsal reduction shortened the nose, her columella became relatively too low, and lateral crural reduction allowed the alar rims to arch higher. Her nasal base is wide, relative to the tip lobule and the upper nose.

SUMMARY OF THE SURGICAL PLAN

1. Limited skeletonization over middle vault, narrow over bony vault

2. Rasp bony vault for graft adherence

3. Transfixing incision, elevating caudal and membranous septa without shortening the nose

4. Septoplasty

5. Asymmetrical spreader grafts, thicker on right than left

6. Dorsal graft

7. Bilateral alar wall grafts

8. Multiple tip grafts with buttress

9. Bilateral alar wedge resections, removing 3 mm of external skin and 2 mm of vestibular skin

---

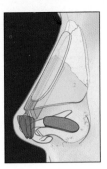

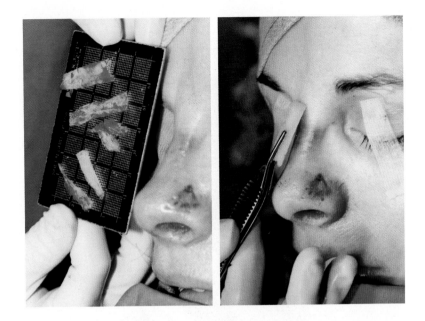

Septoplasty yielded adequate material for the reconstruction. The two pieces at the *bottom* of the image were used for spreader grafts. The straightest and most uniform piece *(top)* was used for the dorsal graft.

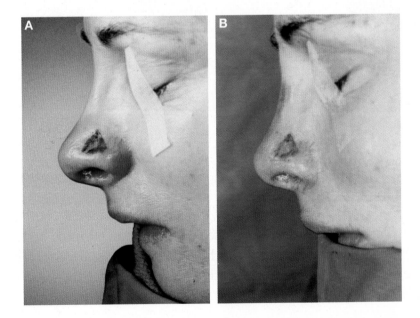

Intraoperatively, remnants of the malpositioned lateral crura were identified, and these were resected and replaced along the alar rims, providing alar wall support and decreasing the need for two additional grafts. Notice the percutaneous sutures coapting the external and vestibular skin *(B)*. Following dorsal graft placement, the nasal base seems smaller.

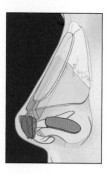

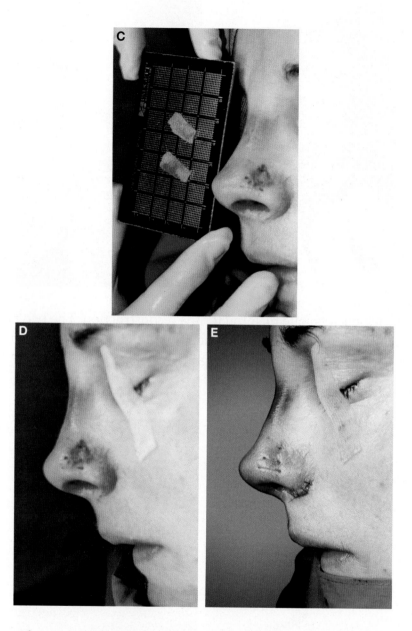

Crushed cartilage tip grafts (C) were placed anterior to an ethmoid buttress, which itself stabilized the angle of rotation in the new tip lobule (D). After the crushed grafts were placed and alar wedge resections were performed, the reconstruction was complete (E).

Postoperative Analysis

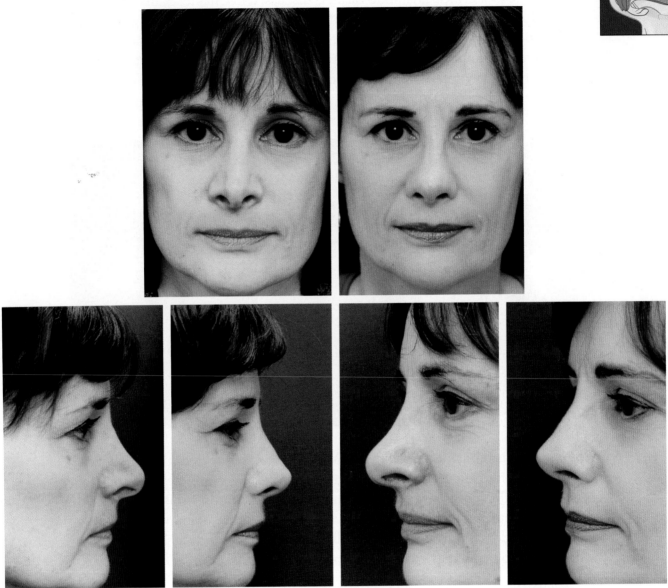

One year postoperatively, the upper and lower noses fit more appropriately. Spreader grafts and dorsal grafts have slightly widened and straightened the upper and middle vaults, lateral crural relocation has corrected the alar hollows, and alar wedge resections have narrowed the base. The thin dorsal graft has filled the dorsal concavity, and tip grafts have recreated a new middle crus and defined the point of greatest tip projection. Geometric mean nasal airflow increased 2.7 times over preoperative values. Alar wall grafts and alar wedge resections have reduced the excessive alar rim arch, and alar wedge resection and tip grafts have improved the tip lobular/nostril length ratio. The patient's skin is sufficiently thin, however, to show not only every preoperative break in the dorsal line and every missing cartilage segment, but also minor irregularities in the postoperative contour.

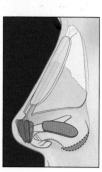

PATIENT STUDY TWO

Among the four critical anatomic variants discussed in Chapter 5, inadequate tip projection most often precedes supratip deformity. Inadequate tip projection cannot be rendered adequate by reduction alone, and any combination of dorsal and tip reduction produces a tip that still seems to hang from the septal angle. If skeletal reduction exceeds soft tissue contraction, supratip deformity develops.

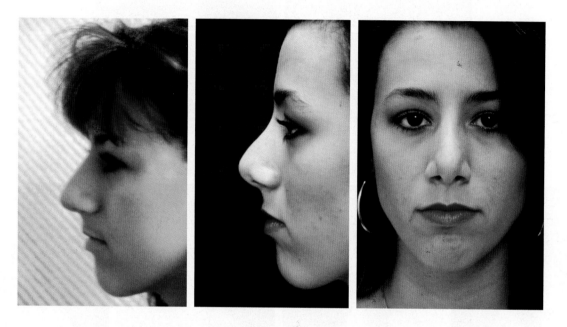

This patient has the same anatomic characteristics as the previous patient, but her soft tissues are thicker. Her alar walls bear the marks of a prior lateral crural malposition. The dorsum is low, the tip is blunt, and the supratip is high. Soft tissues hide middle vault width, but internal valvular incompetence is almost always present following dorsal resection. The alar lobules are heavy, and the base is slightly wide relative to tip lobular width and upper nasal width.

SUMMARY OF THE SURGICAL PLAN

1. Limited skeletonization over bony and upper cartilaginous vaults through a single intercartilaginous incision

2. Septoplasty

3. Dorsal graft

4. Alar wall grafts

5. Multiple tip grafts

6. Bilateral alar wedge resections, removing both external and vestibular skin

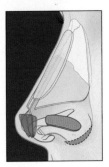

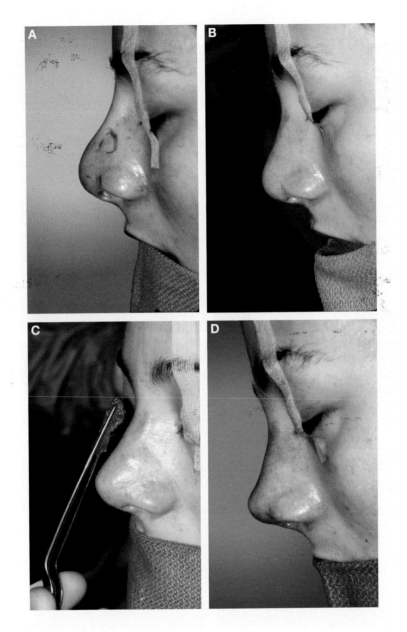

After skeletonizing the dorsum, the supratip flattens (B). As when releasing a burn scar contracture, the soft tissues redistribute. This is the reassuring shape that the first surgeon saw at the conclusion of his operation, but the soft tissues are soft and unsupported. This case was performed in 1990; today I would use a solid dorsal graft, not crushed, for better support under thick soft tissues that are unlikely to show any edges. Tip grafts precede alar resections, which conclude the operation.

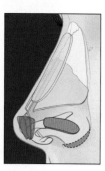
Postoperative Analysis

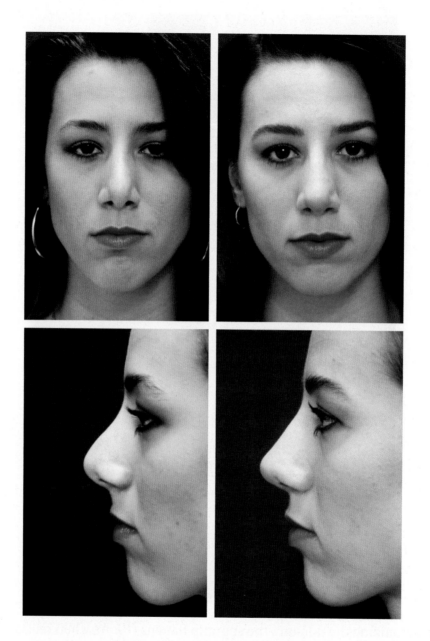

Three years postoperatively, frontal aesthetics have improved. The tip appears differentiated from the dorsum, and grafts have softened the deep alar wall creases. Although the dorsum is higher and tip projection is greater, the overall effect is that of nasal reduction.

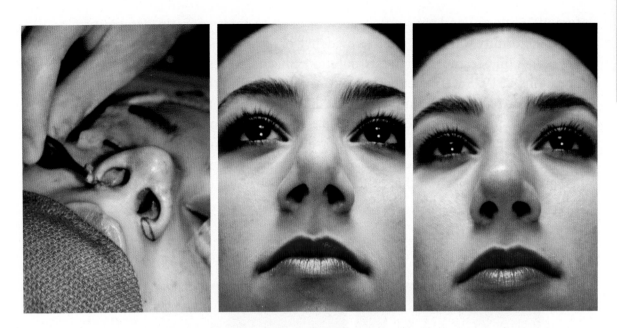

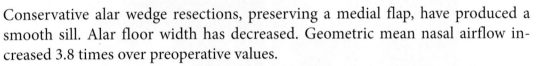

Conservative alar wedge resections, preserving a medial flap, have produced a smooth sill. Alar floor width has decreased. Geometric mean nasal airflow increased 3.8 times over preoperative values.

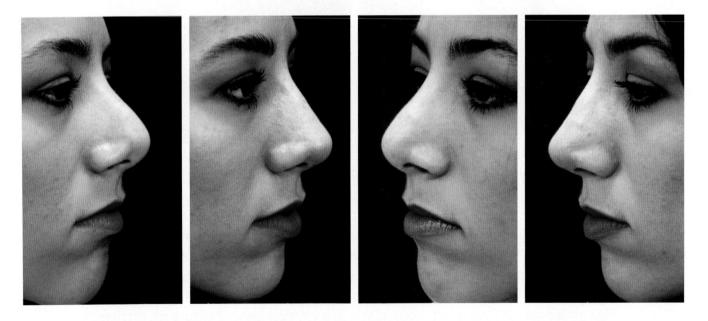

Matching oblique views once again demonstrate that the delicacy of nasal contour is much less a product of skin thickness than it is of the character, volume, and proportion of the skeleton that shapes it. Although no dorsal or tip tissue was resected, the nose seems smaller. This is a right-brain observation, which is why rhinoplasty is such a right-brain operation.

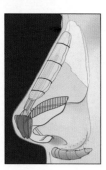

Before 1975, dorsal and tip grafts were not used to treat supratip deformity. Supratip deformity was interpreted as evidence of *insufficient* resection, so additional reduction became the standard solution. Sheen's earliest presentations and publications in 1975 were met with heavy skepticism. But the quality and consistency of his results were unmistakable. Sheen's epiphany that supratip deformity was not a problem of size, but rather of support and proportion, turned the previous conception on its head. And so dorsal and tip grafts redrape the supratip convexity in two directions, cephalad and caudad respectively, to create the dorsal height and tip projection that otherwise may have never existed in a patient.

PATIENT STUDY THREE

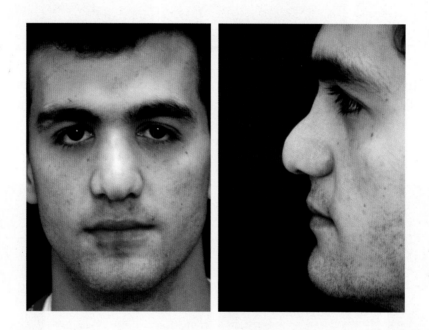

This young Syrian man had undergone a primary rhinoplasty that yielded a supratip deformity. The alar walls bear the footprints of a previous malposition. The supratip is compressible, indicating that it is only possible to offer the patient better nasal shape and function, not a smaller nose. Further soft tissue contraction cannot occur. Previous cartilage septal resection had recessed the vertical position of the upper lip. Septal cartilage was unavailable. A relatively short, asymmetrical defect such as this, beneath a thick soft tissue cover, presents the best circumstance for a rolled ear cartilage graft, particularly in a younger patient whose rib cartilage is likely to be undependable.

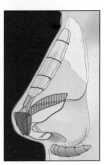

SUMMARY OF THE SURGICAL PLAN

1. Gore-Tex maxillary augmentation
2. Limited skeletonization through a single intercartilaginous incision
3. Reduce cephalic margin, malpositioned lateral crura
4. Rasp bony vault for graft adherence
5. Dorsal graft rolled ear cartilage
6. Ear cartilage tip grafts

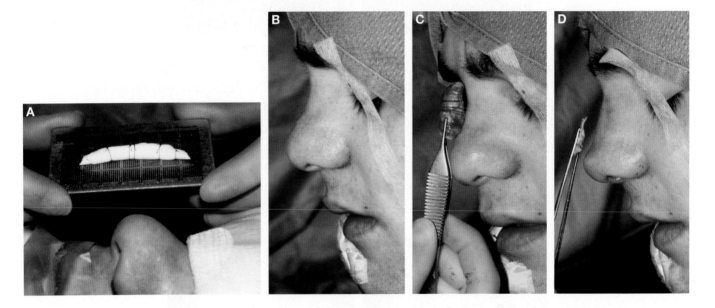

Gore-Tex sheeting was rolled into a maxillary augmentation thickest in the midline. The tapered implant must bridge the perialar areas, and in this case it measured 7 mm at its midpoint *(A)*. Following maxillary augmentation, the vertical position of the lip was corrected *(B)*. A rolled ear cartilage graft was fabricated *(C)*. The beauty of this graft depends partly on the size and shape of the patient's ear, which the surgeon of course cannot control. This dorsal graft had a natural convexity toward the right, which matched the relative concavity in the patient's nasal dorsum (compare with the preoperative frontal view, p. 1248).

Once dorsal and tip grafts redistributed the supratip excess cephalad and caudad, respectively, a small depression appeared in the supratip. This defect was filled with the remaining scrap of ear cartilage, placed beneath the caudal end of the dorsal graft *(D)*. I make this type of final adjustment commonly; the defect is easy to see and correct endonasally because the soft tissues have never been disconnected, so their resting tension has not been altered. It seems paradoxical that a supratip that was too high can actually require augmentation, but this attests to overresection of the anterior septum, despite which the patient developed a supratip deformity.

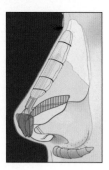

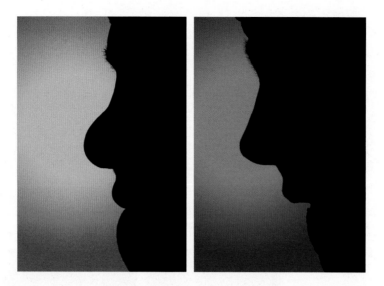

As the tissues became supported, the supratip skin redraped and flattened. The dorsal and tip soft tissues must not be compressible or the deformity will recur. In less experienced hands, insufficient augmentation is more common than excessive augmentation, but either is possible. The surgeon should be able to see and feel the expected result at the conclusion of the procedure.

Postoperative Analysis

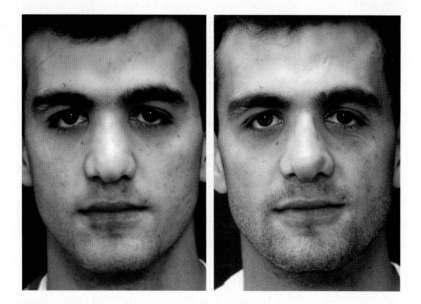

Dorsal grafting has narrowed the nose on the frontal view (no osteotomies were performed). The slight dorsal graft asymmetry has corrected the right-to-left asymmetry in the bony and upper cartilaginous vaults. Tip grafts demarcate the tip lobule from the dorsum. Maxillary augmentation has altered the vertical position of the upper lip, most obvious from the subnasale across to the perialar areas. Repositioning the lip has appropriately reduced the amount of visible upper lip vermilion.

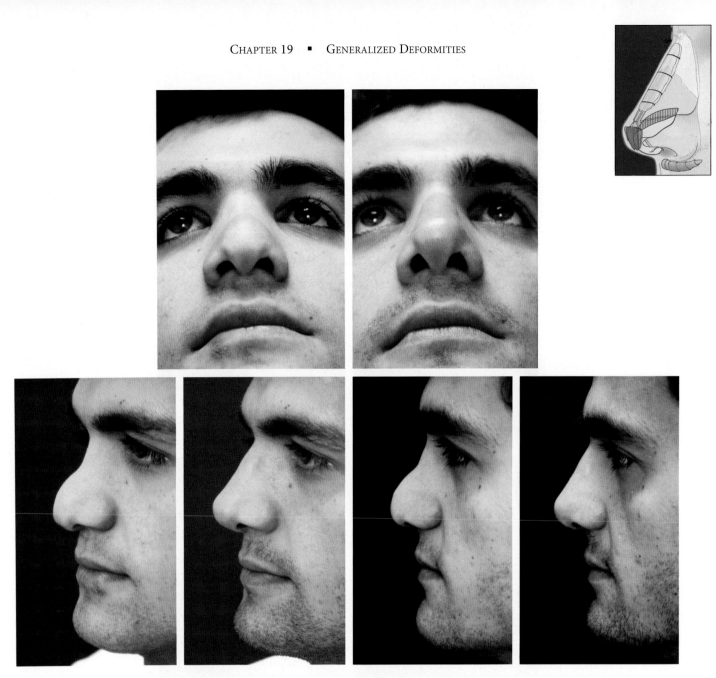

From below, the effect of the dorsal graft on the collapsed middle vault is obvious. Despite the lack of osteotomies, the bony vault appears narrower, because the dorsum has drawn the soft tissues anteriorly. The patient's columella remains unscarred. Fortunately, the patient's original surgery was endonasal: the incidence of lateral or central columellar discontinuities is high in thicker skin when the open approach has been used, and the deformities are difficult to correct.

The dorsum is now straight, the supratip is flat, and the tip grafts have created a normal angle of rotation, separating the tip lobule from the dorsum. Ear cartilage has formed a straight dorsum with a slight convexity, appropriate for the patient's ethnic background. The thinner upper nasal skin, however, shows the edges of the rolled dorsal graft. Although they occur on the lateral edges of the dorsal plane and are not particularly distracting, a rib graft may have produced a smoother result. The patient declined revision.

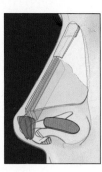

PATIENT STUDY FOUR

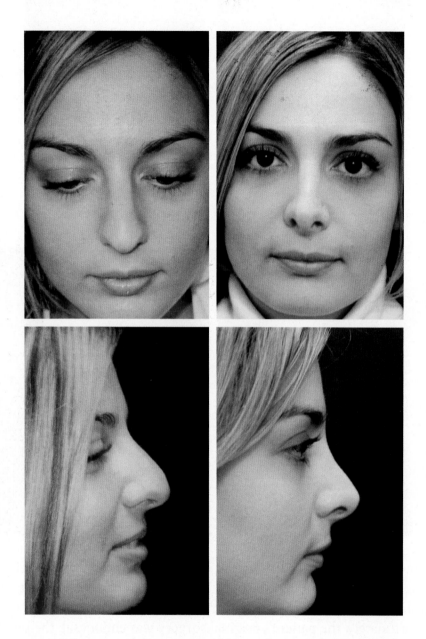

Not all supratip deformities are compressible. In this patient and the next one, the supratip septum seems too high. But in all likelihood it was not too high at the conclusion of the first operation. It is a common misconception that surgeons under-resect the anterior septum, but this would be an unusual omission: excessive reduction is much more common, particularly if the preoperative tip was inadequately projecting.

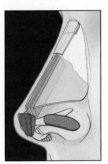

Two things occur postoperatively: the nasal skin contracts, and inadequate tip projection recurs. As the skin envelope reduces, the new sleeve becomes smaller than the original. But the thinner upper nasal skin shrinks more; and when the tip returns to its preoperative position (weakened further by alar cartilage reduction), the supratip septum becomes the highest point in the dorsal line. That is evidently what occurred here, and what has often led surgeons to conclude that the best treatment for supratip deformity was further resection. If the preoperative radix was already low, a high supratip becomes even more likely.

Although the outcome of reduction in this patient with inadequate tip projection can be predicted, the pathophysiology is still interesting. Dorsal reduction has rotated the tip cephalad, pulling the alar rims with it—producing a nose that seems shorter but a columella (pinned down by the caudal septum) that now appears lower. The middle vault is narrower, revealing a high septal deviation toward the left. Lateral crural reduction has flattened the alar sidewalls, producing depressions above the rims. A columellar strut had been placed endonasally, but tip projection remains inadequate.

SUMMARY OF THE SURGICAL PLAN

1. Minimal skeletonization to root

2. Reduce cartilaginous dorsum, deepen radix

3. Transfix, elevate caudal septum without shortening nose and remove columellar strut

4. Resect medial crural footplates

5. Septoplasty

6. Harvest ear cartilage

7. Asymmetrical spreader grafts, thicker on left than right (preoperative asymmetry)

8. Upper dorsal graft

9. Tip graft

10. Bilateral alar wall grafts

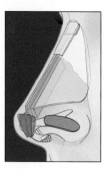

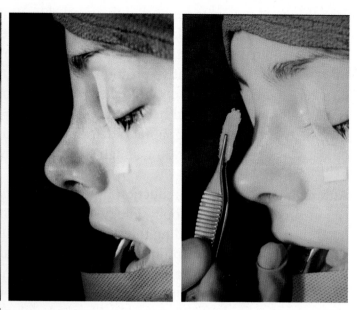

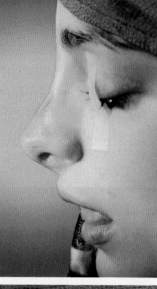

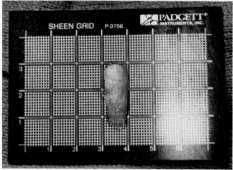

Even after resecting the columellar strut and elevating the caudal septum, the dorsum still began at the level of the lower lash margin. Septal cartilage formed a dorsal graft. A close-up shows a lightly crushed graft, beveled edges, and a distal end tapered to a thin edge. Such fine points are necessary to avoid graft visibility or palpability.

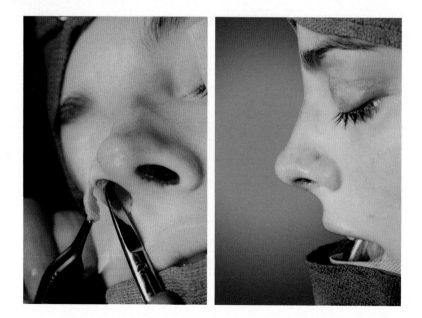

Alar wall grafts were formed from normally convex conchal cartilage, perfect for this purpose, and placed through vestibular incisions exactly in the proper location for lateral crura. Tip grafts completed the reconstruction.

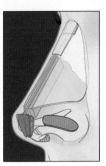

Postoperative Analysis

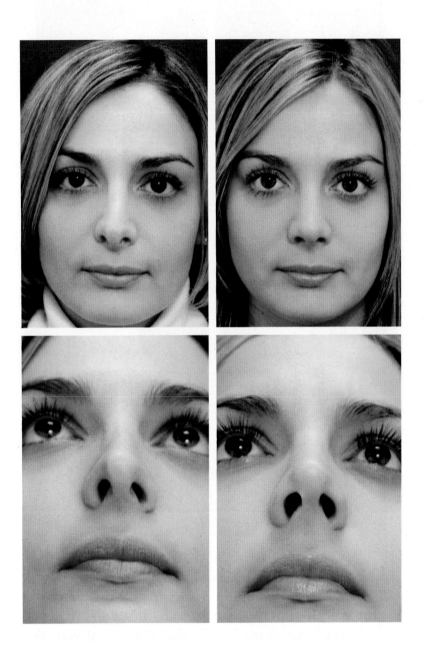

Postoperatively, spreader grafts have straightened the middle vault, and alar wall grafts have created more normal contours. Resection of the strut, caudal septum, and medial crural footplates has reduced columellar width.

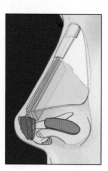

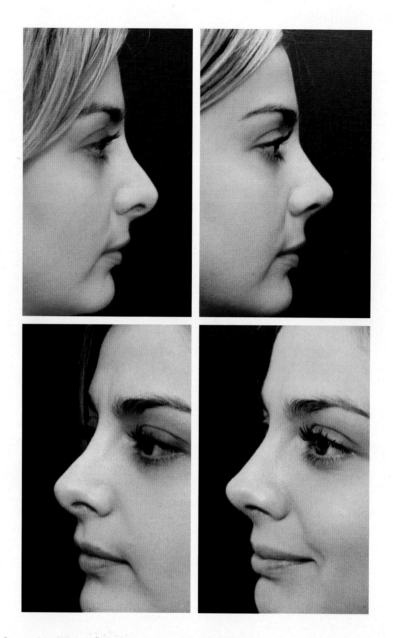

Although the postoperative nose appears shorter, this is an artifact of the change in columellar and tip lobular shape (notice that the frontal view does not show more nostril). The alar walls have a normal convexity; removing the columellar strut and adding tip grafts has created adequate projection.

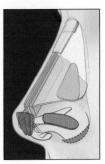

PATIENT STUDY FIVE

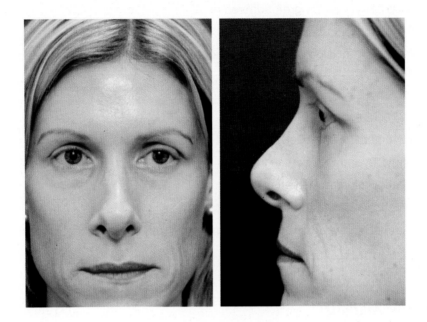

This patient's very thin skin brings each skeletal part into relief. The caudal end of the bony arch demarcates the mid dorsal notch, the central point of the inverted-V deformity, and the cephalic end of the supratip convexity. Below it, the remaining anterior septum protrudes above the tip. Dorsal reduction has allowed the tip to rotate cephalad, producing a columella that is relatively too low; and the reduction of malpositioned lateral crura has allowed the alar rims to arch, creating nostrils that are too visible on the frontal views. There is a high septal deviation toward the left. Only some septal cartilage remains.

The most difficult decision here is what to do with the knuckled lateral genua. If I resect and replace them, can the tip lobule narrow? Should it narrow, or is tip width correct but the upper nose too narrow? Some of these are aesthetic questions and some are strategic. If the lateral crura are resected and replaced, they may not heal symmetrically (particularly true of strong cartilages), and all postoperative asymmetries are likely to be visible. Because of the patient's facial width, I elected to leave the lateral genua where they were and work around them, minimizing the chance of postoperative problems.

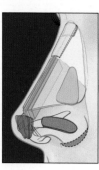

SUMMARY OF THE SURGICAL PLAN

1. Minimal skeletonization over the bony and upper cartilaginous vaults
2. Rasp bony vault for graft adherence
3. Trim cartilaginous dorsum
4. Transfixing incision, shortening caudal and membranous septa, without shortening nose
5. Septoplasty
6. Harvest ear cartilage
7. Asymmetrical spreader grafts, right thicker than left
8. Single layer upper dorsal graft
9. Bilateral lateral wall grafts
10. Ear cartilage tip grafts with ethmoid buttress
11. Bilateral alar wedge resections, removing external and vestibular skin

---

Postoperative Analysis

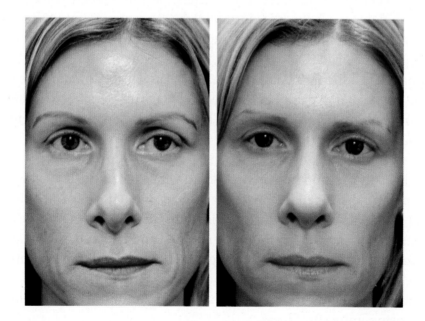

Postoperatively, the middle vault has been expanded, and its asymmetry has been corrected with asymmetrical spreader grafts and onlay grafts. Columellar elevation and alar wedge resections have reduced the gangly appearance of the nasal base, diminishing its apparent size, so that the upper and lower noses fit each other more acceptably. The lateral crura remain undisturbed and symmetrical, but columellar elevation has reduced nostril visibility. Secondary composite grafts are always an option if the patient wishes to reduce alar rim height further.

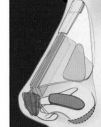

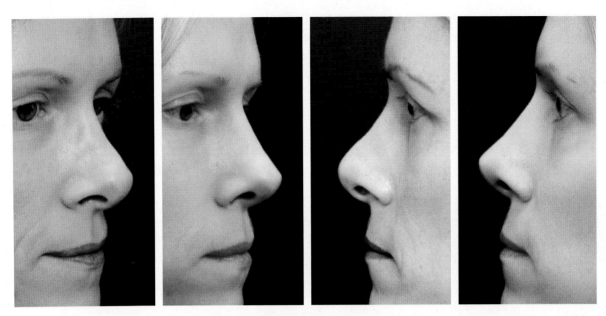

The dorsum is now straight, ending in a tip that projects to the level of the septal angle. The ethmoid buttress has reduced the angle of tip lobular rotation from 80 degrees to a more normal 60 degrees. On the oblique view, the nose is more symmetrical and the supratip has flattened. The caudal edges of the bony vault and the inverted-V deformity are no longer visible, functionally corrected by the spreader grafts and further smoothed by lateral wall grafts placed in specific pockets. Despite an increase in tip projection, the nasal base seems smaller.

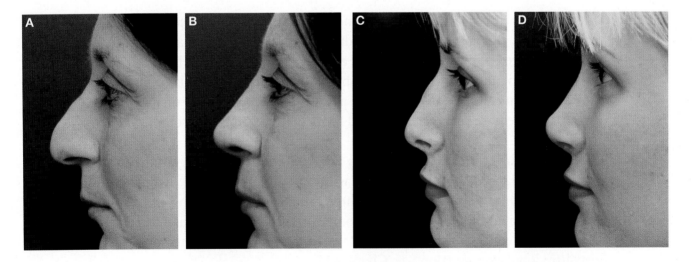

One of the more impressive changes in patients with supratip deformity is their altered nasal balance. The postoperative radix begins at the level of the supratarsal fold (the upper limit of normal). Tip grafts increase the distance from the anterior point of the nostril to the most projecting point of the tip. These changes alter the nasofacial angle, appearing to bring the nasal base closer to the face *(B),* or farther away *(D),* depending on the need.

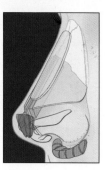

This is the magic that is almost unique to rhinoplasty, and that most patients (and even some surgeons) need to see to believe.

Thick Skin and Thin Skin

PATIENT STUDY ONE

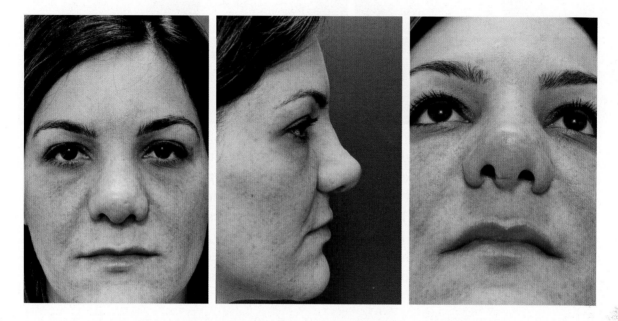

Three previous rhinoplasties have thickened this Latino woman's skin and enlarged her nasal base. Dorsal reduction has reduced her airways, and alar wedge resections have decreased nostril size, adding apparent width to the tip lobule. A previously placed tip graft improved contour but added to the dorsum/base imbalance. The patient wanted to restore her airway, and would consent to any maneuvers that might make the nose seem narrower and more delicate from the frontal view.

This is a difficult strategic problem. Any augmentation will enlarge this nose, yet airway and balance cannot be restored without adding structure. A dorsal graft would decrease frontal width and straighten the dorsal line, but it would also produce a real increase in nasal volume. Composite grafts, placed axially so that the skin island widens the nasal floor, would widen the nasal base slightly but improve nostril/tip lobular proportion (see Chapter 17).

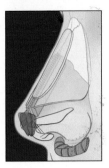

SUMMARY OF THE SURGICAL PLAN

1. Harvest rib cartilage and conchal composite graft
2. Rib cartilage maxillary augmentation, greater on right than left (preoperative asymmetry)
3. Bony vault rasping for graft adherence
4. Rib cartilage dorsal graft
5. Reduction of previous tip grafts and new anterior lobular fill
6. Bilateral axial composite grafts to nostrils
7. Columellar scar revision

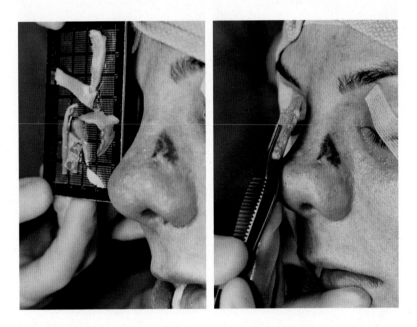

Costal cartilage was harvested and sliced. Notice that thinner pieces with attached perichondrium distort the most (toward the perichondrial side). The dorsal graft was fashioned from an appropriate segment, leaving perichondrium attached; the cephalic end was beveled. Notice the yellowish rib color, indicating calcifications that decrease the chance of warpage.

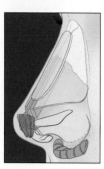

Postoperative Analysis

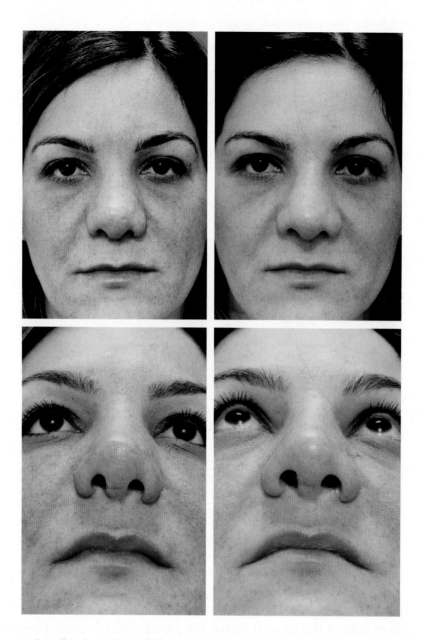

Postoperatively, the dorsal graft has narrowed the bony and upper cartilaginous vaults. Axial composite grafts have widened the nasal base slightly, apparently narrowing the patient's tip lobule. The maxillary arch has become less retrusive, particularly in the perialar areas. The columellar scar unfortunately remains.

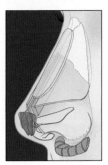

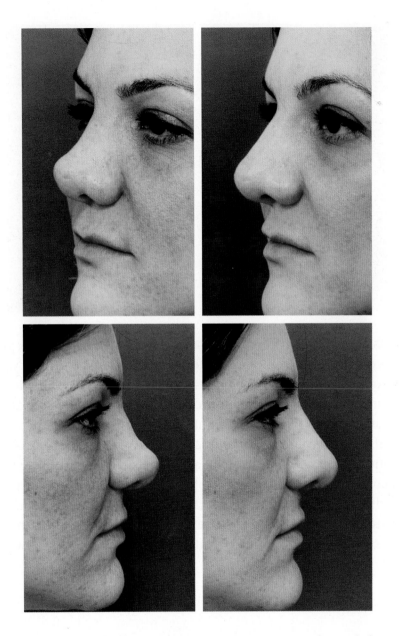

Although the nose is not smaller, the dorsum is now straight and the angle of tip lobular rotation has improved. The position of the radix has not moved.

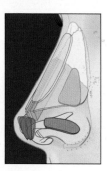
PATIENT STUDY TWO

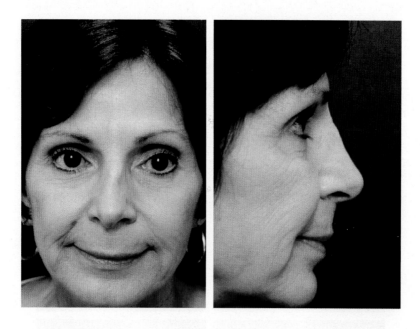

This woman's asymmetries present similar problems as the previous patient's, but her soft tissues are troublesome in a different way. In a prior surgery, a graft had been placed over the left side of the bony vault to smooth a depression, but irregularities remained. The airway was compromised at the middle vault, and the septal partition rotated toward the patient's right. Dorsal contour was good except for the irregularity at the bony vault and an old scar that crossed the upper dorsum. Notice the flat nasofrontal angle associated with a blunted supraorbital ridge: Patients with this type of configuration are unlikely to obtain radixes of appropriate postoperative depth, regardless of what is done to the nasal skeleton. Her tip is asymmetrical, the right side flatter than the left. Previous septoplasty had left a small amount of useable cartilage; I was hoping for one straight piece to be used for a new dorsal roof.

SUMMARY OF THE SURGICAL PLAN

1. Limited skeletonization
2. Removal of the prior dorsal graft
3. Trim the right membranous septum through a hemitransfixing incision
4. Septoplasty
5. Bilateral spreader grafts
6. Onlay graft to left middle vault
7. Crushed cartilage dorsal graft to form new roof
8. Left alar wall graft
9. Crushed tip graft (scraps)

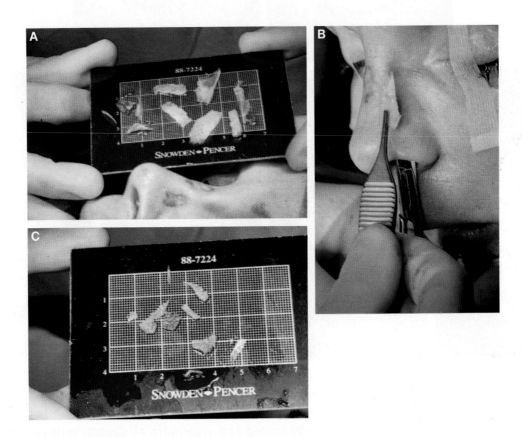

Septoplasty provided a small amount of cartilage and bone for the reconstruction *(A).* The sturdiest pieces were fashioned into spreader grafts, putting nasal symmetry and airway correction first. An additional crushed piece was placed over the left upper cartilaginous vault for symmetry *(B),* and a thin piece smoothed the upper dorsum. The remaining scraps, none of which qualified as a traditional tip graft, were placed into a small pocket high in the tip lobule to maximize their effect *(C).*

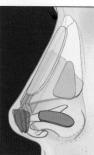

Postoperative Analysis

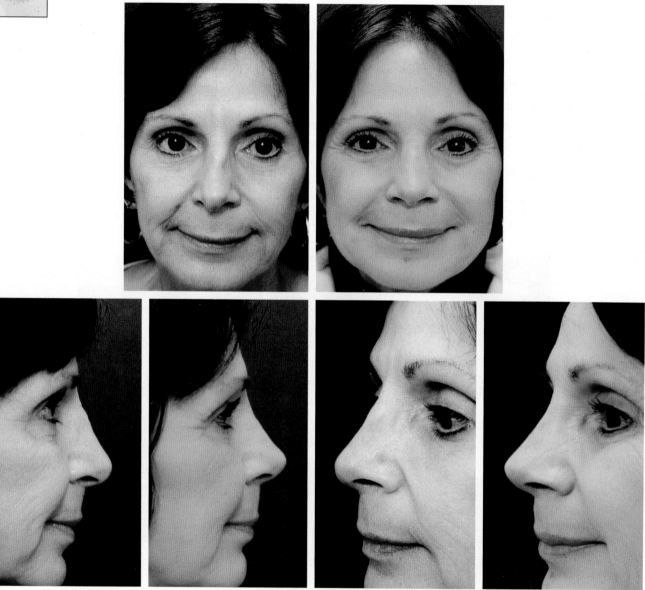

One year postoperatively, spreader grafts and a left onlay have improved symmetry; but a meager septal specimen limited the upper dorsal correction. The airway is widely patent; and the tip is more projecting and symmetrical, despite minimal tip graft material.

PATIENT STUDY THREE

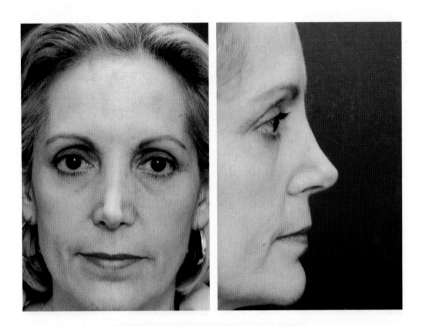

This secondary patient's nose demonstrates the ravages of both thin skin and strong cartilages. A prior dorsal resection collapsed the middle vault, demarcating it from the upper and lower thirds. The narrowed alar cartilages have collapsed medially, closing off the airways and deforming the alar walls. The domes have knuckled. The remaining septal partition has shifted toward the patient's right.

SUMMARY OF THE SURGICAL PLAN

1. Minimal skeletonization over bony and upper cartilaginous vaults

2. Resect the knuckles at the alar domes

3. Septoplasty

4. Harvest ear cartilage for spreader and alar wall grafts

5. Asymmetrical spreader grafts, thicker on left than right

6. Thin upper dorsal graft

7. Bilateral alar wall grafts (conchal cartilage)

8. Multiple crushed tip grafts

9. Columellar graft for contour

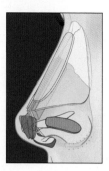

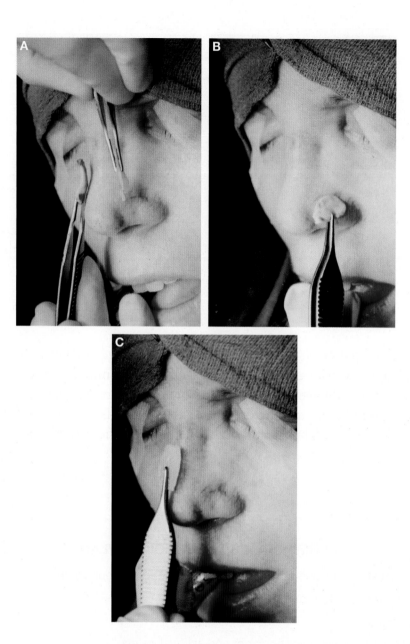

Harvested ear cartilage was split to provide spreader grafts *(A)* and contoured to replace the lateral crura *(B)*. The natural convexity and elasticity of the conchal cartilage make it an excellent lateral crural replacement. Septal cartilage was crushed and placed into the tip, columella, and dorsum *(C)*.

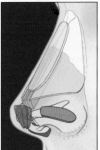

Postoperative Analysis

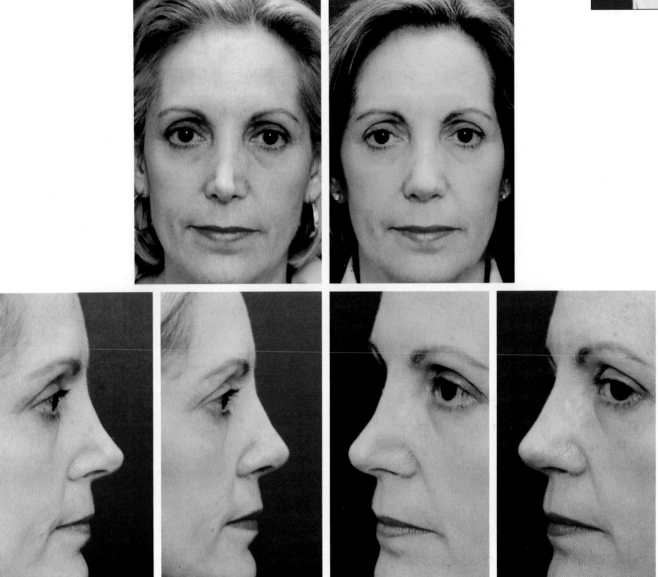

Fifteen months postoperatively, the patient's middle vault is stable, the external valves are supported, and the preoperative alar hollows have been leveled by ear cartilage grafts. The knobby tip deformity has disappeared, recontoured with multiple grafts. The tip remains projecting, but the dorsal discontinuity has improved. Nasal anatomy appears normal, though it has been created by selective, segmental augmentation with septal and ear cartilage. What is critical is not skeletal anatomy, but rather surface anatomy, because that is what the patient sees. Exact skeletal shape is irrelevant, except as it affects surface contour or the airway.

Septal Collapse

The effects of septal collapse are always devastating, and reflect, perhaps better than any other single deformity, the interrelationships among nasal parts and the magnitude of facial change that injury to a single central nasal structure can produce.

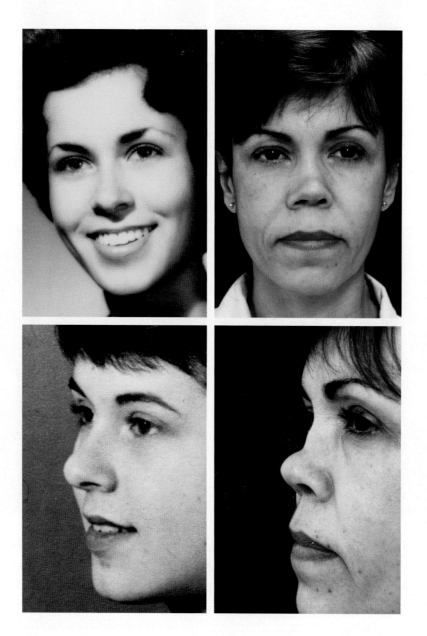

The shape of this patient's nose does not reflect a cocaine-induced polychondritis; it is the result of nasal surgery. Septal resection has allowed the nasal tip to rotate cephalad and has demarcated the caudal edges of the bony vault. The remaining deflected septal partition turns the nasal tip toward the right.

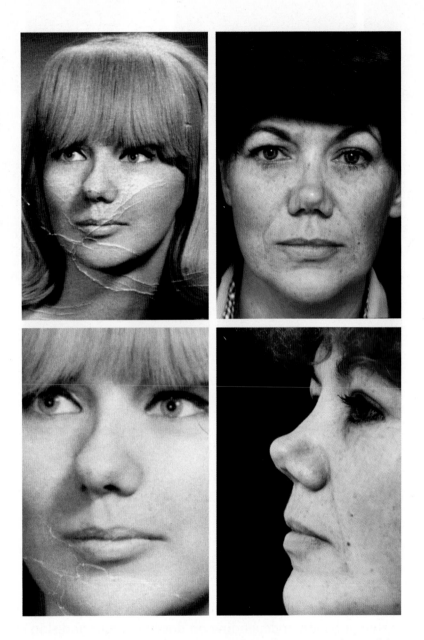

This woman's upper lip has lengthened and fallen posteriorly, and her subnasale has sharpened. Resecting malpositioned lateral crura compounds airway obstruction by rendering the external valves incompetent.

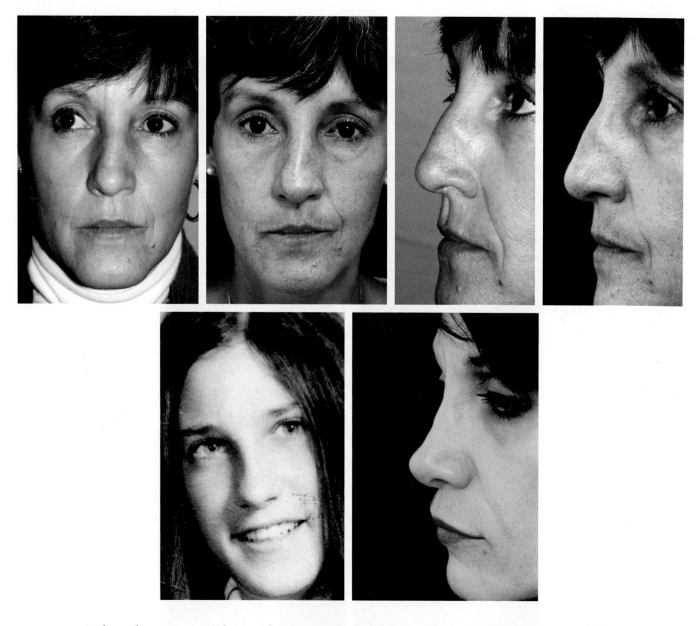

When the septum is deviated preoperatively, collapse worsens the asymmetry. The nose may shorten or lengthen depending on dorsal contour and skin characteristics, but the middle vault always narrows, and the airway always suffers.

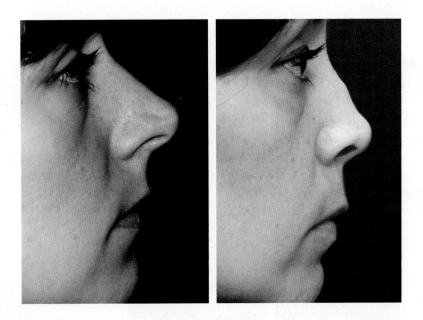

The deformity occurs along a spectrum, but it is important to recognize the more subtle variations. In my experience, a break in the middorsal line (sometimes only a small notch) accompanied by a change in upper lip position are usually two of the earliest signs of septal injury.

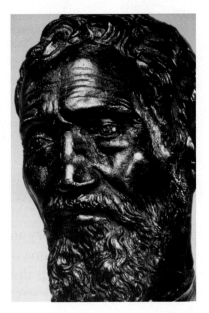

Even Michelangelo's later-life self portrait (reflecting the septal collapse sustained during a fight) accurately shows his own dorsal discontinuity and inverted-V deformity.

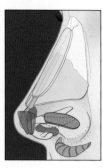

PATIENT STUDY ONE

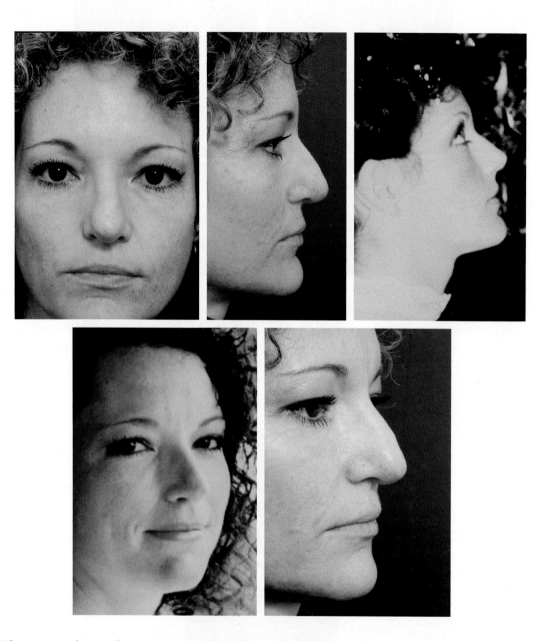

This patient's nasal appearance is deceptive, but history and a previous photograph provide the necessary information. She had undergone three prior surgeries. The first was a reduction rhinoplasty and septoplasty, but the surgeon performed two additional grafts to the dorsum, the second of which was ear cartilage, to correct a supratip depression. The patient developed an airway obstruction after the first surgery, uncorrected by the revisions. Her original goal was a nose with the same shape but smaller and narrower—probably unobtainable. Notice that nasal length has increased, tip projection has decreased, and her upper lip has lost its vertical position.

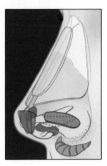

Thicker soft tissues do not reveal the same details as thinner ones, but the changes in lip carriage, tip projection, and upper dorsal height are obvious, although camouflaged by the onlay ear cartilage graft. The lateral crural remnants are malpositioned and bossed, broadening the nasal tip. Because some anterior septal support remained, a cantilevered dorsal graft was not necessary.

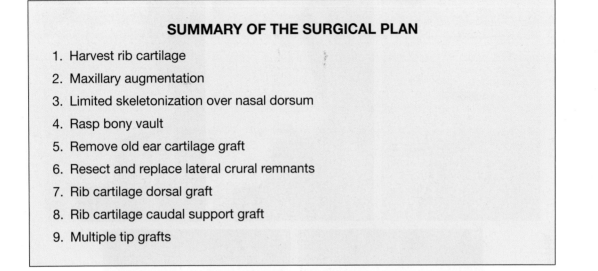

SUMMARY OF THE SURGICAL PLAN

1. Harvest rib cartilage
2. Maxillary augmentation
3. Limited skeletonization over nasal dorsum
4. Rasp bony vault
5. Remove old ear cartilage graft
6. Resect and replace lateral crural remnants
7. Rib cartilage dorsal graft
8. Rib cartilage caudal support graft
9. Multiple tip grafts

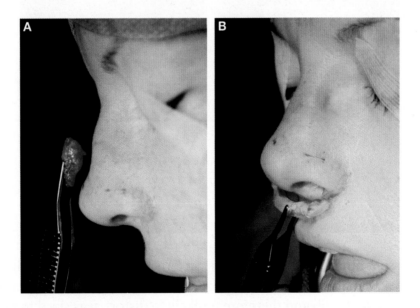

To reduce the number of incisions and ensure good coverage over the dorsal graft, the dorsum was skeletonized through the same infracartilaginous incision used to relocate the malpositioned lateral crura. The old ear cartilage graft was dissected free and removed, revealing the supratip septal depression *(A)*. The tip of the tenth rib was trimmed and beveled to form a single-piece maxillary augmentation, and was placed into the subperiosteal pocket high over the maxillary arch through a short incision in the nasal floor *(B)*.

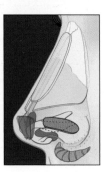

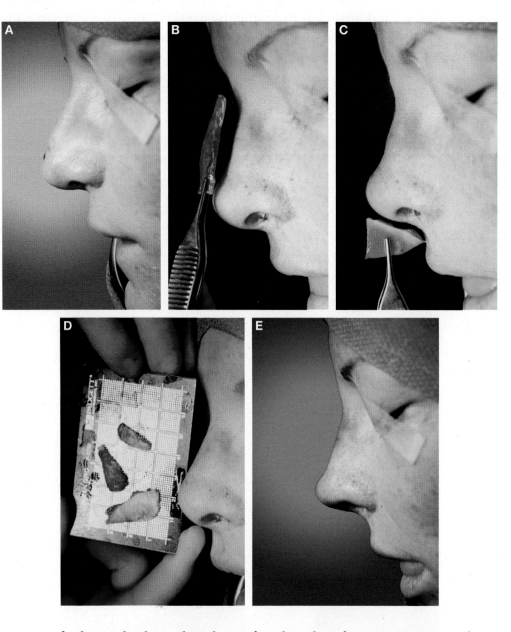

A section of split ninth rib produced a perfect dorsal graft, even containing the correct convexity to match an underlying skeletal asymmetry *(B).* Another graft, cut from the center of the rib and therefore unlikely to distort, was sized to replace the caudal septum, and was slipped into a pocket dissected between the membranous septal flaps, rounding the anterior corners before insertion. Notice its yellow, partially calcified center, typical of this patient's age (*C*; shown before trimming). Thin strips of lightly crushed rib cartilage were rough-cut for tip grafts *(D),* which were then inserted to conclude the reconstruction *(E).*

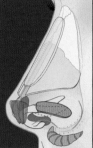

Postoperative Analysis

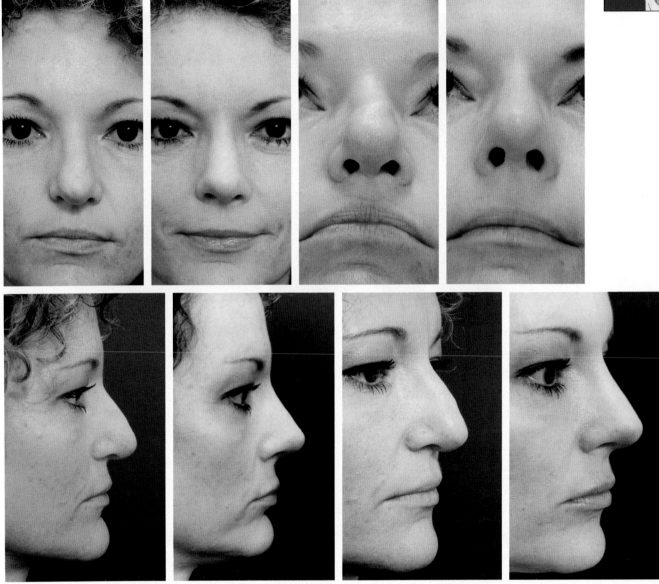

Three years postoperatively, nasal contours are smooth. The rib graft is not palpable. Lateral crural repositioning has normalized alar wall contours. Nostril shape has been improved by correcting dorsal height and tip projection. The columellar scar remains. The dorsum is straight, smooth, and symmetrical, ending in a tip that projects to the dorsal line and approximates the patient's preoperative contours. Notice also that no transfixing incision was made nor was any intranasal soft tissue resected: nasal shortening was produced by better maxillary, caudal septal, and tip support. Geometric mean nasal airflow increased 2.1 times over preoperative values.

PATIENT STUDY TWO

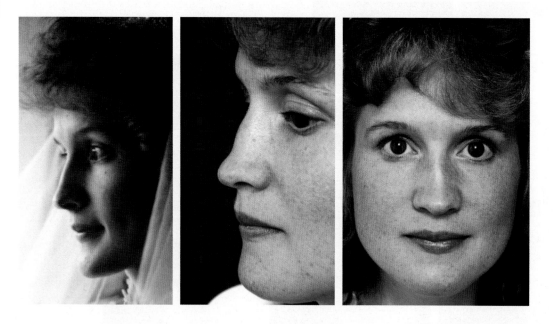

A septoplasty intended to correct airway obstruction collapsed the nose, giving this young woman most of the expected sequelae: increased nasal length, an apparent increase in bony vault height, a supratip depression, retracted columella, decreased tip projection, a sharpened subnasale, and a retrusive upper lip. The remaining septum curved toward the patient's left.

SUMMARY OF THE SURGICAL PLAN

1. Harvest calvarial bone for dorsal, caudal septal, and maxillary augmentation
2. Harvest ear cartilage for tip grafts
3. Limited skeletonization through a right-sided intercartilaginous incision
4. Rasp bony vault to level dorsum
5. No modification of tip cartilages
6. Calvarial bone maxillary augmentation
7. Calvarial bone dorsal graft
8. Calvarial bone caudal support graft
9. Ear cartilage tip grafts

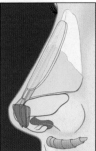

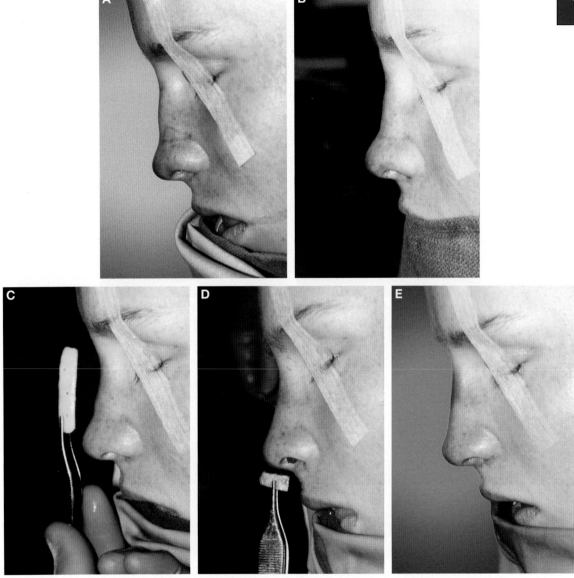

The bony vault was rasped to level the dorsum, bringing the tip into greater relief
(B). The preliminary calvarial bone graft will be shortened before placement *(C)*. A
small section of calvarial bone was used to support the columella *(D)*. Tip grafts
completed the reconstruction *(E)*.

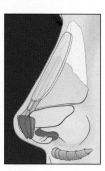

Postoperative Analysis

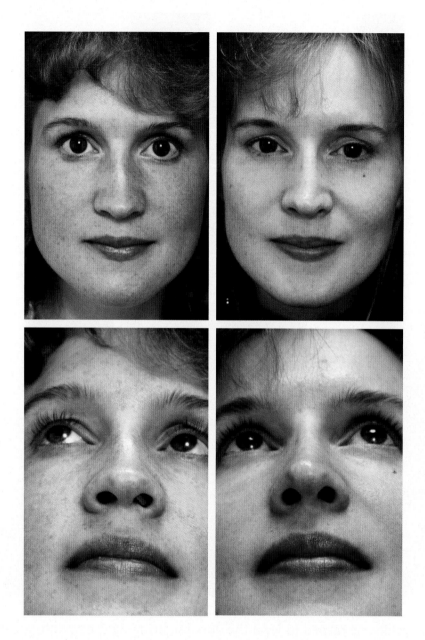

This operation was performed in 1988. Four-and-a-half-year postoperative views show a continuous dorsum, a bony vault that appears narrower, and a middle vault that is no longer collapsed. Upper lip position has improved. Were I performing this case today, I would have added a right lateral wall graft to camouflage the left-sided high septal deviation. Each of the augmentations has played a part in improving nasal base projection and altering nostril contours.

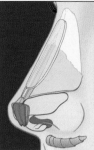

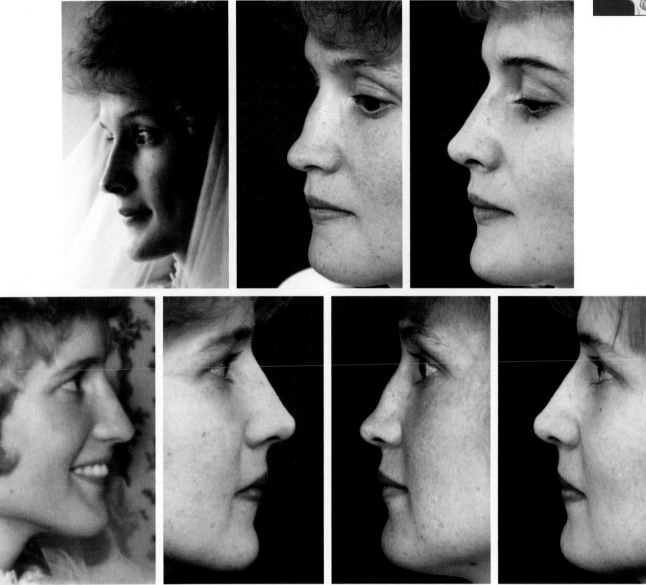

The dorsum remains straight, without any evidence of graft absorption. As seen with the previous patient, restorating underlying support corrects the nasal lengthening that septal collapse produces. Despite the patient's delicate skin, no underlying graft contours are visible. More than four years after surgery, the reconstruction is stable and successfully recreates the patient's premorbid nasal contours.

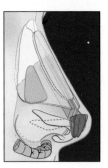

PATIENT STUDY THREE

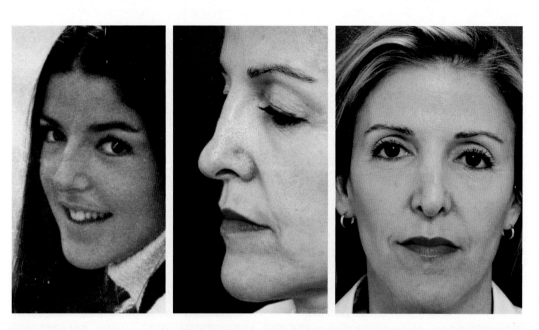

This is a patient whom I misdiagnosed. Thirty years after primary rhinoplasty and limited septoplasty, she sought correction of her airway obstruction and nasal asymmetry. The septal partition was severely twisted internally, obstructing the left airway anteriorly and the right airway posteriorly. The dorsum was stable but distorted toward the left. The reduced, malpositioned lateral crura had retracted her alar rims, and her retrusive upper lip seemed identical to what I had observed so many times in other secondary patients. A basal cell carcinoma resection over the right middle vault had left a depressed scar.

SUMMARY OF THE SURGICAL PLAN

1. Gore-Tex maxillary augmentation
2. Dorsal reduction
3. Resection and replacement of alar cartilage lateral crura
4. Septoplasty
5. Right unilateral spreader graft
6. Onlay over right middle vault
7. Tip grafts

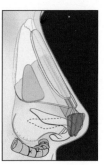

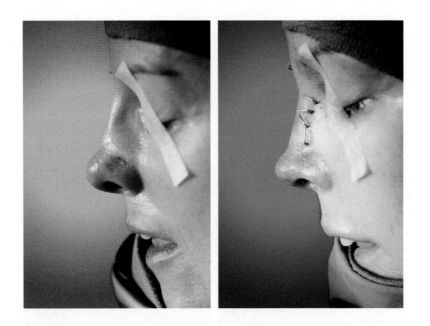

As soon as surgery began, something felt wrong. When I began to rasp the bony vault, the nose felt unstable. There seemed to be too many moving parts. Immediately I presumed an old septal fracture, probably through ethmoid and therefore supported only by a weak fibrous union, even after 30 years.

I was faced with two equally unappealing options. The first was to abandon the airway correction (the patient's primary concern) and treat only the external deformity with onlay and tip grafts. The second was to proceed with the septoplasty, leaving a particularly wide dorsal strut, undissected from its mucoperichondrial attachments, and hope to maintain stability. I chose the latter course.

As the septoplasty proceeded, the dorsal strut became more unstable, and began to settle posteriorly, disconnecting at its ethmoid attachments and producing a saddle nose, despite undissected 25 mm dorsal and 20 mm caudal struts.

I completed the septoplasty, which yielded only small amounts of cartilage but several useful strips of flat ethmoid. I harvested ear cartilage for the tip and right sidewall and placed fine, transcutaneous K wires through the nasal bones and dorsal strut (see Gunter et al, 2006). I then smoothed the dorsal line with ethmoid grafts and reconstructed the tip as planned. Half of the wires were removed at 4 weeks, the rest at 6 weeks.

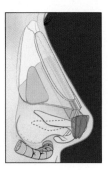

Postoperative Analysis

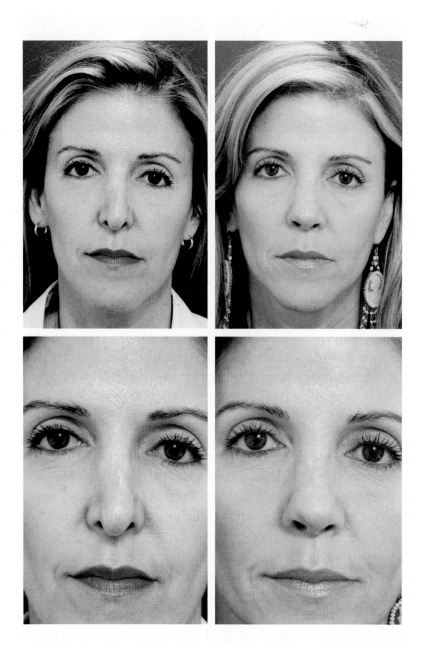

Two years postoperatively, nasal contours remain stable and smooth; and maxillary augmentation has corrected vertical position of the upper lip, most impressively on the frontal view (as is so often the case). The width provided by the onlay grafts and dorsal reduction has improved frontal aesthetics, and repositioned lateral crura support the alar rims. The right nasal scars remain slightly depressed. Geometric mean nasal airflow has improved 12.0 times over preoperative values.

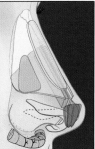

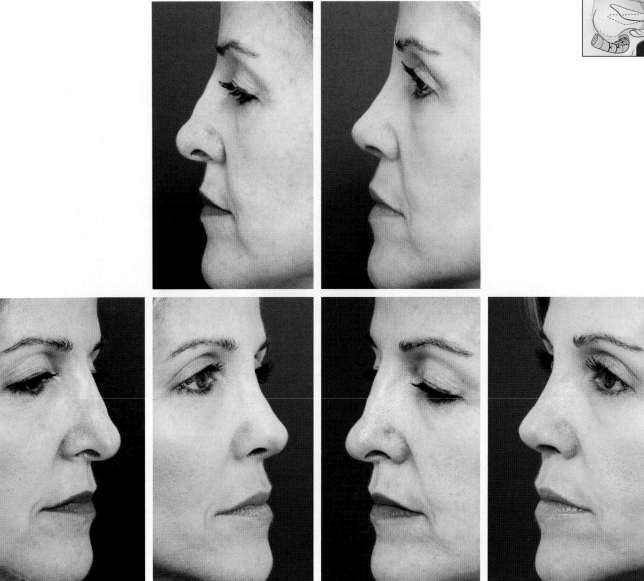

Although this nose is small, it remains balanced; and despite multiple onlay grafts, no disturbing discontinuities are evident. The deepened radix has improved the nasofacial angle. To my knowledge, in the past 30 years I have produced two septal fractures. This was one of them. The other was in a secondary patient in whom I tried to harvest a thin strip from an already-reduced dorsal strut, narrowing its width to less than 10 mm. Although this patient's preoperative appearance could be explained through traditional secondary rhinoplasty pathophysiology, the supratip depression and increased nasal length from her original preoperative photographs might have alerted me to the possibility of septal collapse. Today they would.

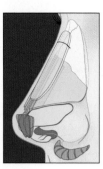

PATIENT STUDY FOUR

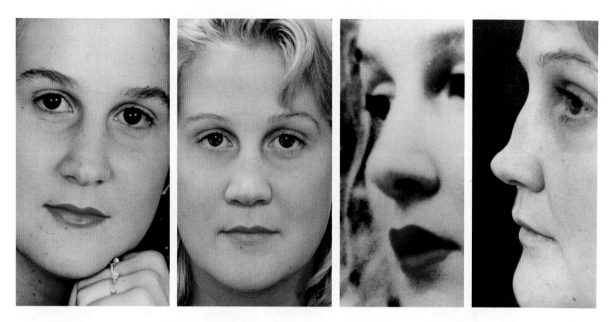

This patient suffered a septal collapse as a result of an infected hematoma following septoplasty and developed many of the signature deformities.

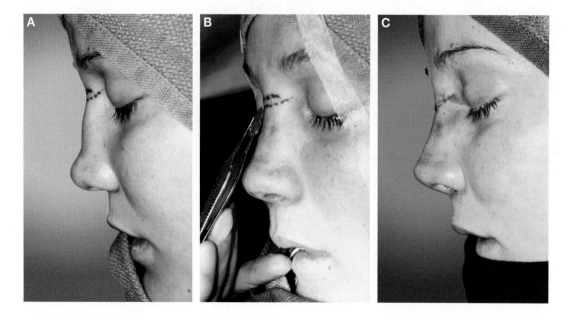

The primary difference in her treatment was a need to cantilever the graft by wire fixation at the bony vault after resecting the roof with an osteotome *(B)*.

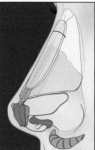

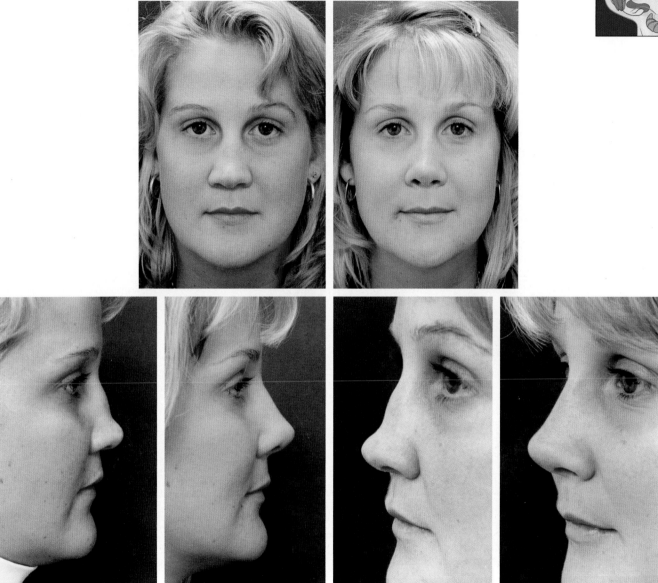

Three years postoperatively, the dorsum remained reasonably straight and stable. Upper lip retrusion and columellar retraction were corrected, and nasal base projection was restored. I published this patient's results after her 3-year follow-up (Constantian, 2001), but her story was not yet over. This patient illustrates the importance of long-term follow-up and the occasional unpredictability of rib grafts in younger patients.

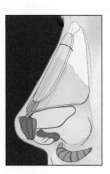

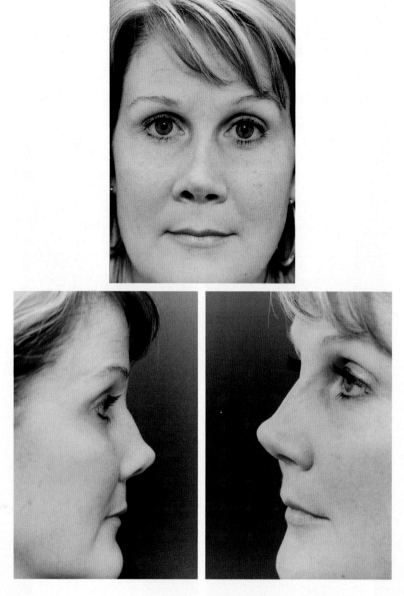

The patient returned 10 years after her first operation, asking to be checked because she sensed that something had changed. Indeed it had. The dorsal graft had warped in all three dimensions, twisting toward her right on the frontal view, bowing anteriorly over the bony vault and buckling into the supratip. In doing so, it elevated the right nostril by distorting the soft tissues above the rim. In addition, the tip lobule had flattened, the tip graft having been partially absorbed. Only the maxillary augmentation had held. Although I had placed an axial, threaded 0.9 mm Kirschner wire to stabilize the dorsal graft (see Gunter et al, 1997), the exceptional forces in the distorting rib had actually pulled the rib away from the wire, which was now palpable subcutaneously.

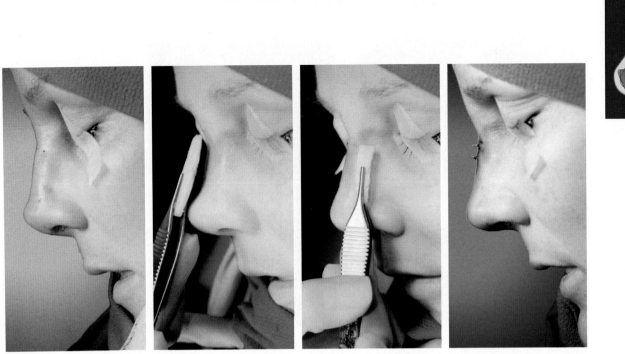

Reasoning that I was 10 years more experienced with rib and the patient was 10 years older (therefore presumably providing more rigid rib cartilage), I reoperated. The new graft was fashioned from the eighth rib, placed through a distal, cartilage-splitting incision to ensure good mucosal cover, fixed at its cephalic end with two smooth K-wires to prevent lateral displacement, and camouflaged at its edges with thin shavings of rib cartilage.

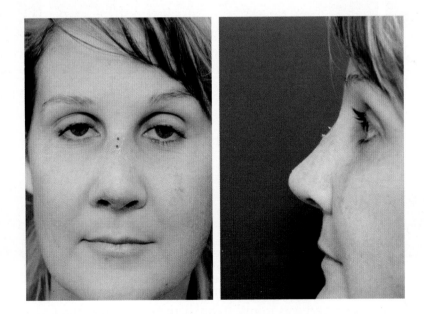

On the day of splint removal the nose was symmetrical, with the contour I had hoped. A few shavings of rib cartilage had been used to expand the anterior lobule, and rounded the tip nicely.

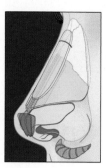

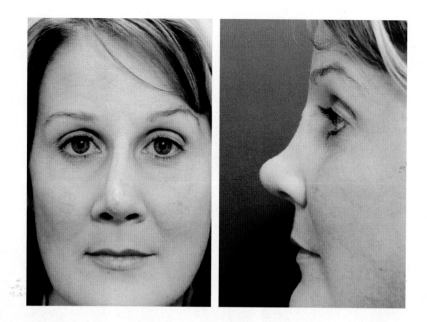

Within 6 weeks the new dorsal graft began to distort. By 10 months (shown here), the graft had curled anteriorly at both ends, lifting the radix and the supratip, and curved once again toward the patient's right. Interestingly, none of the other grafts had distorted.

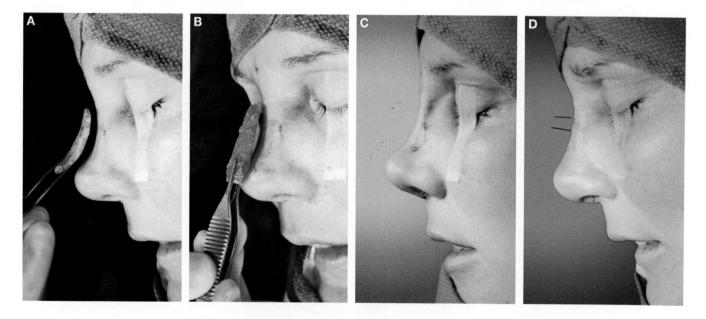

Twelve months later, the dorsal graft was removed through the same unilateral cartilage splitting incision and was found to be distorted as expected *(A)*. Concluding that rib cartilage was unreliable in this patient, I used rib bone instead, trimmed to fit and lightly beveled where necessary *(B)*. The patient is shown at the beginning and end of the correction (*C* and *D*).

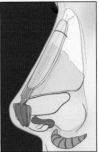

Postoperative Analysis

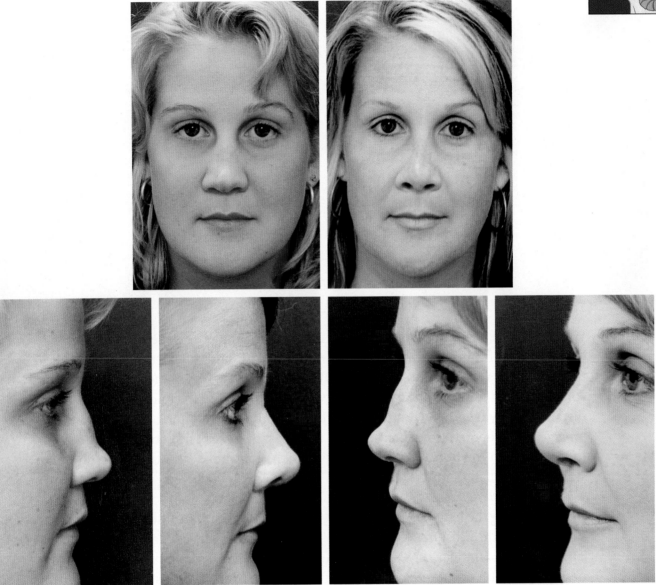

The patient is shown 2 years following her third surgery and 13 years following her first. The dorsal graft has remained midline and straight. Overall nasal balance is good. The upper rib correction has not regressed, and none of the sidewall or tip grafts have become visible. But the future behavior of this patient's unpredictable rib remains unknown. Fortunately, the patient has maintained her equanimity through it all.

Problems of Length and Balance

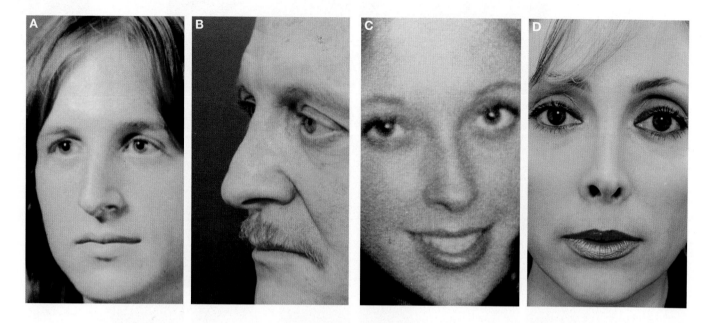

Whether reduction rhinoplasty shortens or lengthens the nose depends on several factors, chief of which are the shape of the preoperative nose (particularly the location of any dorsal convexity) and soft tissue thickness. Noses with medium or thick soft tissues and noses in which the dorsal convexity begins at the midpoint or more distally usually lengthen (*A* and *B*). If they are only reduced, long noses become longer as postoperative edema resolves. In contrast, noses with straight bridges, those in which the dorsal convexity begins high, and those with thinner, tighter skin sleeves usually shorten (*C* and *D*).

Accompanying the lengthening or shortening are the other typical sequelae of dorsal reduction, the most important of which is loss of internal valvular competence. The response of the alar rims to lateral crural reduction also depends on skin thickness: thicker soft tissues respond less or not at all (although a postoperative alar hollow develops), whereas thinner skin retracts cephalad and may require corrective composite grafts to add lining.

Similarly, the degree to which augmentation can shorten or lengthen a nose depends on skeletal and soft tissue factors. As we saw in the section on Septal Collapse, support shortens long noses.

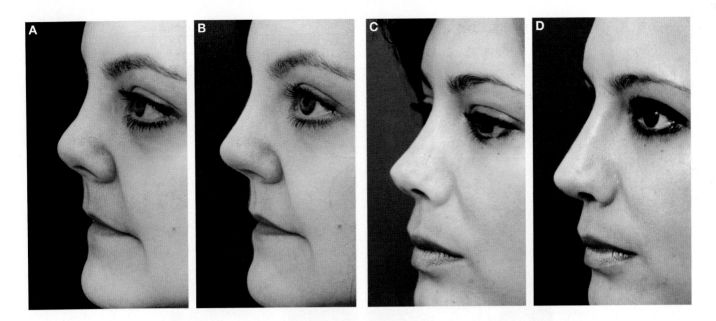

Lengthening is more difficult. A tight, contracted skin sleeve *(A)* only accepts limited expansion safely. A surgeon can augment the dorsum, place caudally-positioned tip grafts, and fill the columella, but soft tissue capacity constrains the results *(B)*. If the soft tissue is slightly more lax *(C)* and a long dorsal graft can be placed (in this case, rib cartilage), the tip lobule will often rotate more completely *(D)*.

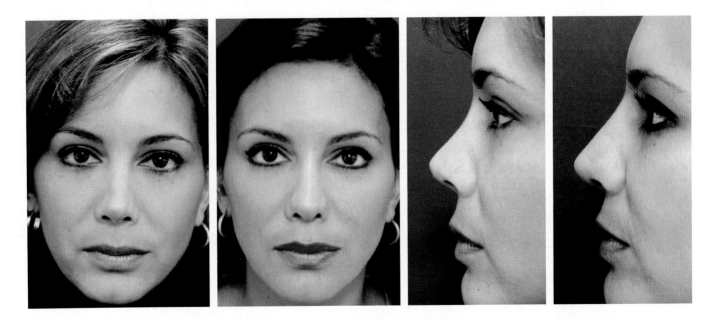

For this tertiary patient, dorsal, tip, and columellar grafts provided only modest improvement. After five other rhinoplasties, her soft tissues had undergone irreversible changes (including the development of unusual grooves along the alar walls) that responded only to a limited degree.

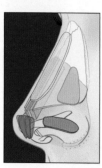

PATIENT STUDY ONE

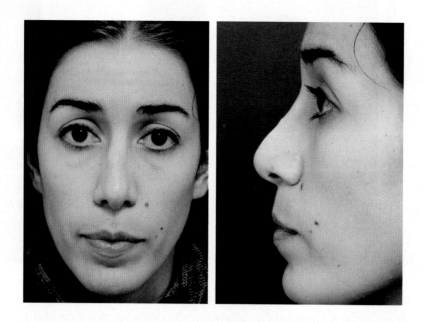

Two previous rhinoplasties and a septoplasty have left his patient with an asymmetrical nose and airway obstruction. The reduction has widened her nose, her middle vault has collapsed, and the septal remnant twists toward her right.

Because of her age and the shallowness of the dorsal defect, I wanted to avoid rib cartilage. If I could obtain one piece from the septum adequate for the dorsum, I could perform the rest of the reconstruction with ear cartilage.

SUMMARY OF THE SURGICAL PLAN

1. Minimal skeletonization over middle vault and dorsum
2. Rasp bony vault for adherence
3. Septoplasty
4. Harvest ear cartilage
5. Asymmetrical ear cartilage spreader grafts, left thicker than right, right graft convexity facing toward left
6. Septal cartilage dorsal graft to cephalic end
7. Ethmoid grafts to left bony vault
8. Crushed cartilage grafts to left lateral wall
9. Bilateral alar wall grafts
10. Crushed tip grafts

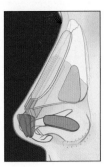

Postoperative Analysis

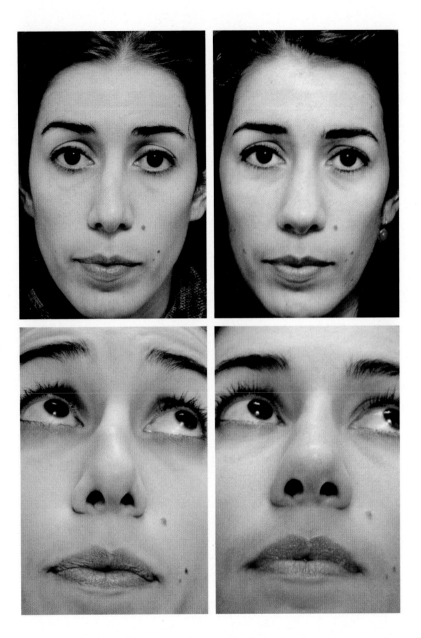

Five years postoperatively, the nose looks slightly longer because dorsal and tip grafts have established dorsal length, and alar wall grafts have decreased nostril visibility. Spreader grafts have opened the middle vault, and lateral grafts have improved symmetry.

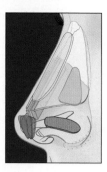

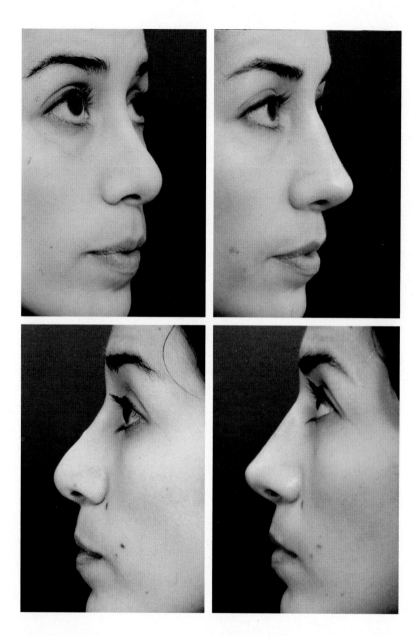

Although the caudal septum remains untouched, notice that the columella has become less visible because of anteroposterior tension provided by the tip grafts.

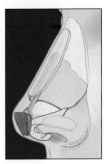

PATIENT STUDY TWO

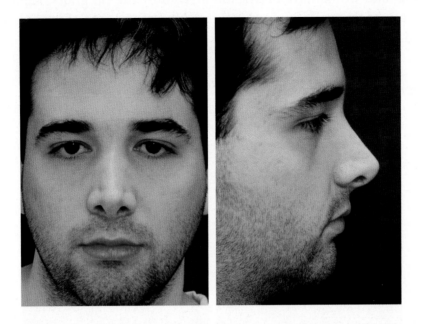

A prior rhinoplasty compromised this patient's airway at the internal and external valves, the latter already weakened by alar cartilage malposition (notice the alar creases and retracted rims). He believed that his lower nose was too large. There was a high septal deviation toward the right, and the lateral genua had knuckled.

SUMMARY OF THE SURGICAL PLAN

1. Resect lateral genua knuckles

2. Limited skeletonization over bony and upper cartilaginous vaults

3. Rasp bony vault for adherence

4. Transfixing incision, elevating caudal and membranous septa without shortening nose

5. Harvest rib cartilage (septum unavailable)

6. Harvest composite grafts

7. Rib cartilage dorsal graft

8. Rib cartilage tip grafts

9. Left lateral wall graft

10. Bilateral, coronally oriented composite grafts

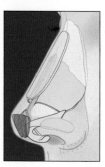

The case was performed in 1997. Were I doing it today, I would not resect the knuckles; this is unnecessary dissection of structures that were not excessively projecting and would have been camouflaged by the tip grafts. Knuckle resection decreased tip projection and increased the complexity of the judgment calls required.

Postoperative Analysis

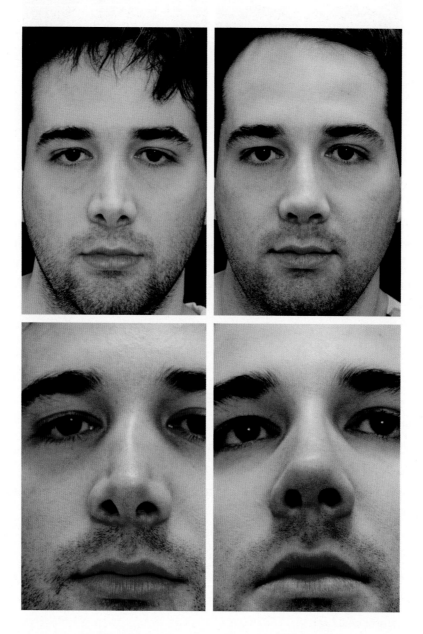

Two years postoperatively, the nose is straight, the tip is symmetrical, and alar retraction has been diminished by the composite grafts. Geometric mean nasal airflow has increased 5.1 times over preoperative values.

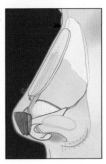

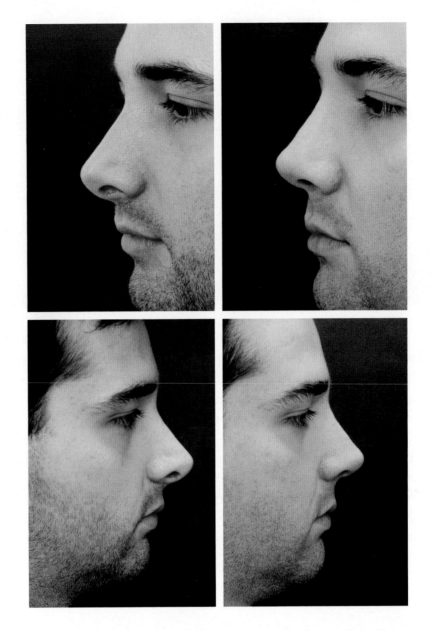

The change in dorsal height and columellar position has reduced apparent nasal base size. Tip projection has not changed but grafts have altered lobular contour. The cartilaginous components of the composite grafts have corrected the alar hollows.

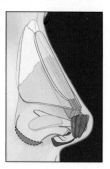

PATIENT STUDY THREE

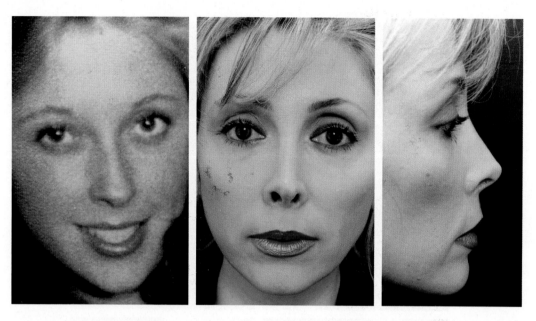

Two previous rhinoplasties created a very narrow nose from a narrow nose, and converted a narrow middle vault and alar cartilage malposition to subtotal airway obstruction with retracted nostrils. Although the patient's profile seems good, imagine, based on the frontal view, what is missing from the inferior tip lobule and the columella. Only a portion of the septum remains.

To avoid a rib cartilage dorsal graft, which would be overkill for such a small defect, the surgeon needs to obtain one nice strip from the septum. Ear cartilage can supply all rhinoplasty needs in most patients (spreader grafts, alar wall grafts, tip grafts, columellar grafts, and composite grafts), but ear cartilage cannot form a thin, long straight dorsal graft that is unlikely to be visible under thin soft tissues.

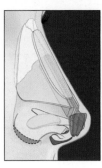

SUMMARY OF THE SURGICAL PLAN

1. Harvest ear cartilage for cartilage and composite grafts
2. Minimal skeletonization through single intercartilaginous incision
3. Resect posterior caudal septum
4. Trim knuckled left genu
5. Septoplasty
6. Asymmetrical ear cartilage spreader grafts, right thicker than left
7. Single layer septal cartilage dorsal graft
8. Crushed cartilage tip grafts
9. Crushed columellar grafts
10. Bilateral coronal composite grafts, left slightly wider than right
11. Right alar wedge resection, removing external skin only

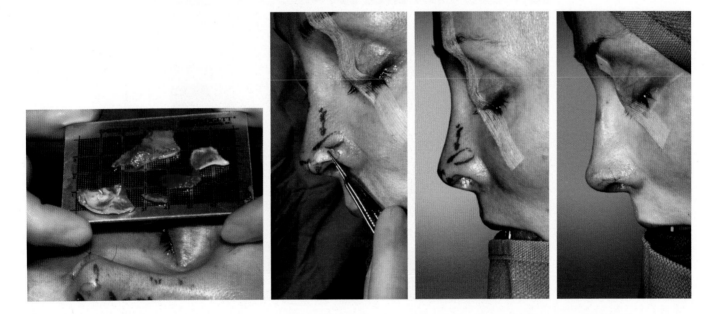

The septum yielded one serviceable piece for the dorsum (top center of grid). The harvested composite graft (skin covering only a portion of the resected cartilage, bottom left of grid) was split to form two pieces, trimmed to the appropriate size, and its cartilaginous component thinned. Comparative photographs from the beginning and the end of the procedure show apparent nasal base rotation and less nostril visibility, largely the result of the caudal septal resection, composite graft, and caudally positioned tip and columellar grafts.

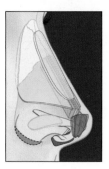

Postoperative Analysis

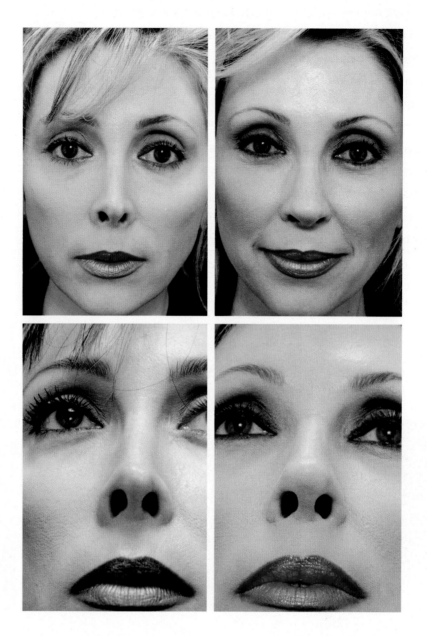

Three years postoperatively, the nose has retained the length achieved at surgery.

Lengthening the nose is not magical. Only so much can be gained by rotating the tip and raising the dorsum. If there is a true lining deficit, it must be replaced. Alar wall grafts will not stretch contracted skin several millimeters to correct a defect of this magnitude.

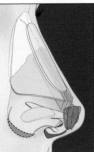

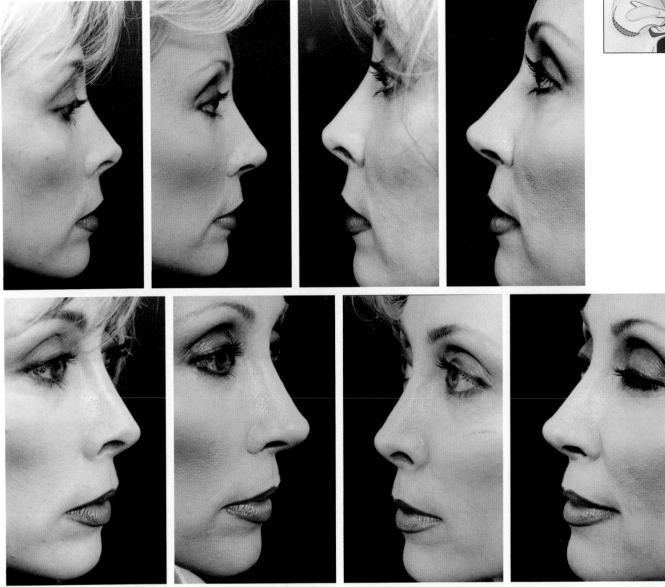

Comparing the lateral views, it should be more obvious now how much of the inferior tip lobule and columella were missing, reconstructed by feeding crushed grafts into separate pockets through vestibular skin incisions, and taking care that the grafts all laid flat and produced no surface irregularities. The postoperative nose is appropriately wider, and the length created by filling the tip lobule and columella can be appreciated best from the oblique view. The cartilaginous components of the composite grafts have created natural convexities in the alar sidewalls. Geometric mean postoperative nasal airflow increased 4.5 times over preoperative values.

Reconstruction in Patients With Prostheses

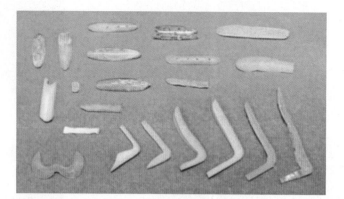

I have never regretted the philosophical decision that I made when I first went into practice to never use nasal prostheses. There are surgeons who do not agree with me, and I am familiar with their argument, because it is echoed by each of the papers that promotes the use of particular implants or nonautogenous material (such as irradiated homograft), correctly citing the problems associated with autogenous materials (such as pain, morbidity, and imperfect predictability). The surgeon who uses a silicone implant knows exactly how the implant will behave intraoperatively—information that the surgeon harvesting rib does not have.

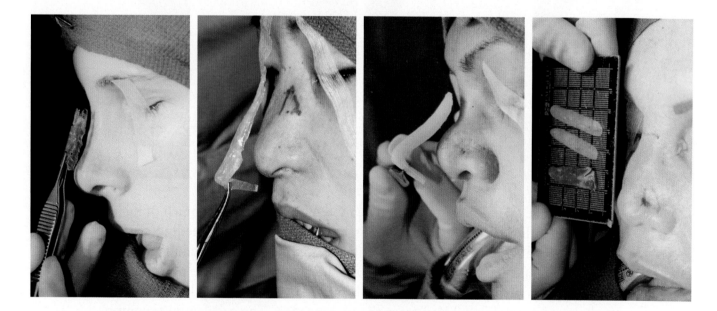

Autogenous materials do involve more pain and recovery for patients and more uncertainty for surgeons, but autografts do not fail in the same ways that alloplastics do. With good surgical technique, infection and extrusion virtually never occur. Instead, suboptimal results from autogenous reconstructions are generally limited to imperfect cosmetic results, which the surgeon can largely (but not completely) avoid.

Some implants placed without tension in primary patients with thick soft tissues can survive for many years. However, many of the patients in whom one would most like to use implants are least suited for them: patients who have undergone multiple prior surgeries, those whose septal and ear cartilage have already been harvested, and others who are understandably exhausted after many failed operations and want only simple solutions. I sympathize with these patients, but they deserve operations that have the greatest chance of long-term success.

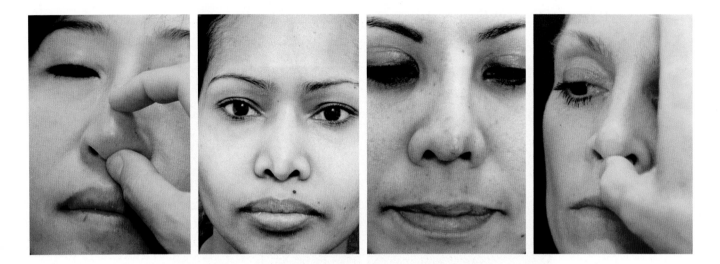

The nasal tissues of these tertiary patients are stiff, scarred, and hypovascular, which is one of the worst possible situations for placing implants, especially under tension. Particularly bad are L-shaped implants, designed to increase tip projection, which put their greatest stresses at the nasal tip.

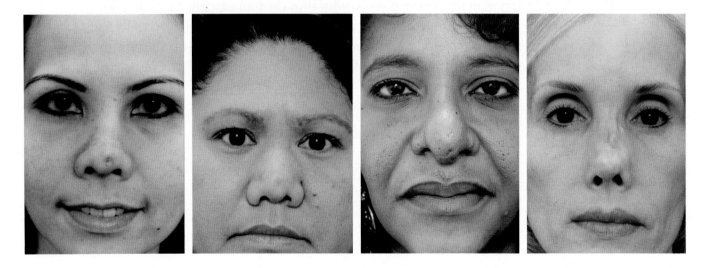

Once implants extrude or are removed, the tip skin may be permanently thinned and damaged from dermal erosion. No one knows the real long-term implant fail-

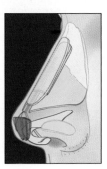
ure rate, the percentage of implants that ultimately extrude, or the number removed because the cosmetic reconstructions were unacceptable.

Nasal prostheses are unquestionably easy to use. A young surgeon's first silicone implant will work, whereas his or her first rib graft may not. But these implants are only easy on the day the surgeon puts them in. Autogenous grafts are the patient's best chance of a lifetime result.

PATIENT STUDY ONE

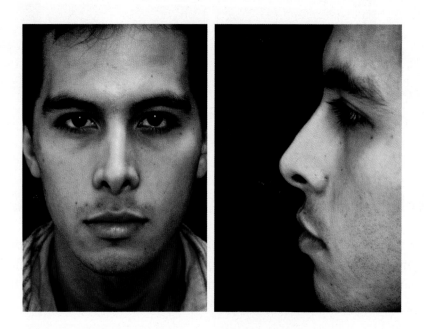

This young Latino man had undergone a reduction rhinoplasty, after which a dorsal silicone implant had been placed to correct an overresection. His frontal view shows the stigmata of previous alar cartilage malposition, recognizable by the creases that used to demarcate the caudal edges of the lower lateral cartilages, and by the nostril retraction.

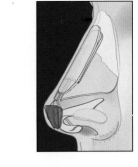

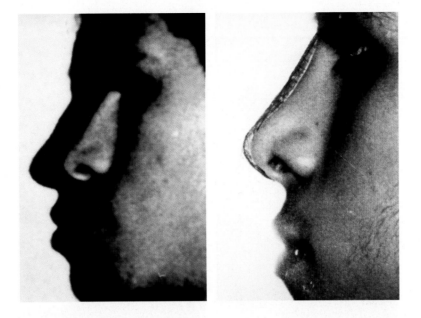

Here is our proof. The patient was able to supply a photograph of his nose prior to any surgery, showing the rotated lateral crural position. He also supplied a photograph of his nose between the first and second procedures (showing a supratip deformity), with an ink overlay tracing what he wanted to accomplish: a higher dorsum with more tip projection and a flatter supratip. The patient instinctively understood skin limitations and the fact that the improvement required augmentation, not further reduction. If the skin could have contracted further, he would not have developed a supratip deformity. Fortunately, septal cartilage was available.

SUMMARY OF THE SURGICAL PLAN

1. Harvest ear cartilage for composite grafts

2. Limited skeletonization through a single intercartilaginous incision

3. Enter silicone capsule on its posterior surface, maintaining as thick a soft tissue cover as possible; remove silicone implant

4. Elevate nasal periosteum, rasp bony vault for graft adherence

5. Transfixing incision, resect an ellipse of membranous septum without shortening nose

6. Septoplasty

7. Layered dorsal graft

8. Tip grafts

9. Coronally-oriented composite grafts

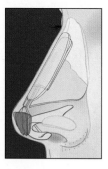

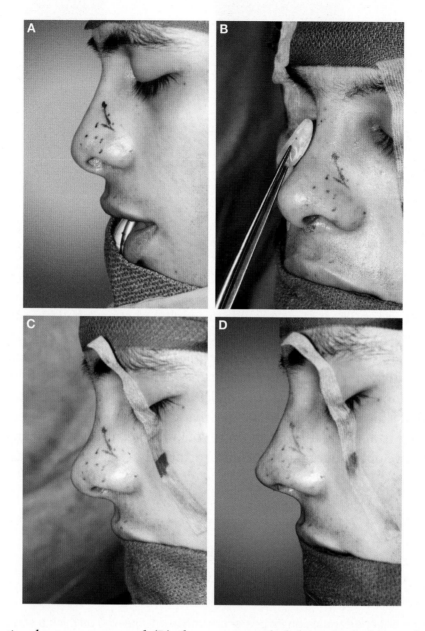

After the implant was removed *(B)*, the nose revealed the same balance alterations seen after any large dorsal reduction: a notch developed at the mid-point of the bridge, the supratip became higher, and the nasal base appeared larger *(C)*. Following dorsal and tip grafts, the nose became straight, with a slight convexity over the bony vault, respecting the patient's aesthetic goal *(D)*.

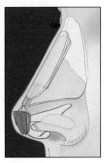

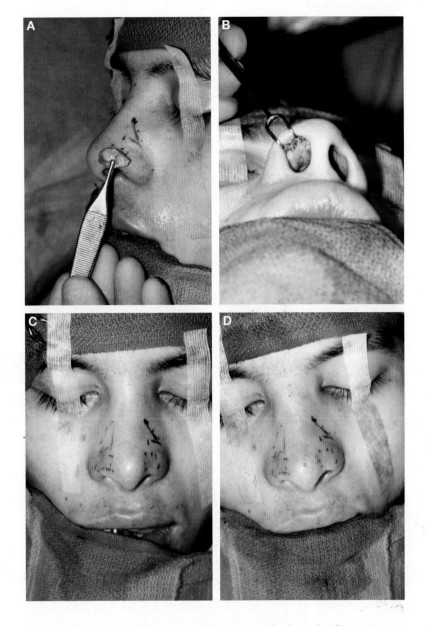

The harvested composite graft was cut to size and placed where preoperative skin markings indicated the greatest deficiency *(A)*. After the right graft was placed *(B)*, the depression in the right alar wall disappeared and rim height dropped *(C)*. After both composite grafts were placed, the nostrils became more symmetrical and the alar hollows disappeared *(D)*.

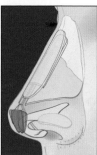

Postoperative Analysis

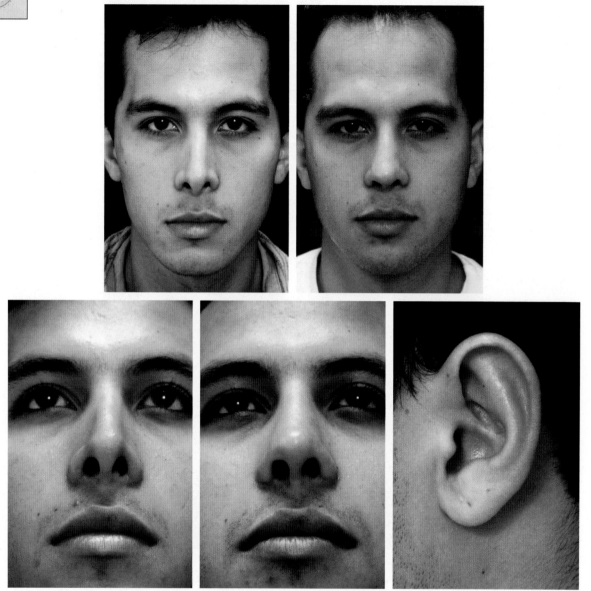

Two and a half years later, the abnormalities of the preoperative nose have decreased. The nasal sidewalls show a gradual, confluent divergence instead of narrow, parallel edges. The alar creases have diminished, and nostril height has improved. The lobulated preoperative inferior view has been softened by composite grafts. The donor ear shows negligible changes from the harvest in the cymba conchae.

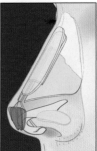

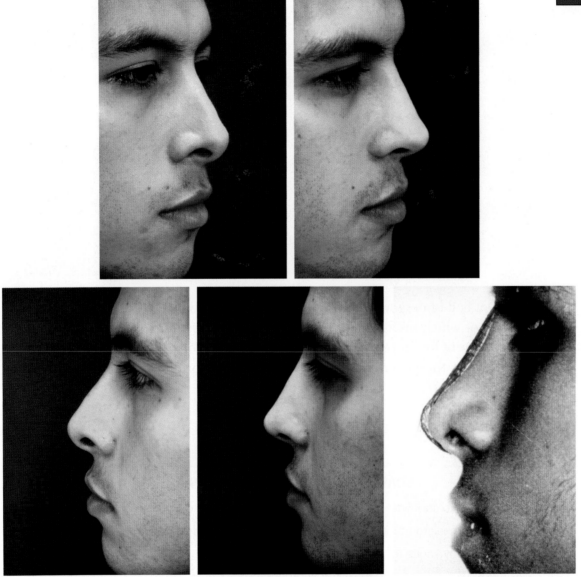

The oblique and lateral views indicate symmetry and separation of the dorsum from the supratip. Columellar elevation and nostril height reduction reduce nostril visibility. The reconstruction is now autogenous and has supplied tip projection not created by the silicone implant. The patient's aesthetic goals have been met.

This part of rhinoplasty is not magic. Most careful surgeons can produce these same results if they understand nasal phenomenology and attend to technical details.

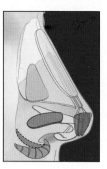

Patient Study Two

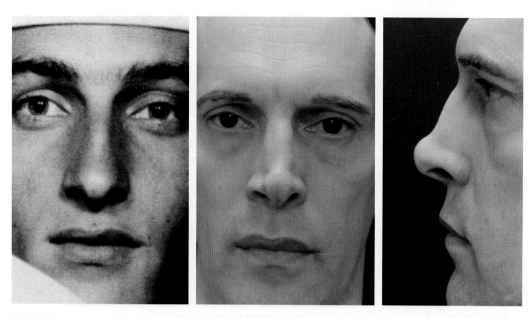

This patient had undergone two rhinoplasties, the first of which reduced his nose, the second of which inserted homograft cartilage. In fairness to the homograft, it had been present for 15 years, but was too small, too short, and too mobile, and it did not correct the patient's airway obstruction. An original preoperative view shows malposition. Septal cartilage was unavailable.

SUMMARY OF THE SURGICAL PLAN

1. Harvest rib cartilage
2. Minimal skeletonization beneath implant, removing old implant
3. Rasp bony vaults for graft adherence
4. Two-piece rib cartilage maxillary augmentation
5. Resect ellipse of caudal and membranous septa without shortening nose
6. Rib cartilage dorsal graft
7. Rib cartilage alar wall grafts
8. Right sided lateral wall graft
9. Tip grafts
10. Right alar wedge resection, removing 3 mm of external skin and 2 mm of vestibular skin

---

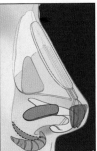

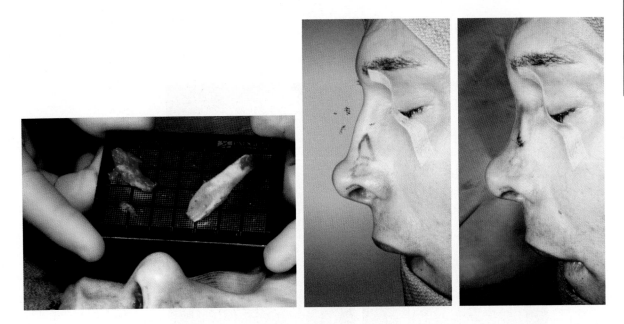

A dorsal graft was fashioned (right of grid), and the homograft was removed (left of grid). Compare lateral views at the beginning of the procedure and following implant removal, and notice the change in apparent nasal base size. The caudal septum was also adjusted.

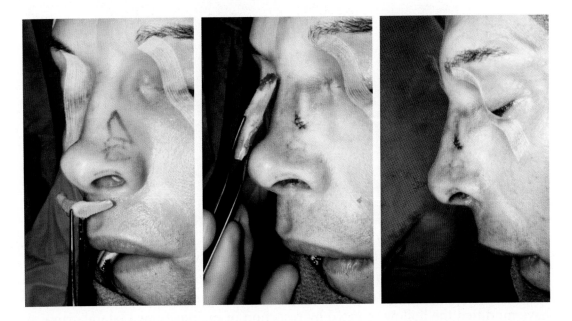

The tip of the ninth rib, with its own nice intrinsic curve, was carved to make a single unit maxillary augmentation, and the carved rib graft was placed into the dorsum, immediately decreasing apparent nasal base size and providing a smooth contour.

A left unilateral composite graft was added 12 months later as an isolated procedure.

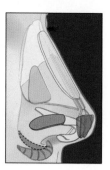

Postoperative Analysis

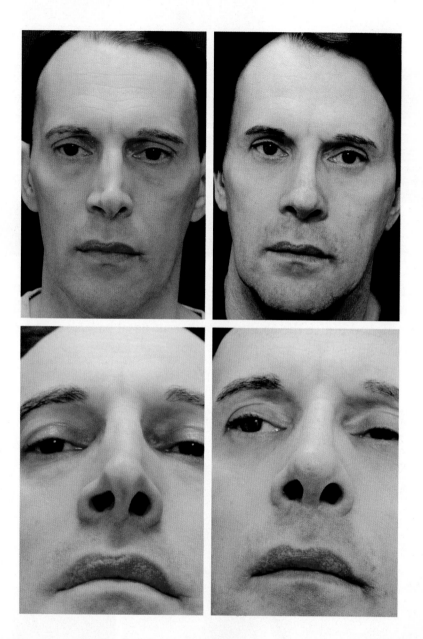

Two years postoperatively, the dorsum remains smooth and straight. The rib graft is not palpable and has fully integrated with the bony arch. The discontinuities created by the narrow, asymmetrical homograft have been corrected. Alar wall grafts have modified the hollows created by resection of malpositioned lateral crura. A right alar wedge resection has improved nasal base symmetry, and tip grafts have diminished the cleft in the patient's tip.

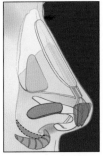

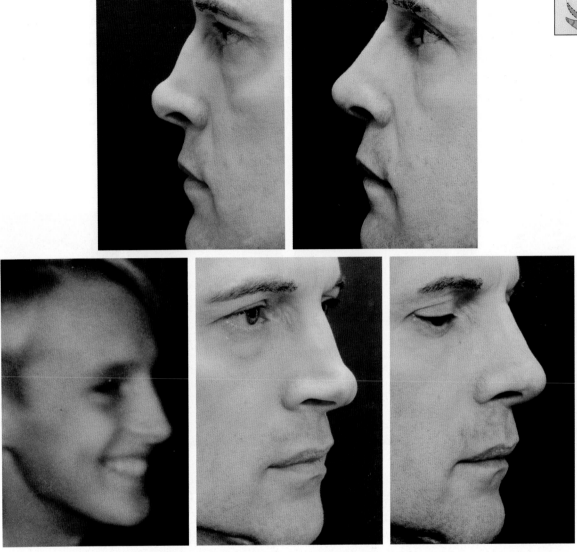

Because the tip and alar wall grafts distribute tip forces, the lateral genua are not as prominent. Geometric mean nasal airflow increased 2.1 times over preoperative values. Maxillary augmentation has improved upper lip position, and the dorsal and tip grafts form an integrated profile without discontinuities, resembling the patient's unoperated nasal shape. The alar wall grafts have filled the hollows and created a normal convexity. Rib is particularly well suited for this purpose, because a shaving of the rib surface naturally produces a curl toward the perichondrial side, which can be used to the patient's advantage.

The operating surgeon should always remember that every implant was inserted for a reason. The surgical plan must include adequate arrangements for a reconstruction that cannot be fully planned until the implant has been removed.

Cleft Lip Nasal Deformity

If there is a most unsolved area of rhinoplasty, it is the cleft lip nasal deformity. Our imperfect progress so far has two causes. First, knowledge is still increasing about cleft deformities and how they change as a child grows. Second, the technical aspects of cleft rhinoplasty must deal with not only deficient or abnormal anatomy and soft tissue changes, but inherently asymmetrical ones (except in bilateral clefts). Like surgery in hands with rheumatoid arthritis, the results (at least my results) are always imperfect. There is always more to do, more to offer the patient, more techniques that might overcome the abnormalities that biology has produced.

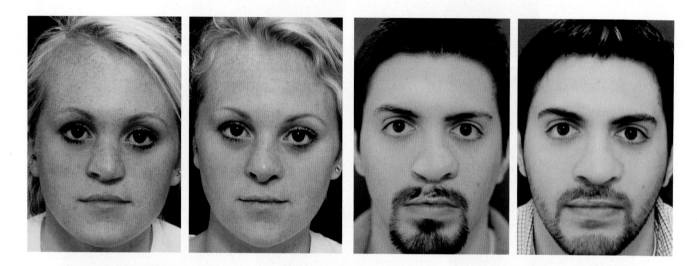

What makes a cleft deformity noticeable? Both of the results shown here are imperfect—works in progress. But there is improvement. Is the change created by a better upper lip contour after maxillary augmentation? Or by a change in nasal tip position? Or by a straighter dorsum? Or by better nostril or alar base position? Or is it the change in the patient's eyes, where the sense of deformity seems to have diminished?

Many surgeons have described elements of the abnormal anatomy that characterizes the cleft lip nasal deformity, which include any or all of the following: the nasal tip and caudal septum deviate away from the cleft side; the septal convexity bows toward the cleft side, obstructing the ipsilateral airway; the left alar dome is depressed; and there is a vestibular web in the cleft side nostril, running from its apex to the pyriform aperture, roughly along the cephalic margin of the alar cartilage.

The cleft side alar rim buckles medially; there is an absent alar/facial groove on the cleft side; and the cleft alar base is laterally displaced. The maxilla on the cleft side is hypoplastic; and the medial crus on the cleft side is positioned inferiorly to its normal mate, abutting a widened nasal floor. The bilateral deformity is characterized by a short columella, an inadequately projecting tip sometimes notched in the midline, lateral displacement of both domes and lateral crura away from the septum, flattened alar rims, flared alar bases, and bilateral maxillary hypoplasia. To these I would add that the lateral crura on the cleft sides of unilateral and bilateral deformities are cephalically rotated and behave exactly like malpositioned lateral crura in noncleft noses.

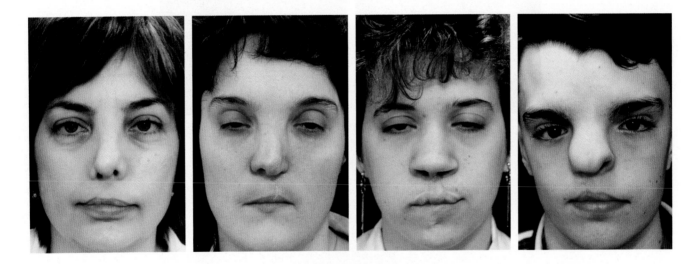

However, most rhinoplasty surgeons see patients with clefts years after the initial repair has been performed, and often after a number of additional surgeries. Frequently complicating the original anatomy (or those elements that remain uncorrected) are nostril stenosis on the cleft side, inadequate tip projection, columellar scars with or without previous forked flaps or other columellar lengthening procedures, residual malpositioned lateral crural remnants, persistent vestibular webs on the cleft side, untreated maxillary hypoplasia, and other causes of airway obstruction or nasal deformity that may have resulted from earlier treatments (such as supratip deformity, internal or external valvular incompetence, or residual septal deviation). With few exceptions, my approach to these patients follows my approach to other tertiary rhinoplasty deformities, remembering that the deformities are usually asymmetrical, that the soft tissues are scarred, and that there are skeletal and soft tissue deficiencies on the cleft side. The phenomenology and logic, however, remain the same.

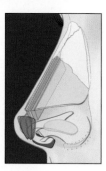

PATIENT STUDY ONE

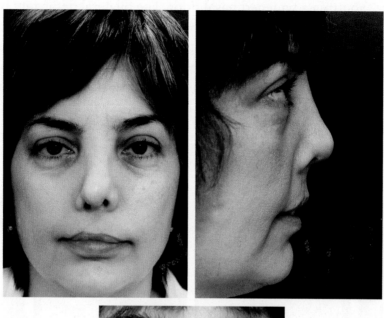

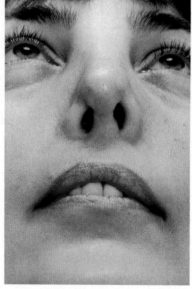

This patient's two prior surgeries had not corrected her airway obstruction from internal and external valvular incompetence. The septum had been previously harvested. The patient was satisfied with her external lip repair but consented to treatment of the modest whistle deformity. She thought that her tip was too flat, her nose too short, and her nostrils too visible.

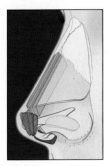

SUMMARY OF THE SURGICAL PLAN

1. Revise lip with V-Y mucosal advancement
2. Harvest composite graft and ear cartilage
3. Resect lateral crural remnants through the same vestibular incisions planned for the composite grafts
4. Minimal skeletonization to root
5. Rasp radix; bilateral ear cartilage spreader grafts, thicker on right than left
6. Bilateral coronal composite grafts
7. Columellar grafts
8. Tip grafts

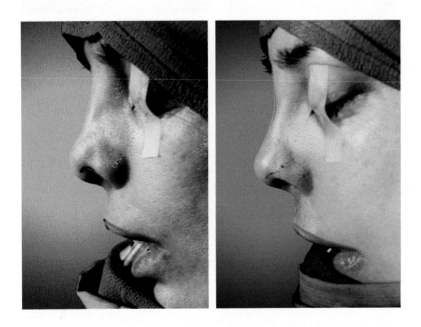

Ear cartilage spreader grafts were placed, the radix reduced, and the tip expanded. The goal was to create a less vertical nasofacial angle.

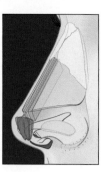

Postoperative Analysis

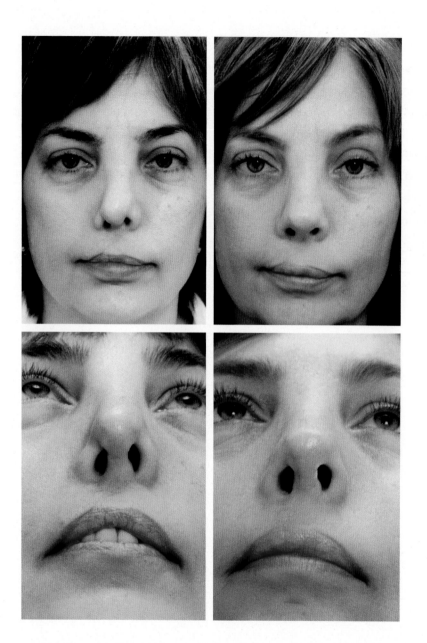

Three years postoperatively, the nostrils remain more symmetrical. Resection of the deformed lateral crural remnants and composite grafting have diminished the asymmetrical alar creases, and asymmetrical ear cartilage spreader grafts have widened the middle vault slightly. Geometric mean nasal airflow increased 4.1 times over preoperative values.

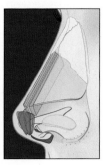

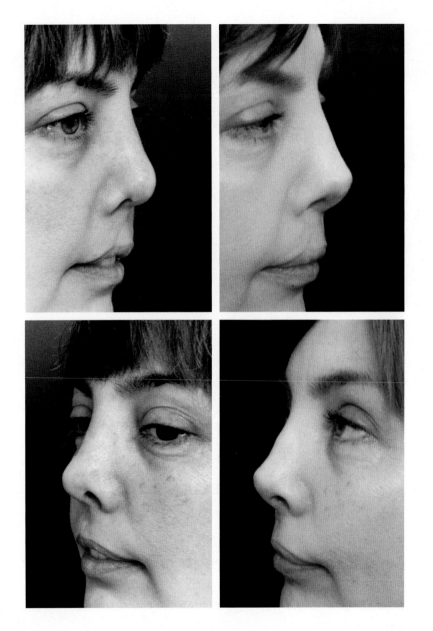

Grafts have separated the tip lobule from the dorsum and displaced the columella caudally. However, the deeper radix obtained during surgery did not persist post-operatively, which is not unusual. When the supraorbital forehead is flat, a change in radix depth is difficult to maintain.

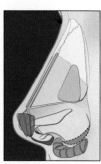

PATIENT STUDY TWO

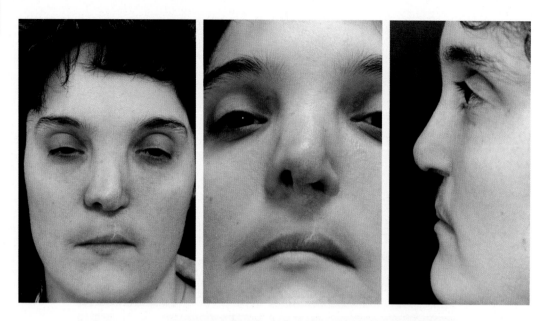

After three nasal corrections (including the repair in infancy) this patient still had valve-related airway obstruction and left-sided nostril stenosis. Only a small amount of septal cartilage was available. She declined lip revision.

SUMMARY OF THE SURGICAL PLAN

1. Harvest ear cartilage
2. Minimal skeletonization through single intercartilaginous incision
3. Minimal rasping and trim of nasal dorsum
4. Septoplasty
5. Maxillary augmentation (vomer and ear cartilage scraps only)
6. Tip grafts
7. Columellar grafts
8. Left lateral wall graft
9. Left alar base flap

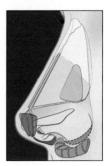

Because the patient's donor materials were limited to a small amount of septal cartilage and one unused ear, the residual building materials not needed for other areas were used for maxillary augmentation. These were insufficient for the job, but rib cartilage was not warranted and alloplastics are always contraindicated under a scarred gingivobuccal sulcus.

Postoperative Analysis

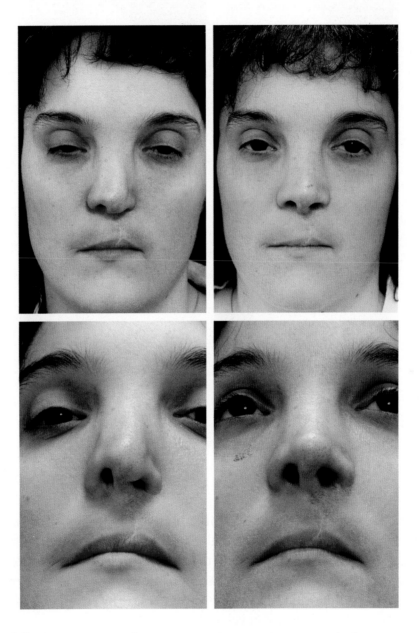

One year following surgery, the nose remains more symmetrical.

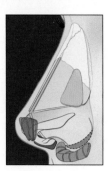

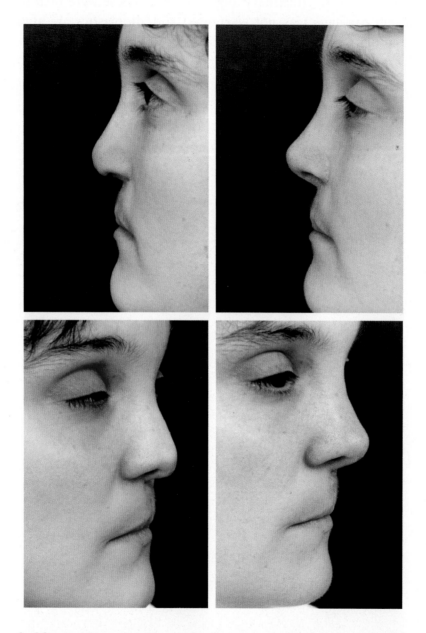

Lateral and oblique views show a modestly improved upper lip carriage, with better tip and columellar position. The left alar crease remains appropriately deep, although slightly flatter when compared to the normal side. Because the left alar base was displaced medially, an alar base flap repositioned the base and opened the stenotic nostril. It is important to recreate an alar crease by advancing the cheek, so that a flattened contour does not develop.

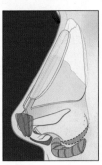

PATIENT STUDY THREE

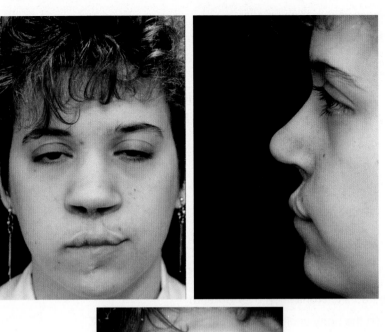

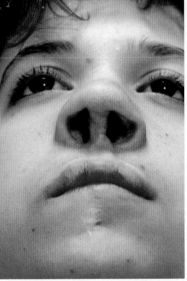

Besides repair of her bilateral cleft lip in infancy, this young woman had undergone two columellar lengthening procedures using a forked flap and cartilage strut. Despite columellar lengthening, the patient's tip lobule remains small, and the nasal base has taken on a gangly, unnatural appearance. It is too wide from the front, and the nostrils are large, triangular, and notched laterally. The columella is symmetrical but scarred and too narrow at its posterior end. In terms of overall nasal balance, the dorsum is straight but too low in relation to a relatively large nasal base, and the tip is undefined.

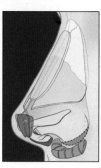

SUMMARY OF THE SURGICAL PLAN: FIRST STAGE

1. Ear cartilage maxillary augmentation
2. Resect posterior columella
3. Alar wedge resections, removing 3 mm of external skin and 2 mm of vestibular skin

SUMMARY OF THE SURGICAL PLAN: SECOND STAGE (6 MONTHS LATER)

1. Revise lip repair
2. Harvest ear cartilage
3. Additional maxillary augmentation
4. Additional columellar grafts

SUMMARY OF THE SURGICAL PLAN: THIRD STAGE (1 YEAR LATER)

1. Limited skeletonization over dorsum
2. Rasp the bony vault for graft adherence
3. Septoplasty
4. Harvest ear cartilage (limited donor material from previous septoplasty)
5. Dorsal graft
6. Additional columellar grafts
7. Tip grafts, solid and crushed

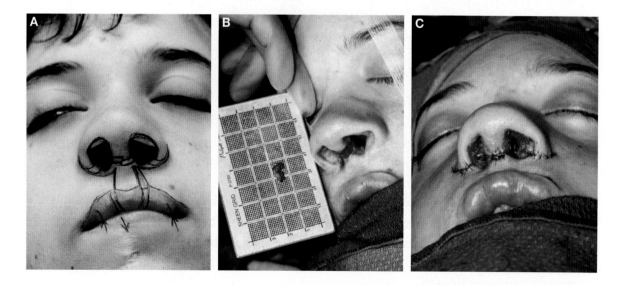

The needed columellar resection is often disarmingly small. My preoperative plan can be seen in *A.*

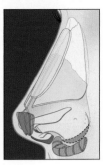

Postoperative Analysis

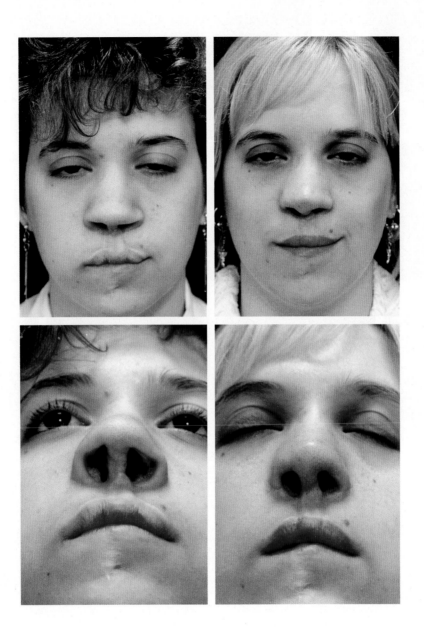

Three and a quarter years after the final procedure, frontal balance has improved. Although scar maturation is slow during the teenage years, lip contour is better, the whistle deformity has been improved by mucosal advancement, and the left Cupid's bow notch has been corrected. The philtral column, however, is not symmetrical, but the patient declined further surgery. Alar rim excisions have improved nostril contour; and the combination of the dorsal graft and alar base resections has brought the frontal view into better balance by narrowing the upper and lower noses, respectively. The nasal base shows an overall improvement, though covered with objectionable scars, some of which are from me. Nostril size has decreased and tip lobular size has increased; nostril contour is more normal, but could benefit from further revision. The lower lip scar is the vestige of an Abbé flap performed by the previous surgeon.

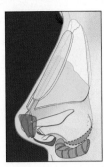

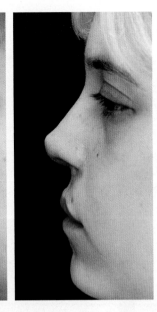

Autogenous maxillary augmentation (using ear cartilage) has improved the vertical position of the upper lip. The columella is no longer retracted. Tip grafts have improved contour, and the dorsal graft has improved the balance between nasal base size and bridge height.

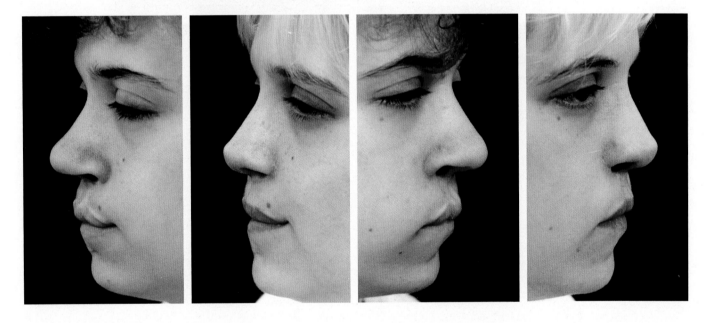

On the oblique views, the improvement in balance is perhaps more obvious. A slightly higher dorsum and grafted tip have corrected the profile.

Recall the size of the columellar resection, which was less than 3 mm and could not by itself have caused the improvement in nasal balance. Columellar and alar wedge resections merely corrected the view from below; dorsal and tip grafts improved the relationships among the dorsum, middle vault, and nasal base on all other views.

Despite a reduction in nostril size, geometric mean nasal airflow increased 4.8 times over preoperative values, indicating the combined effect of septoplasty and the dorsal graft, which strengthened the internal valves.

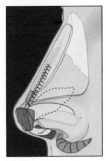

PATIENT STUDY FOUR _____

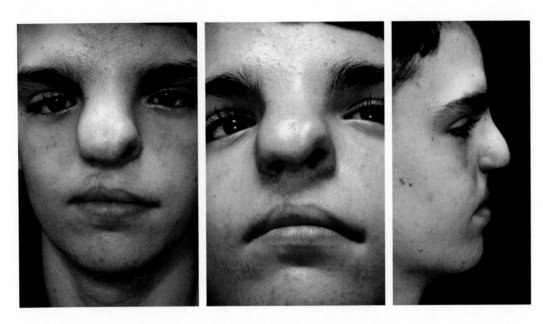

Despite the frontonasal dysplasia spectrum with a right unilateral cleft lip and palate, the family remained uninterested in correcting the patient's mild hypertelorism, which caused no visual disturbance. His speech was good. Nevertheless, the nose was broad, the dorsum bifid, the tip undefined, and the nostrils asymmetrical.

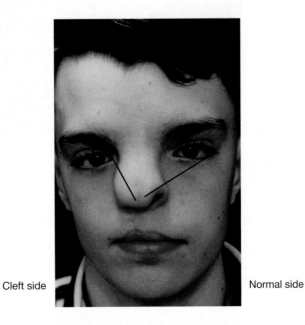

Cleft side   Normal side

Notice that the lateral crural axes are not symmetrical: the normal (left) side is orthotopic (its axis points toward the lateral canthus), but the cleft (right) side is cephalically rotated, (its axis points toward the medial canthus).

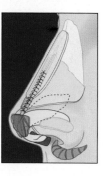

SUMMARY OF THE SURGICAL PLAN: FIRST STAGE

1. Harvest rib cartilage

2. Rib cartilage maxillary augmentation

3. Midline skin excision

4. Rib cartilage dorsal graft, placed through midline incision

5. Columellar grafts

6. Tip grafts

SUMMARY OF THE SURGICAL PLAN: SECOND STAGE (1 YEAR LATER)

1. Composite graft, left nostril

2. Excise skin, right rim

3. Revise lip

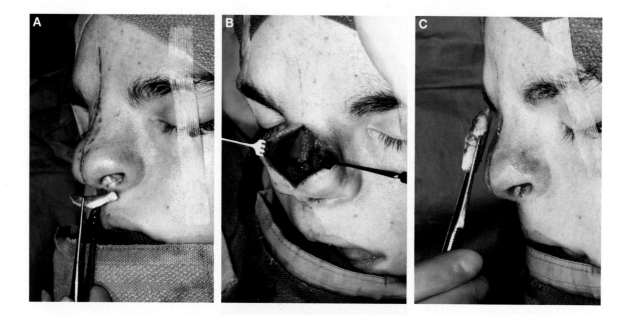

Rib cartilage was carved into a single piece maxillary augmentation, its limbs deliberately asymmetrical to compensate for maxillary hypoplasia on the cleft side. Notice the midline mark and planned middorsal excision *(A)*. The dorsum was split and the malpositioned right lateral crus rotated into proper position, symmetrical with the left side *(B)*. The rib graft was carved, sized, and placed into the dorsal defect, where it was immobilized with fine absorbable sutures *(C)*.

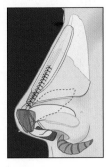

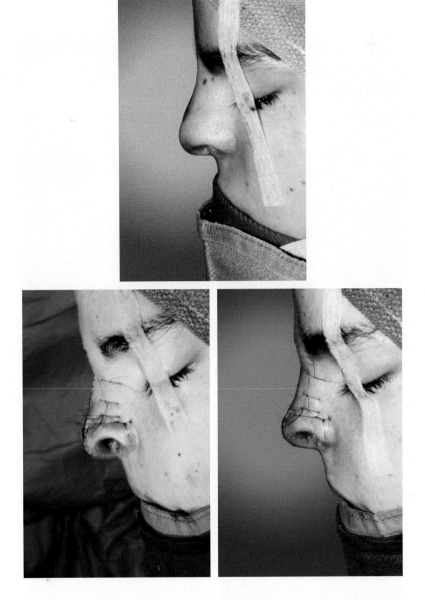

The patient is shown at the beginning of the procedure and following the dorsal graft. Notice that the skin has been coapted to the thinned underlying soft tissue with basting sutures, advancing the skin medially under very gentle tension. The basting sutures were removed in 24 hours. Although the dorsum is straight, tip projection is still inadequate, common in many clefts. Tip grafts complete the reconstruction. No cast was placed.

During the following year, a large composite graft was added to the left side, the right nostril rim was excised, and lip revision was performed.

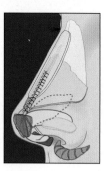

Postoperative Analysis

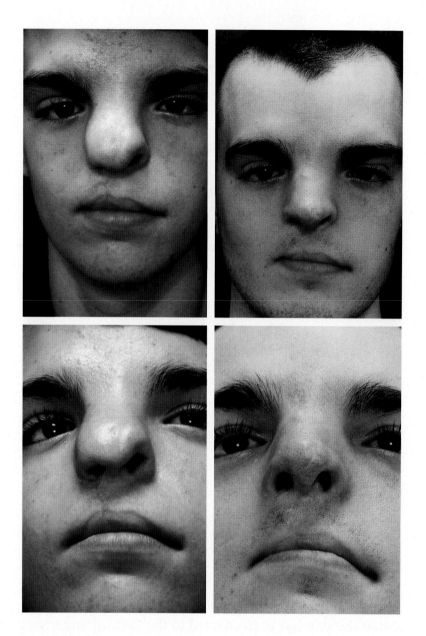

Seven years postoperatively, the dorsum remains straight and midline.

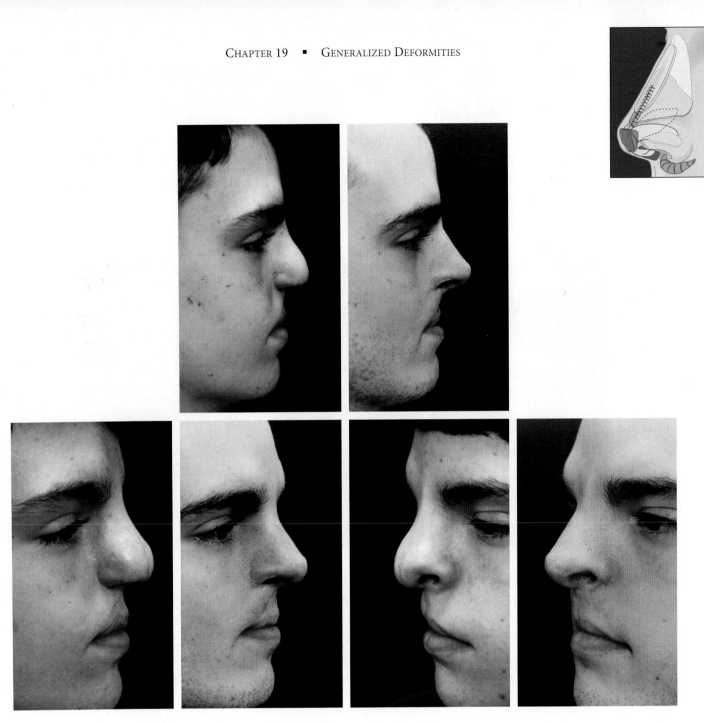

The nasal base is less asymmetrical. Excision of nostril skin on the right and the left composite graft have improved symmetry, but the dorsal and tip scars are still suboptimal. A second composite graft would improve left alar rim height, but the patient has declined further surgery. The amorphous nasal shape has improved with dorsal, tip, and columellar grafts. Although disparate preoperatively, the postoperative oblique views match more closely. Geometric mean nasal airflow increased 4.1 times over preoperative values.

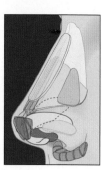

PATIENT STUDY FIVE

Aside from the lip scars and frequent whistle deformities, I have often thought that the maxillary hypoplasia and flat tip make a cleft deformity most obvious. Other surgeons may disagree, but two of my primary goals in patients with clefts are to improve both vertical lip position and tip projection.

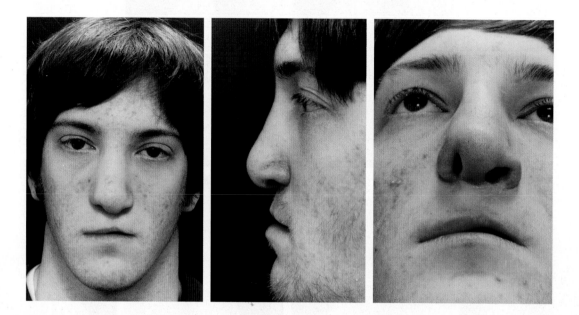

Like so many patients with clefts who are treated in their teens, this man had already undergone several surgeries, including a septoplasty that failed to clear an airway obstructed at the internal valves. His dorsum was straight, but his maxillary arch was characteristically retrusive, his tip was inadequately projecting, and nasal base projection was poor. The unsupported base seemed to drip off the dorsum. Although the cleft nostril was not stenotic, the floor was depressed, and the normal right alar rim was higher than the left.

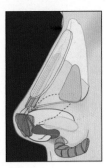

SUMMARY OF THE SURGICAL PLAN: FIRST STAGE

1. Harvest rib cartilage
2. Rib cartilage maxillary augmentation, thicker on the left than right (preoperative asymmetry)
3. Moderate skeletonization over bony and upper cartilaginous vaults
4. Retrograde reduction of left lateral crus
5. Rib cartilage spreader grafts
6. Rib cartilage dorsal graft
7. Rib cartilage left middle vault onlay
8. Rib cartilage caudal support graft
9. Tip grafts
10. Left lateral wall graft
11. Excision left alar rim

SUMMARY OF THE SURGICAL PLAN: SECOND STAGE
(1 YEAR LATER)

1. Harvest rib bone
2. Harvest composite graft
3. Revise lip
4. Dorsal graft, rib bone
5. Coronal composite graft, right nostril
6. Right osteotomy

SUMMARY OF THE SURGICAL PLAN: THIRD STAGE
(1 YEAR LATER)

1. Left alar wedge resection
2. Repeat right composite graft (partial loss) using left alar wedge as graft
3. Revision of left alar rim

Unfortunately, the dorsal graft distorted, as detailed in Chapter 14. One year later, that graft was removed and replaced with tenth rib bone, the lip was revised, and a right composite graft and right osteotomy were performed. Small revisions were done the following year.

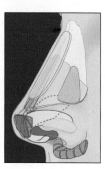

Postoperative Analysis

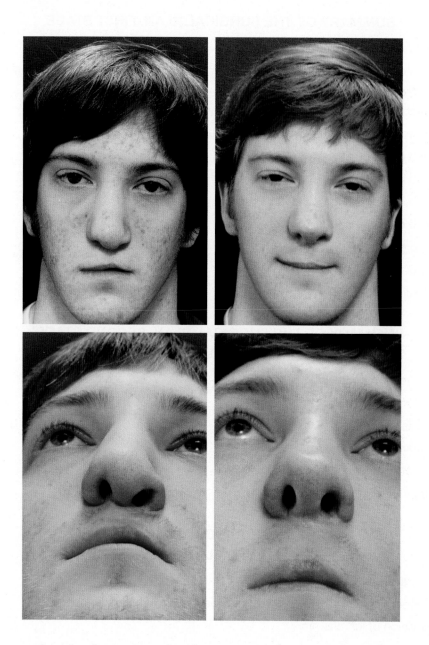

Three years after the first stage, the dorsum remains smooth, symmetrical, and straight, and the bone graft edges are not palpable. Maxillary augmentation, columellar grafts, and tip grafts have rotated the nasal base cephalad, and have improved the nasal base/upper lip complex, reducing the cleft stigma.

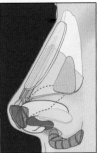

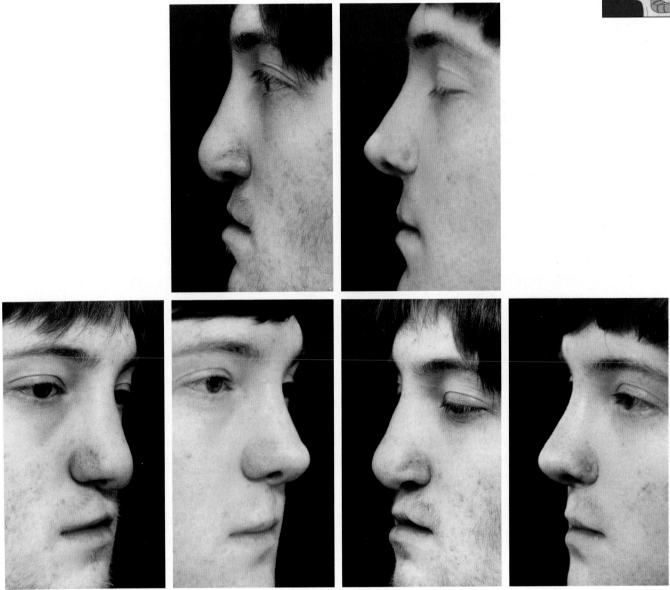

The oblique views match more evenly. The combination of left alar wedge resection, left nostril rim excision, and right coronal composite graft have improved nostril symmetry, but multiple attempts to correct the left nostril have produced a lining that is thick and almost stenotic. Despite that, geometric mean nasal airflow increased 2.5 times over preoperative values.

Deformities Resulting From Previous Open Rhinoplasty

Open rhinoplasty is an operation nearly without complications. I know this because there are almost no papers on the subject. One of the larger open rhinoplasty series indicates no complications. Another series notes an occasional hypertrophic scar, but says that other complications were "comparable to those seen after the endonasal approach." In several series reviewing successes, the incidence of suboptimal scars was listed at 1% to 3%, with rare exceptions: Daniel's report (1995) of 22 patients indicated a 9% rate of objectionable scars, and a group of 50 patients was reported to have a 44% rate of unsatisfactory scars (Bafaqueeh and Al-Qattan, 1998).

However, the columellar scar that results from open rhinoplasty is not the real issue. Every surgeon needs access. My objection to the open approach is not the exposure that it provides, but rather the exposure that it does not provide—one that reveals the proportion, contour, and nuance of the nasal surface, which is what the patient sees.

The putative advantages of the open approach—wider exposure, and the ability to fix grafts, set columellar struts, and place sutures—become liabilities when the result is not what the surgeon had intended. Although I have seen many very good open rhinoplasty results from my colleagues and in the literature, no one knows how often suboptimal results occur, even in the best hands, or how they compare to those seen in patients treated endonasally. Are there differences in surgical outcome? Does the access route chosen by the surgeon place patients at risk for particular postoperative consequences?

To answer some of these questions, I performed a review of 100 consecutive secondary or tertiary rhinoplasty patients (66 women and 34 men) on whom I operated between 1997 and 1998 (Constantian, 2002). Their mean age was 35 years (range, 14-68 years). Of these patients, 64 had previously undergone only endonasal rhinoplasty (45 women and 19 men), and 36 had undergone one or more open rhinoplasties (21 woman and 15 men). Most of the open rhinoplasty patients had undergone *only* open procedures; at the very least, the most recent rhinoplasties had been performed through the open approach. There was no significant difference in the proportion of men to women among those patients who had undergone either rhinoplasty approach (chi square = 1.47; $df = 1$; $p > 0.05$).

At the time the survey was conducted, the popularity of the open approach had been increasing progressively for several years. In 1996 and 1997, 21% and 23% of my secondary and tertiary patients had previously undergone open rhinoplasty, respectively; by 2000, the number was 50%; and currently it is more than 80% (with a higher proportion from United States surgeons relative to those patients undergoing surgery overseas).*

There were provocative differences between the two patient groups. Open rhinoplasty patients had undergone more previous operations (3.1, versus 1.2 for closed rhinoplasty patients) and had a larger number of presenting complaints (5.8, versus 2.6 for closed rhinoplasty patients).

Relative Frequency of Presenting Complaints in 100 Consecutive Secondary Rhinoplasty Candidates After Closed or Open Approaches

Presenting Complaint	Previous Closed Approach	Previous Open Approach
Airway obstruction (internal valve)	42%	64%
Alar distortion	16%	64%
Bridge too low	50%	64%
Tip too blunt	33%	61%
Nose asymmetrical	27%	50%
Airway obstruction (external valve)	11%	50%
Tip too narrow	28%	47%
Nose too short	14%	39%
Nose too long	20%*	3%
Bridge too high	17%*	11%
Nose too narrow	8%	31%
Columella wider	0%	36%
Columellar scar	0%	25%
Hard struts	0%	19%

*Higher incidence following closed approach.

The nature and rank order of complaints differed in each of the groups. Although both patient groups complained of bridges that were too low, airway obstruction at the *internal valves,* tips that were too blunt, or postoperative asymmetry, patients previously treated by open rhinoplasty also frequently complained of nostril and alar distortion, airway obstruction at the *external valves,* noses that were too short or too narrow, or unacceptably wide columellae. Of all complaints presented in both groups, only excessively long noses and bridges that remained too high were more common in previously treated closed rhinoplasty patients.

*A Z test comparing the difference between proportions for independent samples indicated significant prevalence for most presenting complaints individually and as a whole.

Surgical Problems More Frequent After Open or Closed Rhinoplasty (100 Consecutive Secondary Patients)

Surgical Problem	Relative Occurrence (Times More Frequent)
More Frequent After Open Rhinoplasty	
Excessive columellar width	36
Hard columellar strut	19
Excessively narrow tip	11
External valvular obstruction	4.5
Chronic rhinitis	4.5
Alar/nostril distortion	4.0
Excessively narrow nose	3.9
More Frequent After Closed Rhinoplasty	
Nose excessively long	6.7
Bridge too high	1.5

With those two exceptions, patients previously treated by the open approach voiced more complaints in every other category than their closed rhinoplasty counterparts. Complaints related to the columella ranged from 19% to 36%. Interestingly, the columellar scar, widely assumed by open rhinoplasty critics to be its major drawback, troubled only 25% of the open rhinoplasty patients.

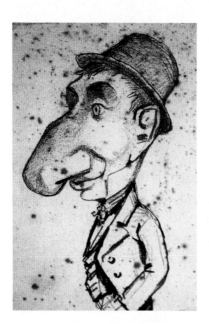

The complaints registered by these two groups of patients are not difficult to interpret. When a surgeon resects a dorsum like the one Monet has caricatured here, a skin sleeve that cannot contract will often lengthen, accounting for the "nose excessively long" complaint, as well as complaints traceable to internal valvular incompetence. When tip reduction decreases tip support (or when inadequate tip projection existed before rhinoplasty) the tip hangs further, creating a patient belief that the bridge is now too high (when in fact the tip is too low).

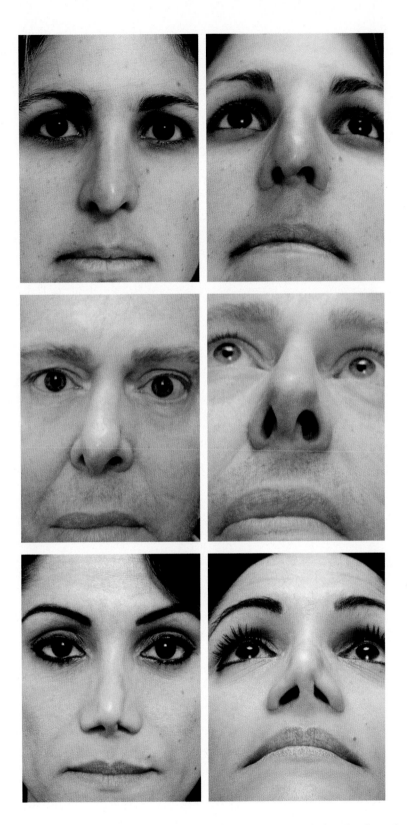

Unlike the closed group, however, alar distortion, external valvular obstruction, and a too-narrow tip ranked high among previous open rhinoplasty patients.

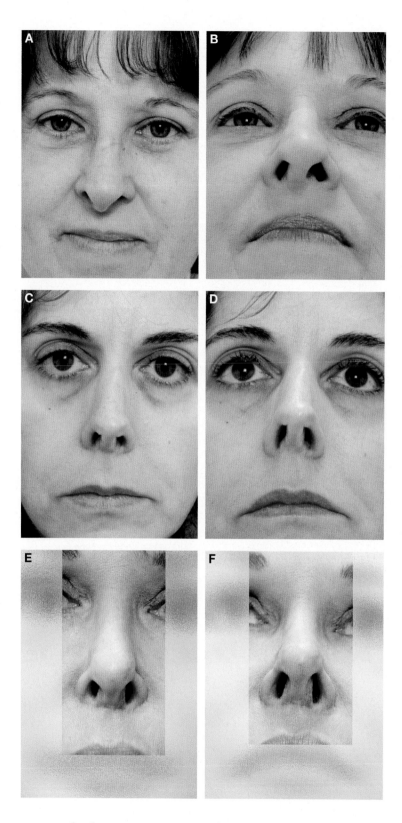

Columellar struts, which are very easy to place, can create their own deformities: columellae that are too wide with displaced medial footplates (*B* and *D*), or columellae that are overrotated and broad (*F* and *H*).

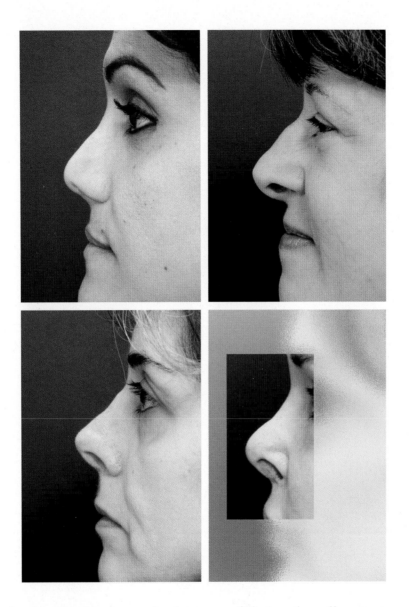

Interestingly, despite the size and substance of their columellar struts, notice that each of these patients still has inadequate tip projection. Adequate tip projection results from adequate middle crural length, not from direct pressure transmitted from the maxilla or medial crural extensions.

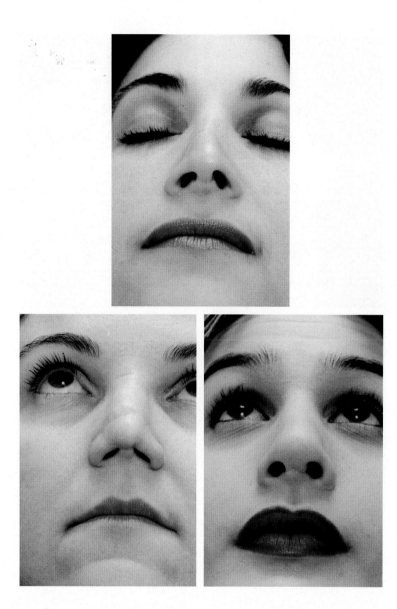

The columellar scar was a relatively infrequent complaint among the open rhinoplasty patients (ranking eleventh out of 15 complaints), but it was distressing to 25% of the patients in this group. Particularly unfortunate deformities can occur when the surgeon resects a portion of the columella, leaving incongruous surfaces with missing normal tissue. Such resections are performed in an effort to reduce large nasal bases or decrease tip projection; but the procedure rests on an anatomic misdiagnosis and creates a deformity for which I currently know no adequate correction.

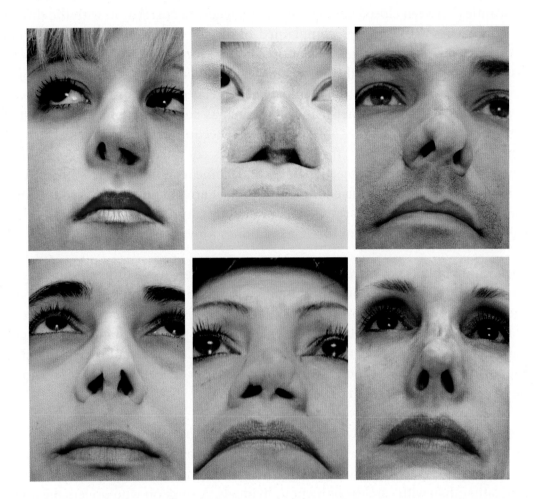

The most severe deformities occur after multiple surgeries, compounded by aggressive dissection, devascularization, deliberate resection, and inadvertent tissue loss. It is here that the concept of using the open approach in a tertiary reconstruction can be most dangerous. Much safer are techniques that allow improvement with limited dissection, limited danger for the patient, and limited access. As should be apparent from inspection alone, the investing nasal tissue is not inviolable.

Comparisons of my review with any previous studies are obviously difficult and must be approached cautiously. However, one report of revisionary surgery on 22 previous open rhinoplasty patients does document related deformities (Daniel, 1995). In that report, nasal base problems occurred with similar frequency to my study (columellar scar: 18%, nostril asymmetry: 27%, excessive infratip lobular fullness: 18%, or distorted nostril apices: 27%). Only 9% of the patients in that study objected to their columellar scars, which contrasts with the 25% in my group.

Although none of this data should be over-interpreted, the divergent spectrum of deformities between closed and open results suggests a correlation with the different approaches. Both groups complained of airway obstruction at the internal valves, an overresected bridge, loss of tip contour from alar cartilage resection, or nasal asymmetry. However, the open rhinoplasty patients were more likely to complain of deformities and functional impairments related to the structures most easily accessed by a transcolumellar incision (such as complaints of alar and nostril distortion or external valvular obstruction) or to techniques that can be performed more readily or aggressively through it (such as complaints of rigid columellar struts, wide columellae, or objectionable scars). Some techniques that would be difficult or impossible using the endonasal approach are of course provided by open rhinoplasty access: columellar resection, or directly suturing the upper or lower lateral cartilages to each other or to the nasal bones for valvular stability.

Open rhinoplasty is not merely a different access route—it is a different operation. Surgeons who prefer the open technique must acknowledge not only the advantages that it affords but the restrictions that it imposes on nasal circulation, accurate surface study, interpretation of dynamic intraoperative changes, and right brain analysis. Despite the volume and enthusiasm of the relevant literature, open rhinoplasty has its own unique catalog of unintended consequences. No one knows the prevalence of these results, even in expert hands.

It is not my aim here to criticize any operating surgeons. When a similar set of preoperative conditions produces the same unintended consequences by different surgeons, the inescapable conclusion is that we are dealing with an error-prone situation, rather than with careless or inept individuals. A surgeon who prefers the open approach should perform it with eyes open to the limitations that it imposes, and be prepared to minimize the potential for the nasal base deformities that are easier to create through the access, exposure, and techniques advocated for this approach.

The surgeon revising open rhinoplasty results must remember the tip suturing or strut techniques that previous surgeons may have used. Tip sutures are only reversible on the day they are placed; once healed, the deformed structures often require repositioning or resection and reconstruction.

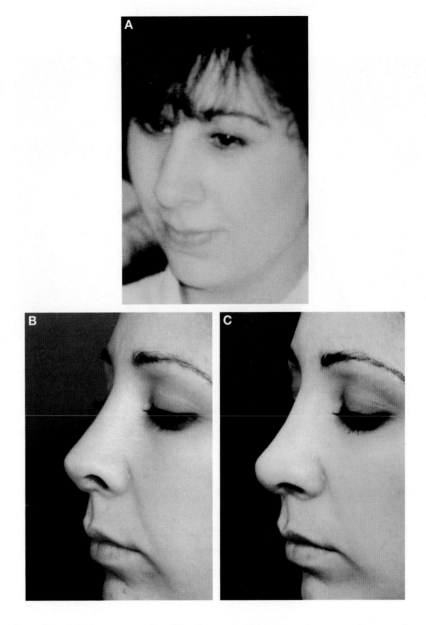

It is true that the open approach affords a surgeon an opportunity to place and secure a columellar strut and determine the angle of tip rotation; but because the strut is not an anatomic correction, it can also broaden and distort the columella and create excessive tip rotation (compare *A* and *B*). Resecting the strut, thinning the columella, and grafting the tip corrects this deformity *(C)*.

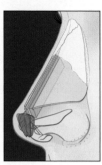

PATIENT STUDY ONE

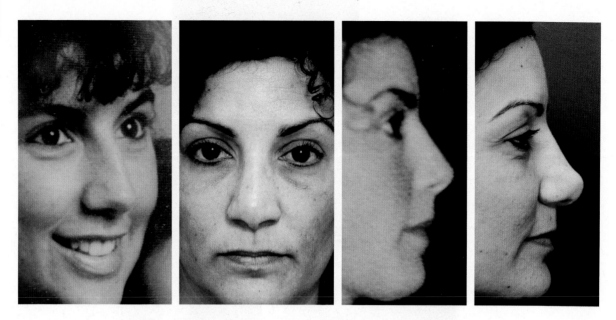

Thick skin creates additional complexity for surgeons performing open rhinoplasty. Although the same can be said for endonasal surgeons, the wider dissection of the open approach, the columellar struts used, and the difficulty of producing a beautiful columellar scar in heavier tissues place thicker-skinned patients at special risk.

This patient's preoperative nose was not especially wide, but two rhinoplasties, reducing dorsal height and tip projection, have allowed the soft tissues to thicken so that surface landmarks have become invisible. The columellar strut has distorted the angle of rotation, raising it to 80 degrees; and relative nasal base size, very difficult to assess during open rhinoplasty, has increased. Dorsal reduction uncovered a high septal deviation toward the right. No septal cartilage was available.

SUMMARY OF THE SURGICAL PLAN

1. Harvest ear cartilage

2. Minimal skeletonization

3. Dissect and remove columellar strut

4. Bilateral ear cartilage spreader grafts, thinner on the right (with a convexity toward the left), thicker on the left

5. Tip grafts

6. Thin crushed graft to supratip

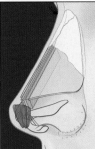

Postoperative Analysis

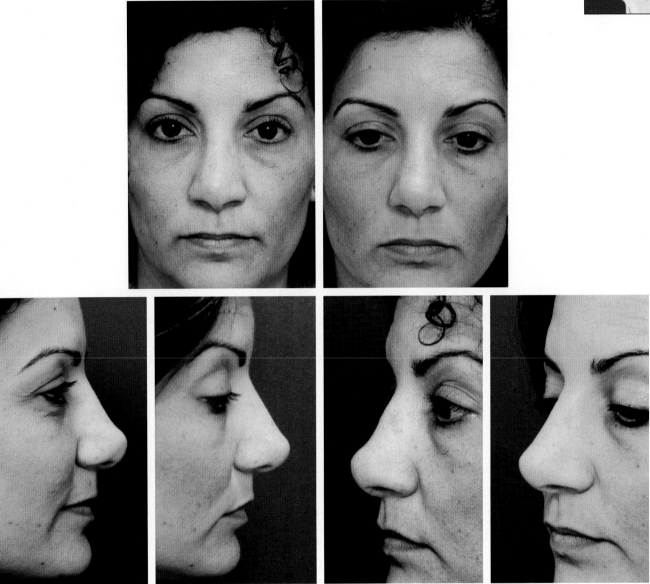

Even 18 months postoperatively, there is very little difference on the frontal view, although the distortion produced by the strut has diminished. Heavy soft tissues hide the airway improvement created by spreader grafts. Pliable ear cartilage will not straighten a high septal deviation as vigorously as stiffer septal or rib cartilage, but the functional improvement is the same. Strut resection and tip grafts have altered the angle of rotation. Rebalancing a nose like this is difficult, because dorsal grafting is not possible; as always, the surgeon is limited by the volume and distribution of the preoperative skin sleeve.

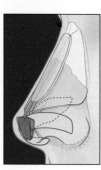

PATIENT STUDY TWO

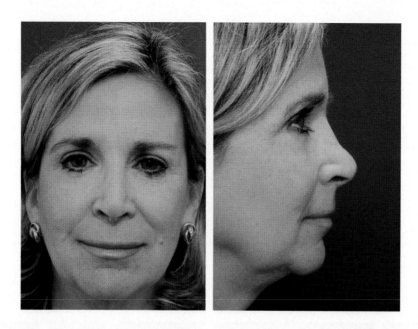

This patient's columellar scar was good, and was located at the junction of the columella and upper lip; but the external valvular and alar wall deformities typify most common adverse open rhinoplasty results. Despite the columellar strut, supratip deformity was present.

SUMMARY OF THE SURGICAL PLAN

1. Minimal skeletonization over bony and upper cartilaginous vaults
2. Rasp dorsum for graft adherence
3. Resect and relocate malpositioned lateral crura
4. Transfix, resect ellipse of posterior membranous septum, remove columellar strut
5. Septoplasty
6. Dorsal graft
7. Tip grafts

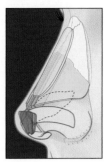

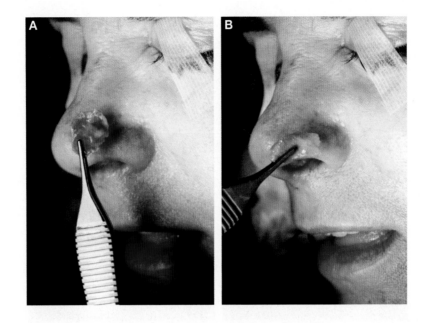

The malpositioned lateral crura were recovered through vestibular skin incisions placed 3 mm above the rims. They were resected at the lateral genua *(A)*, crushed, and replaced *(B)*.

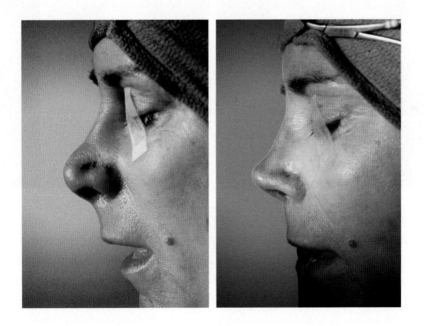

Yellow and blue card photographs show the contour change created only by redraping the soft tissues cephalad and caudad. Dorsal and tip reduction create supratip deformity; dorsal and tip grafts correct it.

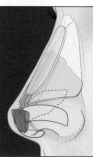

Postoperative Analysis

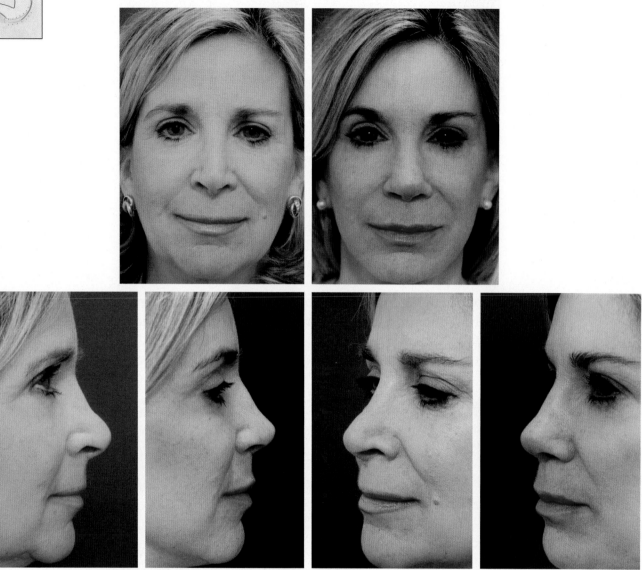

Three years later, the supratip deformity remains corrected. Adequate tip projection is present. The airway has been improved by the dorsal graft (internal valves) and the repositioned lateral crura (external valves). In combination with the septoplasty, geometric mean nasal airflow increased 13.4 times over preoperative values, an unusually high response because of the patient's significant preoperative obstruction.

However, she was unhappy because her postoperative nose remained wider than it had been. She did not see the preoperative tip and alar walls as pinched and collapsed, but rather as narrow. Although she liked her postoperative profile, her new alar wall contour improvement, and her better airway, none of this overcame her dissatisfaction with the postoperative frontal width.

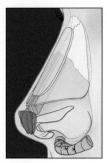

Aside from patient selection issues, one other point must be made. Maximally contracted skin can only redistribute itself—it cannot shrink. Although the alar wall grafts may have bowed postoperatively, some of the patient's postoperative width is attributable to this redistribution, for which I know no acceptable alternative.

PATIENT STUDY THREE

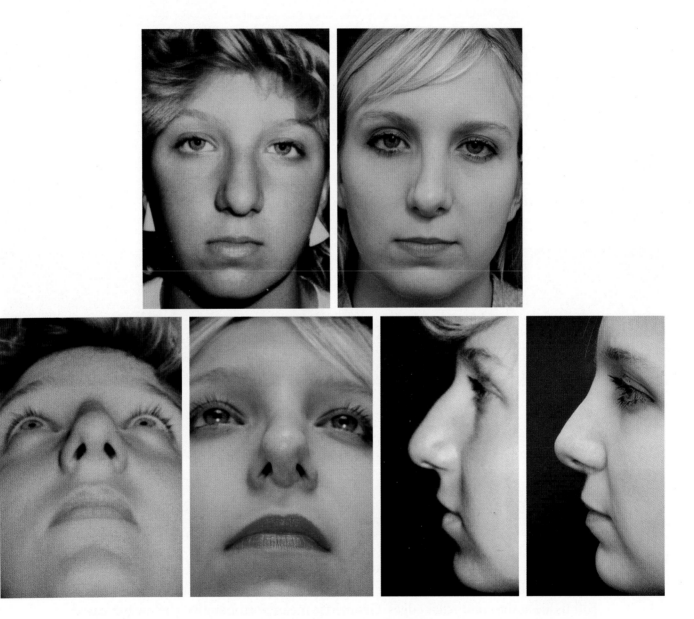

Thick skin may obscure underlying skeletal deformities, but the deformities are nonetheless present. Dorsal and tip reduction have created supratip deformity in this patient; inadequate tip projection remains, despite a columellar strut; and collapse of the internal valves now outlines a high septal deviation toward the patient's left. Only a small amount of septal cartilage was available.

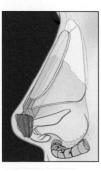

SUMMARY OF THE SURGICAL PLAN

1. Harvest ear cartilage (change gloves)
2. Two-piece Gore-Tex maxillary augmentation
3. Limited skeletonization over bony and upper cartilaginous vaults
4. Resect columellar strut
5. Trim supratip septum
6. Septoplasty
7. Asymmetrical spreader grafts (thicker on right than left)
8. Dorsal graft
9. Tip grafts
10. Excise columellar edges

Postoperative Analysis

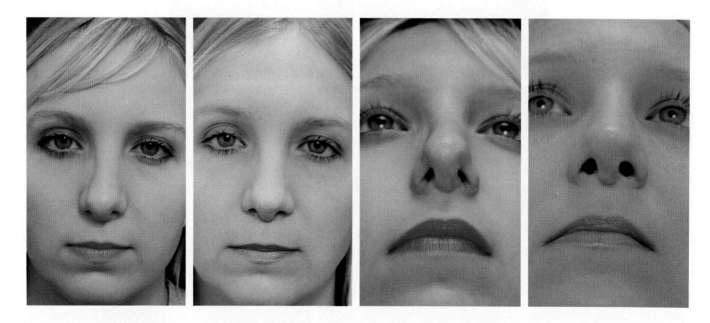

Three years postoperatively, the nose remains more symmetrical. The patient's columella has been narrowed by strut removal and excision of subcutaneous scar and soft tissue at the columellar edges. Geometric mean postoperative airflow increased 4.1 times over preoperative values.

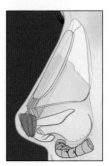

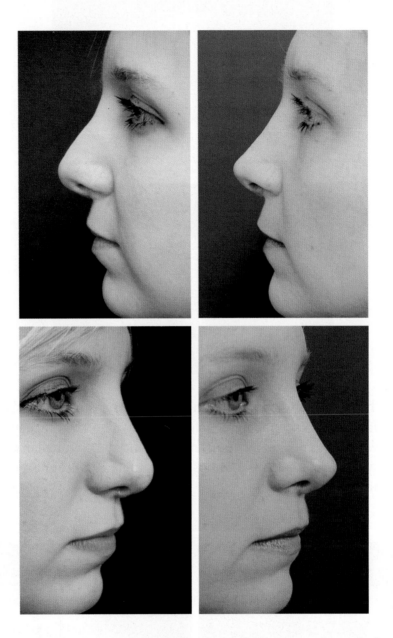

On the lateral view, the dorsum is straight, the radix begins at the right level, and the nose looks less bottom-heavy, even though tip projection has increased. When absolute reduction is not possible, balance and proportion are the surgeon's best allies.

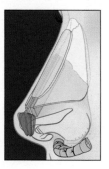

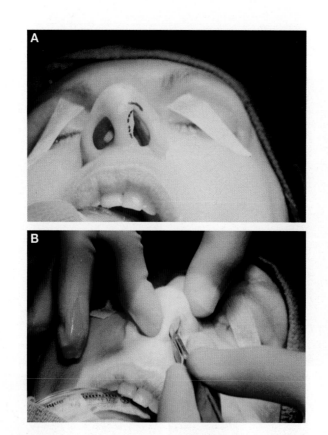

Columellar thinning is shown here in another patient who previously underwent open rhinoplasty. She had a unilateral deformity and a notch at the left soft triangle (to be filled with a composite graft). After removing the columellar strut, I drew a dotted line symmetrical with the opposite columellar contour *(A)*, and incised along this line *(B)*.

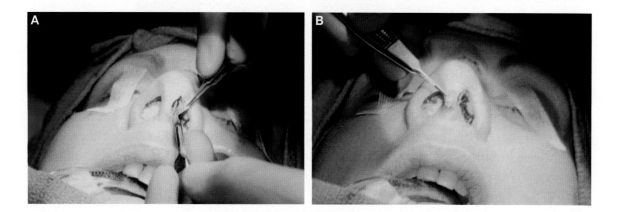

The membranous septal flap was elevated, but no tissue had yet been removed *(A)*. Excess soft tissue was removed from beneath the membranous septal flap *(B)*. In many patients reduction is produced by thinning and rearrangement rather than skin excision.

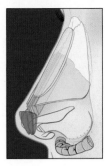

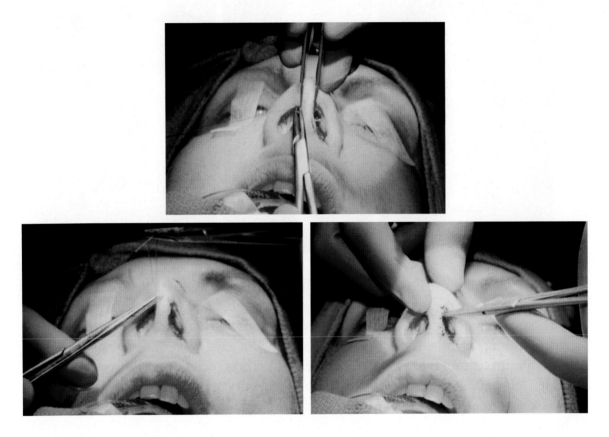

Once thinned, the membranous septal flap redundancy was conservatively sized, and absorbable transfixing sutures closed the dead space. Fine nylon sutures repaired the wound.

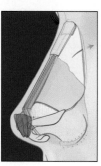

PATIENT STUDY FOUR

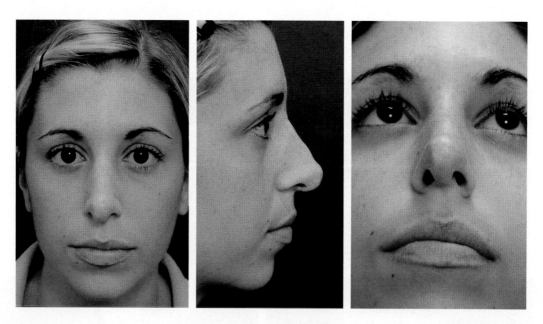

This is a difficult nose because it is so unbalanced and because skeletal distortions, produced by a strut and cartilage suturing, have created knuckles and asymmetries that have attenuated the skin sleeve. There is a high septal deviation toward the right, with tip asymmetry in that direction. The internal valves are compromised, the supratip septum is high, but the lower nasal skin is distended. The bony vault is wide. The best alternative is to reduce the deformity and rebalance, trying to decrease apparent nasal base size by shortening the nose and maintaining dorsal height.

SUMMARY OF THE SURGICAL PLAN

1. Wide skeletonization over upper cartilaginous vault, narrow over bony vault

2. Rasp bony vault for graft adherence; trim anterior septal edge

3. Shorten caudal ends upper lateral cartilages submucosally

4. Transfix, shorten caudal and membranous septa

5. Deliver middle crura through vestibular incisions; resect knuckles

6. Septoplasty

7. Asymmetrical spreader grafts, thicker on left than right

8. Upper dorsal graft

9. Crushed cartilage tip grafts

10. Bilateral osteotomies

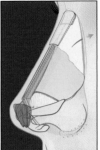

Postoperative Analysis

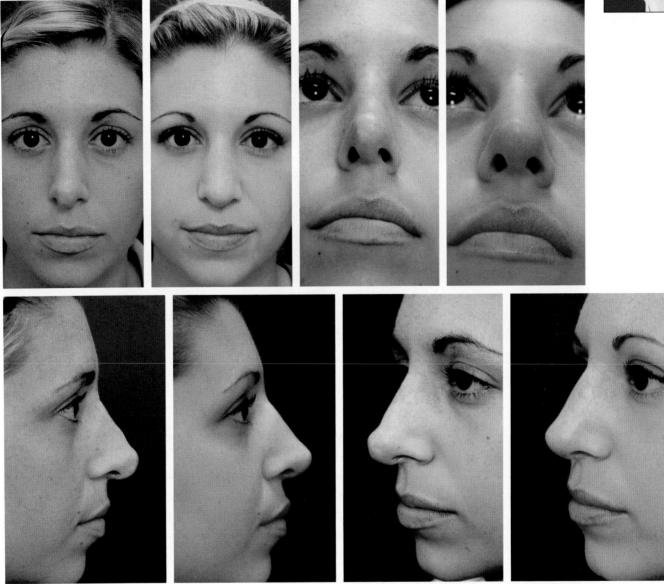

Twenty-two months postoperatively the nose is more symmetrical, and the tip deformities have disappeared. Notice the expression in the patient's eyes. Unfortunately, this is still a bottom-heavy nose. Although only two crushed grafts were used for the tip, the tissues have been sufficiently stiffened by previous surgery to limit their ability to contract further. The dorsum, however, is straight and the angle of tip rotation has improved. Apparent nasal base size has diminished slightly, assisted by nasal shortening, dorsal elevation, and a change in tip lobular contour.

PATIENT STUDY FIVE

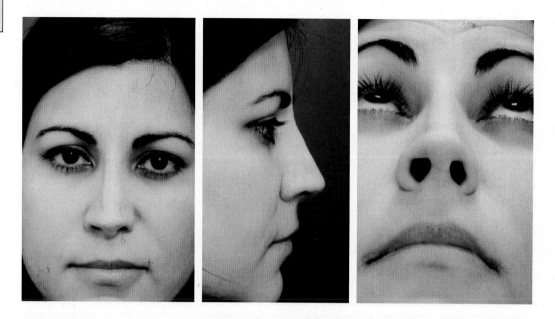

After three rhinoplasties, this patient's two concerns were her nostril shape and the rigidity of her lower nose. She recognized that her alar walls had uneven contours, and was unhappy that each nostril was shaped differently.

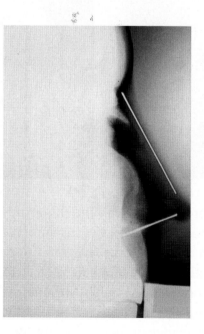

A radiograph shows why the nose was so rigid. Dorsal and columellar grafts fixed to one another and to the facial skeleton are as uncompromising as an L-shaped silicone strut. Although such constructions create stability and can produce very good cosmetic results, they are nonanatomic solutions and do trouble some patients. The normal tip moves independently of the bony and upper cartilaginous vaults, a fact that is related to its anatomic investiture between the external and vestibular skin. As such, the alar cartilages float like a cap anterior to the remaining nasal skeleton, which explains why the nose shortens when the dorsum is reduced and lengthens when it is raised (see Chapter 1).

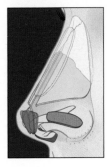

SUMMARY OF THE SURGICAL PLAN

1. Harvest ear cartilage
2. Resect columellar strut and maxillary wire
3. Shorten lateral crural grafts
4. Trim caudal end, dorsal graft
5. Alar wall grafts (to simulate lateral crura)
6. Tip grafts
7. Columellar grafts

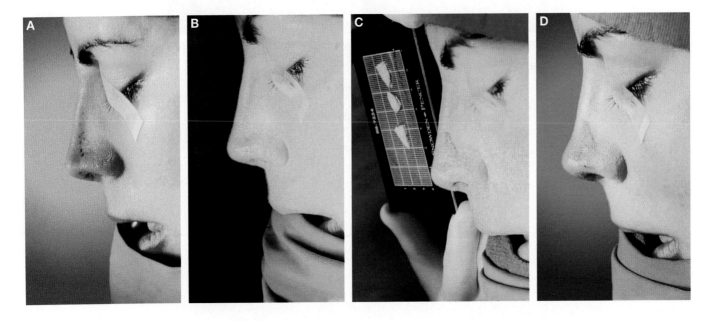

The wire was exposed through a short intraoral incision and pulled forward out of the maxilla after the columellar strut had been cut. As expected, very little immediate change in tip projection occurred *(B)*, but the tip lobule and columella were now soft. The lateral crural grafts were cut short so that they no longer extended so far posteriorly and now floated in the alar soft tissues, enough to support the rims but no longer braced against the pyriform aperture edges. Crushed ear cartilage was used for the tip and columella, and to create the surface markings of the missing lateral crura *(C)*.

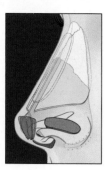

Postoperative Analysis

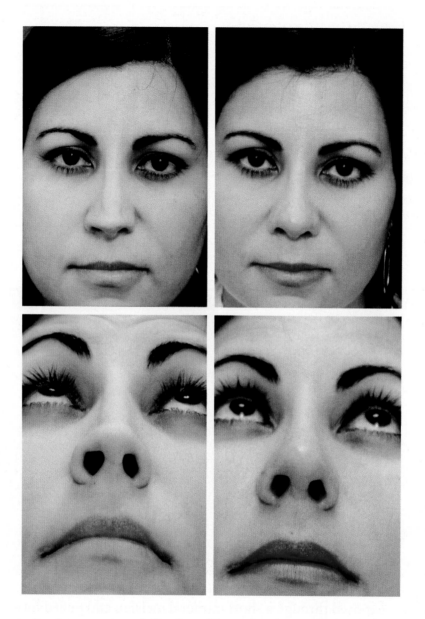

Postoperatively, the severity of the dorsal lines has been diminished, partly by releasing the soft tissues from the dorsal, columellar, and lateral crural struts, and partly by grafting the tip to form a discrete, independent lobule. The alar rims have become more symmetrical, no longer tethered by long lateral crural grafts. The columellar/lobular angle is softer, and the tip is slightly less angular and now projects beyond the septal angle. The alar walls are smooth and slightly convex.

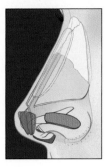

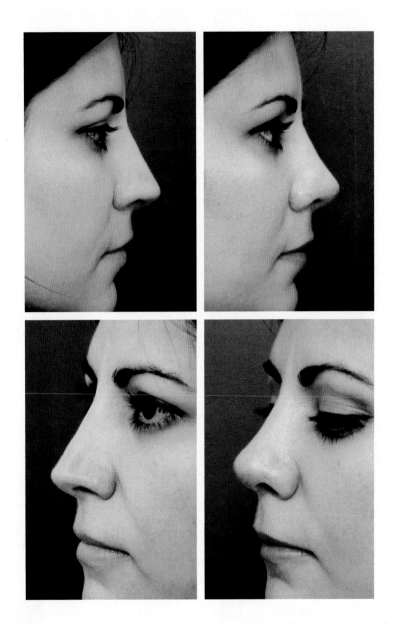

Of all the open rhinoplasty examples in this section, this was certainly the best preoperative result. Contour lines were smooth, the airway was open, and the columellar scar was very good. Yet the mechanisms used to support the nose created an artifactual rigidity and contour that this patient could not accept.

Complex Deformities

By using the phrase *complex deformities,* I mean to indicate anything out of the ordinary: unusual patient requests, combinations of donor sites, or deformities limited by cutaneous scars and multiple surgeries.

The management principles, however, do not change. Identify the visible deformity, the airway obstruction, and the important anatomic variants and their sequelae. Select the best donor sites. Remove or reposition the deforming structures. Augment to restore function, to improve contour, and also to create proper proportion.

PATIENT STUDY ONE

Body image is a personal issue. I do not believe that a surgeon must decide whether a patient's goal is justifiable, whether it seems right to the surgeon, or whether the surgeon would want the same goal for himself or herself. What is important is *whether the goal is achievable for the surgeon who is going to provide the result, and whether the surgeon believes that the patient will be happy with the result.*

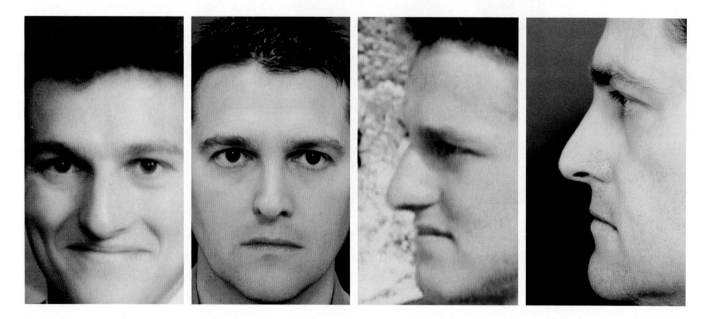

This gentleman had undergone airway surgery, and at the last minute agreed to small external changes. The result upset him greatly. Not only was his airway newly diminished, but he was disconcerted by the reduced nasal size. He could not accept the straight, narrow dorsum or the tapered tip, and wanted as much of his preoperative appearance restored as possible.

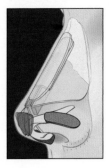

In these circumstances, it is important for the surgeon to explain that the skin sleeve itself has also changed, and therefore restoration of exact nasal dimensions is not possible. Yet a great deal can be done. Fortunately for this man, his septum was untouched.

SUMMARY OF THE SURGICAL PLAN

1. Limited skeletonization over bony and upper cartilaginous vaults
2. Rasp bony vault for graft adherence
3. Septoplasty
4. Asymmetrical spreader grafts (right thicker than left)
5. Layered dorsal graft, placed deliberately low to produce a notch at the radix
6. Tip grafts placed caudally (to produce inadequate tip projection)
7. Columellar grafts
8. Alar wall grafts

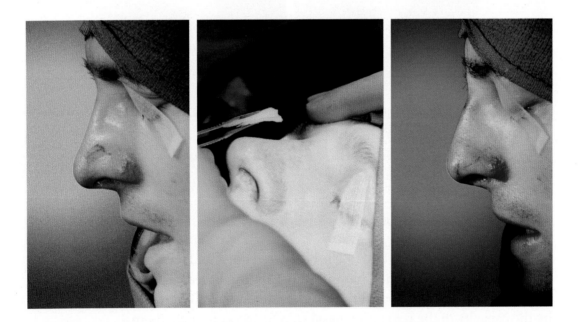

The patient's septum provided ample cartilage for a layered dorsal graft to rebuild his preoperative convexity.

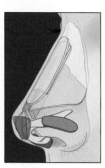

Postoperative Analysis

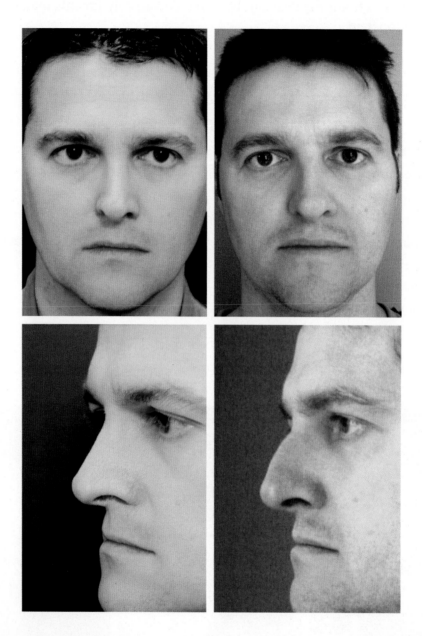

One year postoperatively, the nose is broader, higher, and longer. Restoration of internal valvular competence has substantially increased airflow. Layered dorsal grafts reconstructed the patient's considerable preoperative arch, fortunately aided by the capacity of the remaining nasal skin to accommodate them.

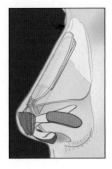

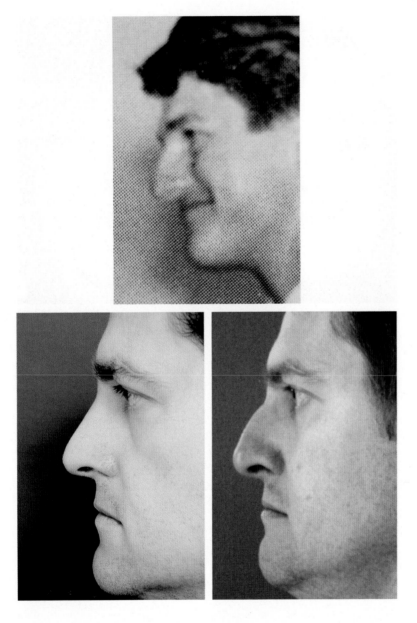

Augmenting the caudal tip lobule and columella has increased nasal length slightly and recreated the bow of the preoperative columella. There is a subtle but real expression change in the patient's eyes.

PATIENT STUDY TWO

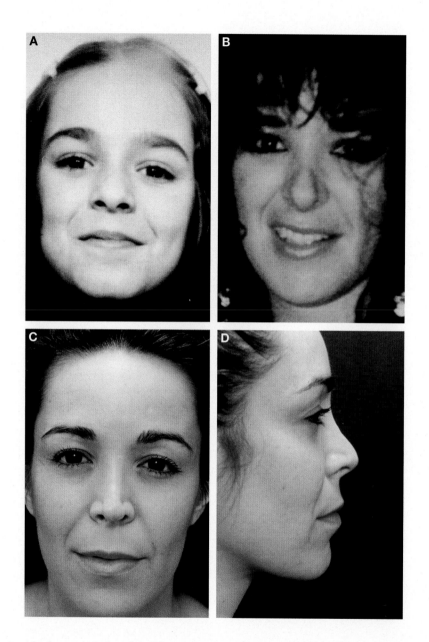

The personal photographs that this young woman supplied trace the evolution of her deformity. As a teenager, malpositioned lateral crura are easily visible *(A)*. Following the first rhinoplasty, dorsal and tip reduction collapsed the sidewalls *(B)*. An additional surgery produced the preoperative appearance with notched alar rims and almost no ability to breathe through the nose *(C)*. The patient's thin skin had contracted, producing a tight supratip deformity *(D)*.

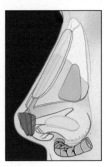

SUMMARY OF THE SURGICAL PLAN

1. Harvest calvarial bone
2. Harvest composite grafts
3. Harvest conchal cartilage
4. Gore-Tex maxillary augmentation
5. Minimal skeletonization over bony and upper cartilaginous vaults
6. Dorsal graft of calvarial bone
7. Lateral wall calvarial grafts
8. Alar wall calvarial grafts
9. Conchal cartilage tip grafts with calvarial buttress
10. Conchal cartilage grafts to anterior columella
11. Bilateral composite grafts, coronal orientation

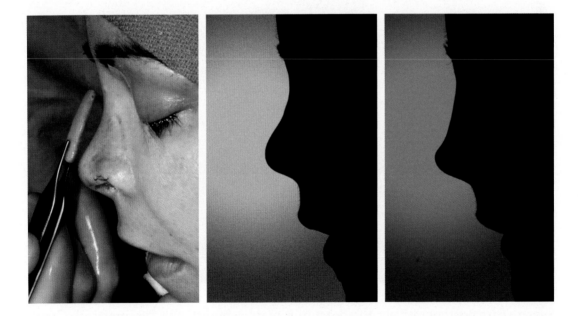

A longer dorsal graft than usual has been created to recover maximum nasal length. Silhouettes dramatize the intraoperative changes achieved.

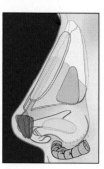

Postoperative Analysis

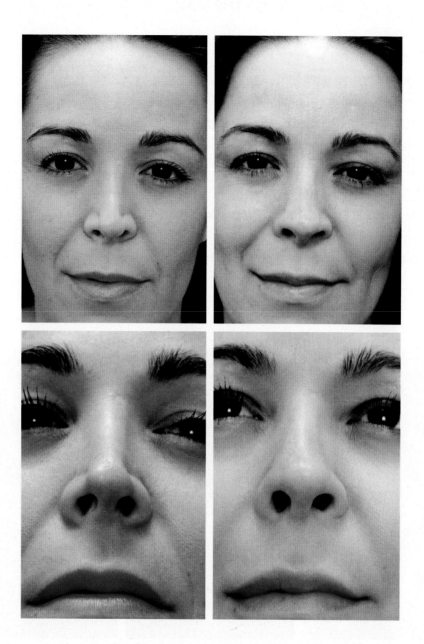

Seven years postoperatively, the dorsum remains smooth and symmetrical. Composite grafts have recreated the alar walls and corrected the retraction. Multiple tip grafts form a smooth lobule. The columella has been displaced caudally and occupies a more normal position, although a notch remains at the previous scar site.

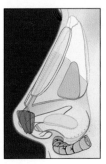

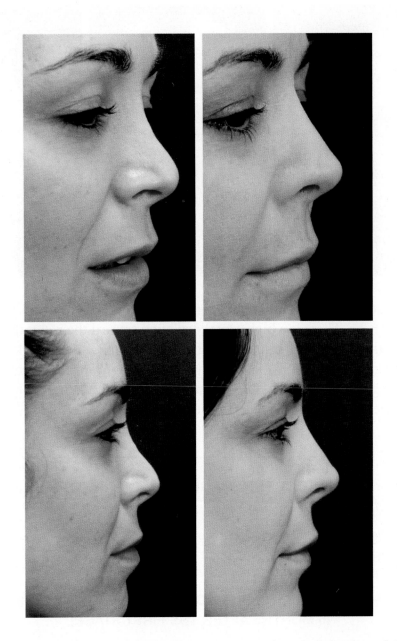

A combination of dorsal grafting and augmenting the caudal sides of the tip and columella has increased apparent nasal length, even in this tight skin sleeve. Geometric mean nasal airflow increased 3.8 times over preoperative values.

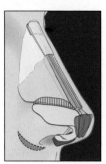

Patient Study Three

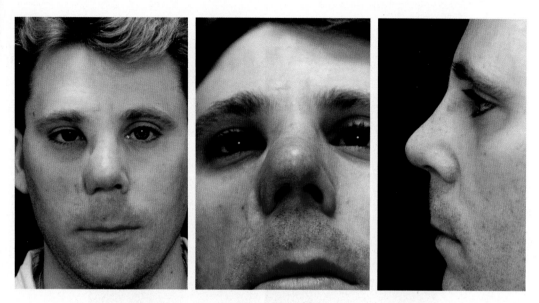

The combination of a childhood hemangioma and previous trauma has distorted this patient's nose. There is a high septal deviation toward the right, the dorsum is slightly low, the supratip is high, the soft tissues are thick, and the right alar base is malpositioned. Previous surgeons had thinned the right medial cheek and upper lip, improving contour but effacing the nasolabial fold. Previous alar base scars are apparent. The correction will be performed in stages

---

SUMMARY OF THE SURGICAL PLAN: FIRST STAGE

1. Thin soft tissues, right sidewall; place percutaneous sutures
2. Right alar base flap, repositioning base cephalad
3. Excise right alar rim skin

SUMMARY OF THE SURGICAL PLAN: SECOND STAGE
(6 MONTHS AFTER THE FIRST STAGE)

1. Minimal skeletonization over bony and upper cartilaginous vaults
2. Harvest ear cartilage
3. Septoplasty
4. Asymmetrical spreader grafts, left thicker than right (preoperative asymmetry)
5. Layered upper dorsal graft
6. Tip grafts
7. Columellar grafts
8. Revise right alar crease scars

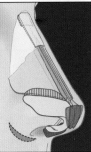

Postoperative Analysis

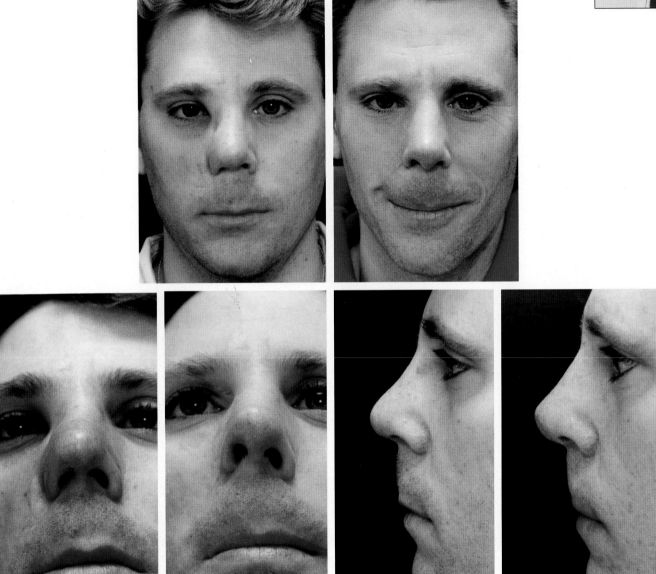

Five years postoperatively, the alar bases remain symmetrical. Some hypertrophy has occurred at the cephalic end of my right nasolabial fold scar revision. Dorsal and spreader grafts have aligned the upper nose; the right sidewall remains flat following thinning procedures. Tip grafts separate the tip lobule from the dorsum. The right alar crease is reasonably well defined, but when soft tissue deficits are present, this landmark often becomes effaced as time passes. Dorsal and tip grafts have flattened the supratip and added nasal length. Geometric mean nasal airflow increased 4.0 times over preoperative values.

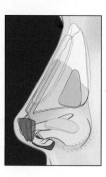

PATIENT STUDY FOUR

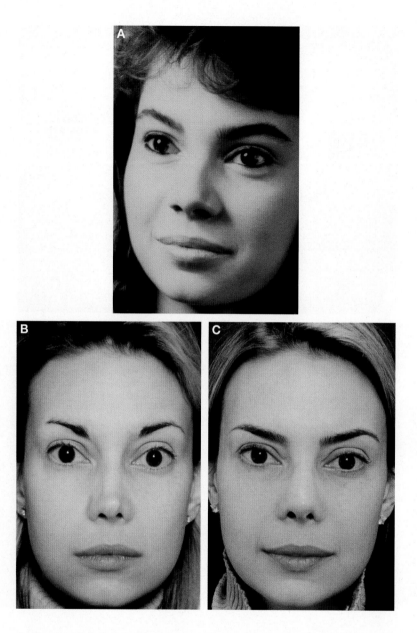

This patient's desire to have a slightly smaller nose in the same shape started a cascade of unhappy experiences. She was treated by multiple experts and underwent septal surgery and rib grafts, and then sought treatment from Dr. Sheen *(B)*. He placed new rib grafts *(C)*, then referred her to me when he retired.

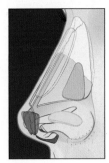

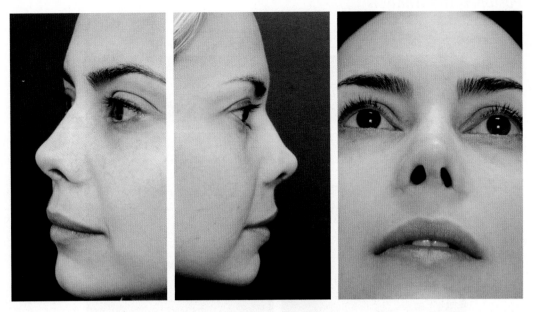

A number of problems remained. The patient thought that her nose was still too short. The alar rims were high, notched, and uneven. The deficit produced by alar wedge resections had created hypertrophic scars. Dorsal asymmetries remained, with the left supratip lower than the right. Repeated open rhinoplasties had left a notched columellar scar; nostril diameter was uneven, the left side was stenotic, and the columellar base pulled toward the patient's left. No septal cartilage was available. Fortunately, parts of both conchae remained.

SUMMARY OF THE SURGICAL PLAN: FIRST STAGE

1. Crushed ear cartilage grafts to left upper vault, adjacent to dorsal graft

2. Coronal composite grafts to alar rims

3. Tip grafts to caudal lobule and columella

SUMMARY OF THE SURGICAL PLAN: SECOND STAGE (1 YEAR LATER)

1. Axial composite graft left nostril

2. Revise columellar scar; crushed ear cartilage grafts to columella

SUMMARY OF THE SURGICAL PLAN: THIRD STAGE (1 YEAR LATER)

1. Revise old alar wedge resection scars

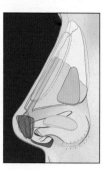

Postoperative Analysis

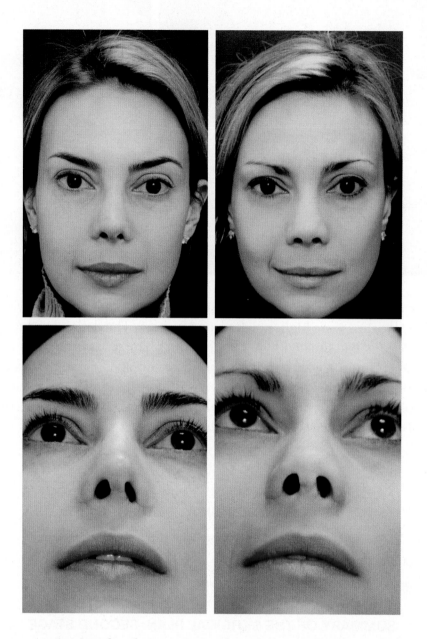

Five years postoperatively, alar retraction has decreased. When tension was reduced at the alar bases, the patient's scar hypertrophy self-corrected. The vestibular stenosis has improved, although the columella still veers toward her left. The nose seems longer and more symmetrical.

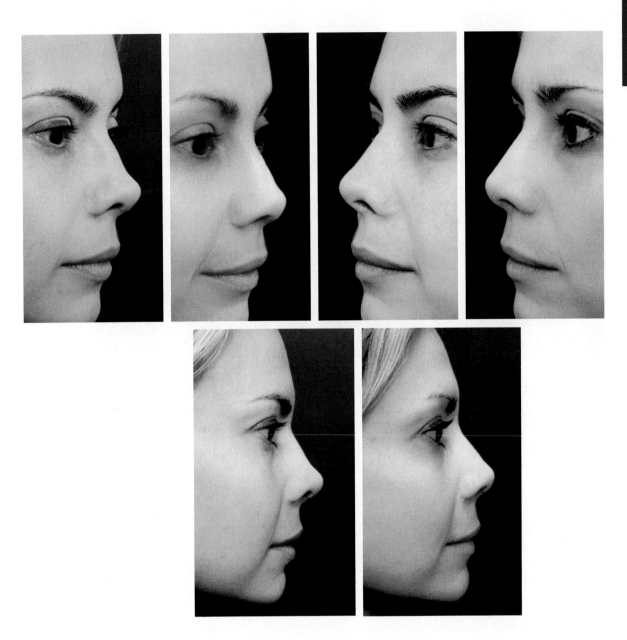

Crushed ear cartilage grafts must be used cautiously. Uncrushed ear cartilage is not flat. Even crushed, it retains asymmetrical stresses on its two surfaces, and can deform postoperatively, bowing the grafted area outward, providing a bonus augmentation that the surgeon and patient do not want. These grafts must be crushed sufficiently (remembering to protect their survival), trimmed to fit, and placed accurately. Slight undercorrection is often wise.

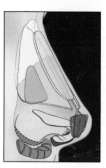

PATIENT STUDY FIVE

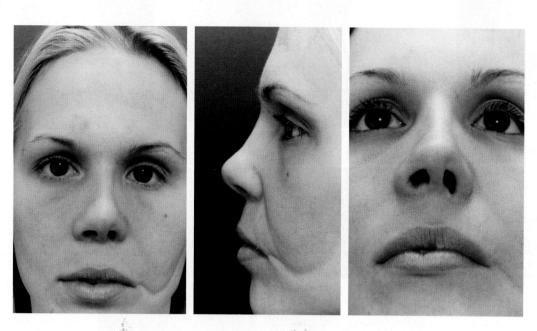

A severe motor vehicle accident followed by three rhinoplasties (the last of which included a rib graft) had left this patient with a distorted nasal base, airway obstruction, and a nose that she believed was too short. The rib dorsal graft had shifted toward her left. Her maxillary arch remained retrusive, and her tip blunt.

SUMMARY OF THE SURGICAL PLAN

1. Harvest rib cartilage
2. Two piece maxillary augmentation, thicker on left than right
3. Minimal skeletonization over bony and upper cartilaginous vaults
4. Remove old rib graft
5. Rasp dorsum for graft adherence
6. Rib cartilage dorsal graft
7. Right lateral wall graft
8. Multiple tip grafts
9. Columellar grafts
10. Composite graft from right alar lobule to left nasal floor

---

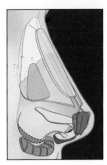

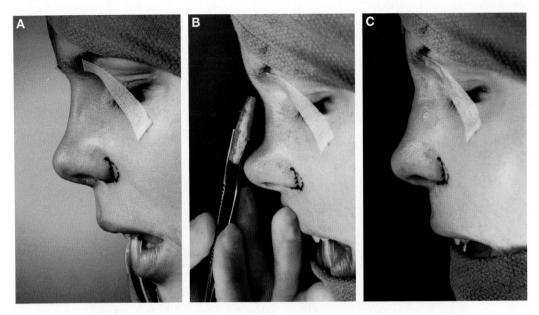

Once the old rib graft was removed, the nose shortened (compare *A* and *B*). A thicker, longer rib graft was prepared and placed, which immediately regained nasal length, reduced apparent nasal base size, and created internal valvular competence *(C)*.

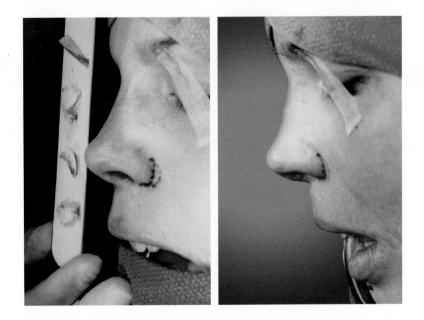

Shavings of rib cartilage were used for the nasal tip and columella. They increased real and apparent nasal length.

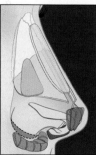

Postoperative Analysis

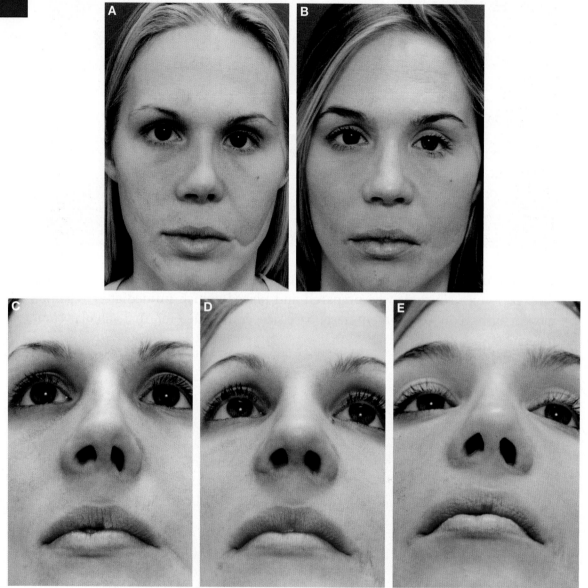

At 28 months postoperatively, the nose remains more symmetrical. The dorsal graft has added real length. The upper lip retrusion has improved. Inferior views reveal that the improvements seen in the left nasal floor at two months *(D)*, produced by a composite graft taken from the alar lobule, have diminished by 50% at 2 years. A skin/cartilage composite graft from the ear may have produced a longer-lasting result, but the patient declined further surgery.

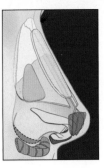

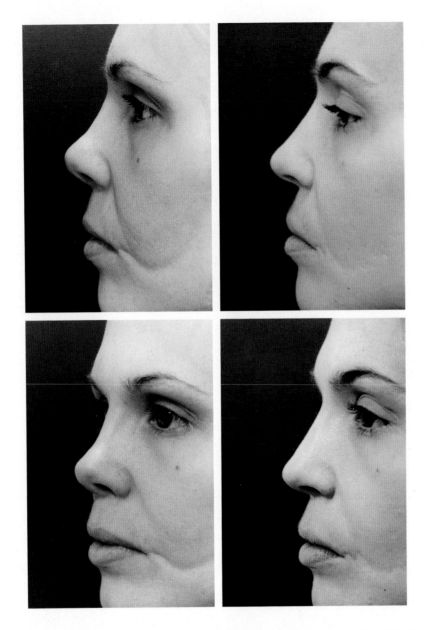

Of all the techniques for increasing nasal length, the most predictable is a significant dorsal graft—and the effect can be further augmented by also filling the undersides of the tip lobule and columella. However, the length achieved always depends on the pliability of the investing nasal skin and lining.

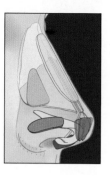

PATIENT STUDY SIX

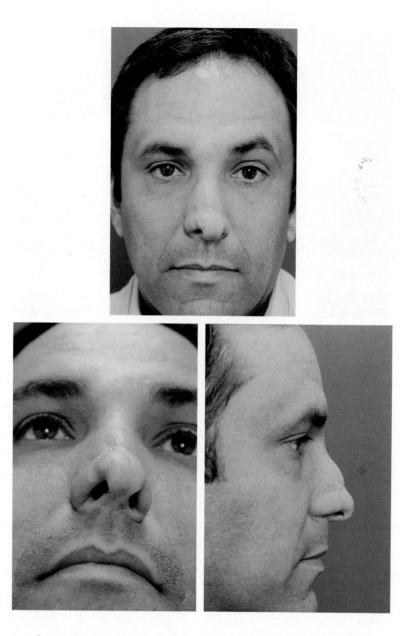

Four previous rhinoplasties had left this patient with a grossly distorted nose and a diminished airway. The patient's septum had been resected. Previous surgeons, in haste to revise early, had perforated the dorsal skin, leaving a nearly circumferential scar that encircled the tip lobule. The alar walls were flaccid, and the combination of the constricting scar and lack of support had allowed the nasal base to collapse toward the patient's left.

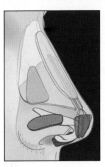

SUMMARY OF THE SURGICAL PLAN

1. Harvest rib cartilage
2. Limited skeletonization through a single cartilage-splitting incision
3. Trim dorsum of residual cartilage and scar
4. Rib cartilage dorsal graft
5. Fillet left alar wall through vestibular incision, releasing contracture
6. Left alar wall grafts
7. Right-sided lateral wall graft
8. Tip grafts
9. Columellar grafts

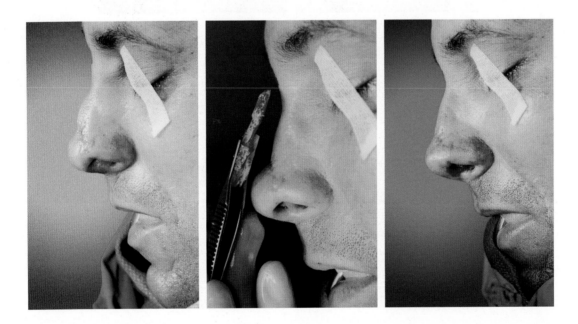

The patient's rib cartilage was typically rigid for his age. However, the underlying skeleton was so irregular, and the dermis was damaged so unevenly that the graft had to be contoured so that its center was thinner than either its cephalic or caudal ends. A second layer was added in the supratip. Only the proximal and distal ends of the graft were covered by perichondrium. Once in place, notice that the tension supplied by the dorsal graft seemed to smooth even the cutaneous scars. As I dissected the left alar sidewall, the contracture unfurled, and the tip rotated toward the midline. An alar wall graft stabilized the correction.

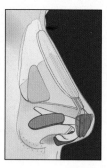

Postoperative Analysis

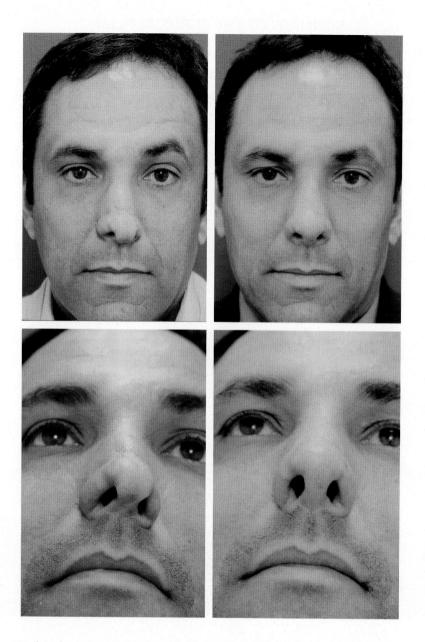

Postoperatively, the nose remains stable and symmetrical. Airflow has improved significantly. The rigidity supplied by mature costal cartilage worked in the patient's favor. Almost more interesting than any of the other configurational changes is the improvement in the cutaneous scars, visible even early in his postoperative course, and a reminder that the dynamic equilibrium of many scars can be modified by stress. Although this man had held a high level executive position for 20 years with his deformity, his eyes show a gratifying change in expression.

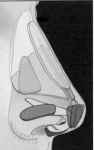

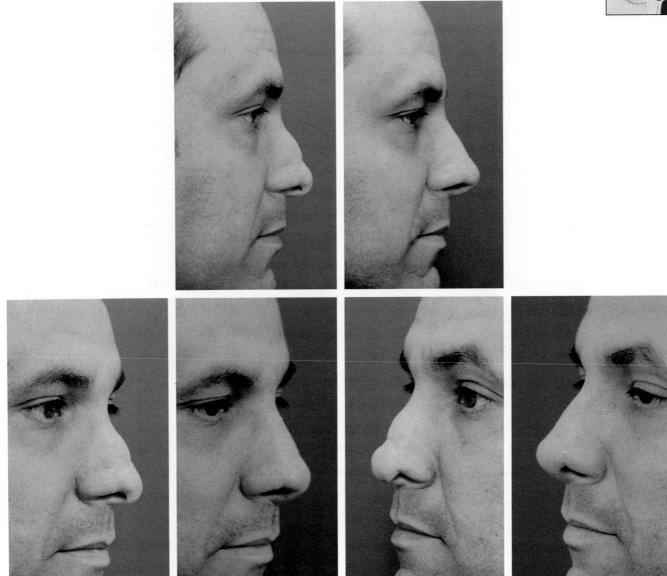

PATIENT STUDY SEVEN

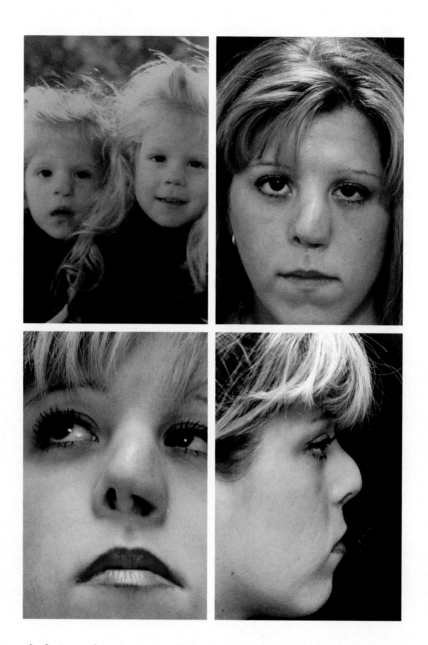

This woman's fraternal twin sister did not share her congenital anomaly. When I first saw the patient, she had undergone three surgeries, and septal cartilage was unavailable. Her airway was significantly compromised. Her original alar rim asymmetry persisted, and the columella had been broadened with a strut and was crisscrossed by scars.

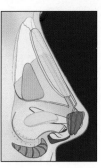

SUMMARY OF THE SURGICAL PLAN: FIRST STAGE

1. Harvest rib cartilage
2. Single stage maxillary augmentation
3. Harvest composite graft
4. Limited skeletonization through a single cartilage-splitting incision
5. Rasp bony vault; remove old septal cartilage graft from supratip
6. Rib cartilage dorsal graft
7. Right composite graft, coronal orientation
8. Excise left alar rim
9. Tip graft
10. Columellar grafts

SUMMARY OF THE SURGICAL PLAN: SECOND STAGE (1 YEAR AFTER FIRST STAGE)

1. Harvest ear cartilage
2. Remove and reposition dorsal graft
3. Thin and contour left alar wall
4. Augment tip further
5. Thin columella
6. Graft right lateral wall

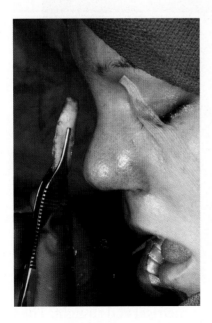

The dorsal graft was carved to fit the asymmetrical defect.

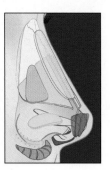

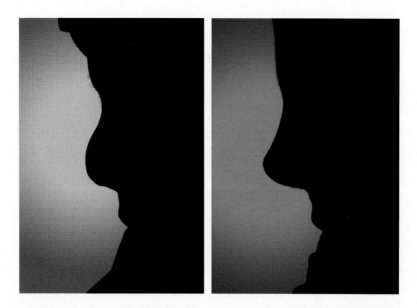

The combination of dorsal grafts, tip grafts, maxillary augmentation, and columellar augmentation altered the nasal profile dramatically. The patient's dorsal graft shifted toward the right after the first procedure and was repositioned during the second stage. When the underlying bony platform is asymmetrical or the nose is extremely short (so that the tight skin sleeve might displace the dorsal graft proximally), I immobilize the dorsal graft with one or two 0.7 mm smooth Kirschner wires, which are removed at 7 days. Further immobilization has not been necessary.

Postoperative Analysis

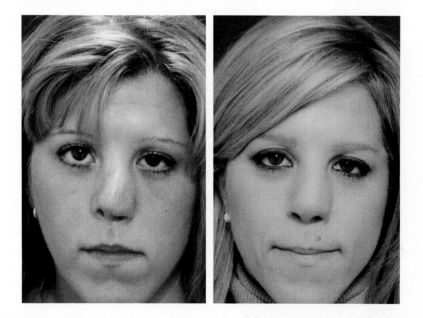

Ten years postoperatively, the nose remains symmetrical and straight. The left alar rim excision and the right composite graft have improved nostril symmetry.

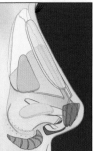

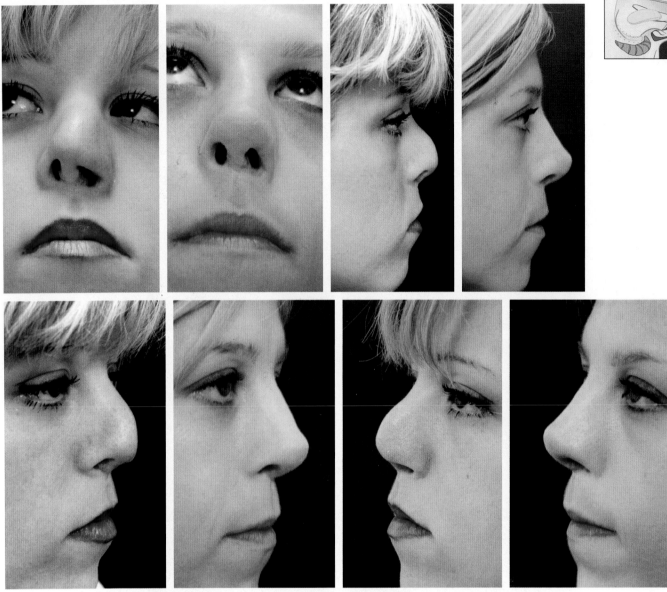

The columella has narrowed, but remains too wide. Geometric mean nasal airflow increased 5.1 times over preoperative values. The dorsal line is straight, with adequate tip projection and a good relationship of the columella to the alar rim.

This patient's preoperative tip lobule was small and tight, but the combination of her age and staged surgery allowed me to achieve normal projection. It is important not to press the tissues too far: not every reconstruction can be performed in a single session, particularly when tip or columellar augmentations are required beneath tight, scarred tertiary tissues.

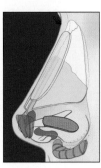

PATIENT STUDY EIGHT

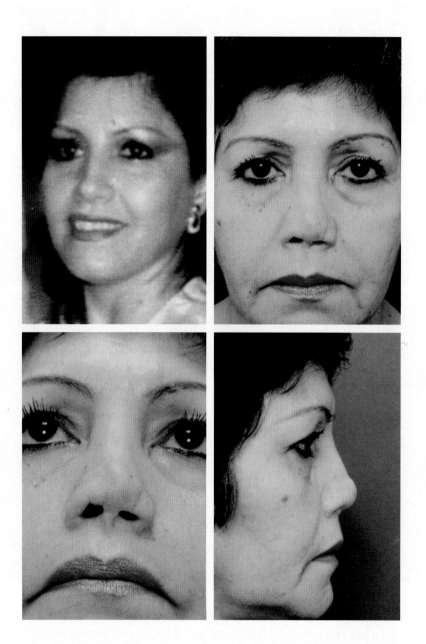

This woman had undergone five rhinoplasties that used all available septal and ear cartilage. Her dorsal strut had collapsed, producing a soft supratip and a nose held distally only by a small ear cartilage graft in the supratip. A large septal perforation left only 12 mm of intact vestibular lining above the columella. Her maxillary arch was retrusive. The tissues were rigid with scars.

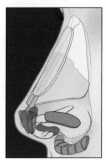

This patient's reconstruction must be staged, and the surgeon must be careful not to raise patient expectations too high. My goal in the first procedure was only to restore the airway and a stable nasal dorsum. I anticipated that two additional procedures would be needed, each separated by at least 1 year. Incisions must be planned cautiously, because this patient cannot afford another unsuccessful procedure or further soft tissue loss. The entire operation will be done through four short incisions.

SUMMARY OF THE SURGICAL PLAN

1. Harvest rib cartilage

2. Maxillary augmentation

3. Excise ear cartilage grafts in supratip through vestibular incision, left

4. Dorsal graft, placed through transverse incision at nasal radix, immobilized with two 1.6 mm by 6 mm self-tapping screws

5. Left alar wall graft

6. Caudal support graft

7. Tip graft

Postoperative Analysis

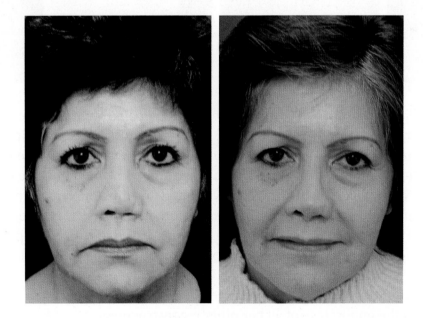

These images were taken 7 months after the successful first stage. The airway correction is complete. The dorsum and alar rims are stable.

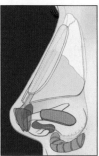

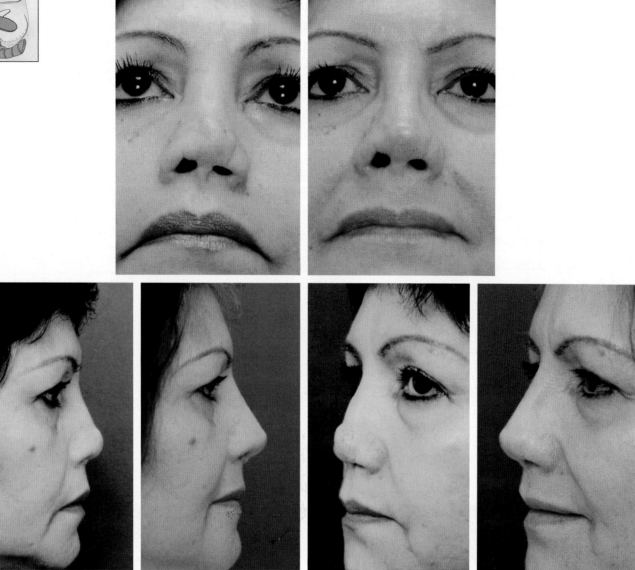

Her maxillary retrusion has been corrected, her caudal septum is braced, and her tip contour has improved. No soft tissue was lost. Limited access, limited dissection, and autogenous augmentation provided this patient's best chance for a lifetime solution. However, her nostrils remain asymmetrical: the right side requires a composite graft if one can be harvested without deforming the remaining ear. Her heavily scarred tip skin, still pink after expansion, needs time to recover. The columella will never expand normally under the transverse scars. As healing proceeds, more problems may develop. Adequate long-term follow-up is required.

Yet something else indefinable has happened here, seen in the patient's eyes, that may exceed the importance of all her other reconstructions.

The magic never stops.

BIBLIOGRAPHY

Adams WP Jr, Rohrich RJ, Gunter J, et al. The rate of warping in irradiated and nonirradiated homograft rib cartilage: a controlled comparison and clinical implications. Plast Reconstr Surg 103:265-270, 1999.

Adams WP Jr, Rohrich RJ, Hollier LH, et al. Anatomic basis and clinical implications for nasal tip support in open versus closed rhinoplasty. Plast Reconstr Surg 103:255-261, 1999.

Adamson PA, McGraw-Wall BL, Morrow TA, et al. Vertical dome division in open rhinoplasty. Arch Otolaryngol Head Neck Surg 120:373, 1994.

Adamson PA, Smith O, Tropper GJ. Incisional and scar analysis in open (external) rhinoplasty. Arch Otolaryngol Head Neck Surg 116:671, 1990.

Agarwal R, Bhatnagar SK, Pandey SD, et al. Nasal sill augmentation in adult incomplete cleft lip nose deformity using superiorly based turn over orbicularis oris muscle flap: an anatomic approach. Plast Reconstr Surg 102:1350-1357, 1998.

Ahuja RB. Primary definitive nasal correction in patients presenting for late unilateral cleft lip patients. Plast Reconstr Surg 110:17-24, 2002.

Ahuja RB. Radical correction of secondary nasal deformity in unilateral cleft lip patients presenting late. Plast Reconstr Surg 108:1127-1135, 2001.

Bafaqeeh SA, Al-Qattan MM. Open rhinoplasty: columellar scar analysis in an Arabian population. Plast Reconstr Surg 102:1226-1228, 1998.

Baran CN, Tiftikcioglu YP, Baran NK. The use of alloplastic materials in secondary rhinoplasties: 32 years experience. Plast Reconstr Surg 116:1502, 2005.

Bassichis BA, Thomas JR. Foreign-body inclusion cyst presenting on the lateral nasal sidewall 1 year after rhinoplasty. Arch Facial Plast Surg 5:530-532, 2003.

Becker H. Nasal augmentation with calcium hydroxylapatite in a carrier-based gel. Plast Reconstr Surg 121:2142-2147, 2008.

Beekhuis GJ. Silastic alar-columellar prosthesis in conjunction with rhinoplasty. Arch Otolaryngol 108:429-432, 1982.

Bejar I, Farkas LG, Messner AH, et al. Nasal growth after external septoplasty in children. Arch Otolaryngol Head Neck Surg 122:816-821, 1996.

Berghaus A, Mulch G, Handrock M. Porous polyethylene and Proplast: their behavior in a bony implant bed. Arch Otorhinolaryngol 240:115-123, 1984.

Berman WE. Balancing the nasal tip height with a potential pollybeak. Ear Nose Throat J 73:854, 1994.

Bikhazi NB, Chow AW, Maas CS. Nasal reconstruction using a combination of alloplastic materials and autogenous tissues: a surgical alternative. Laryngoscope 107:1086-1093, 1997.

Boccieri A, Pascali M. Open rhinoplasty without transcolumellar incision. Plast Reconstr Surg 97:321-326, 1996.

Botti G. Thick skin and cosmetic surgery of the nasal tip: how to avoid the cutaneous polly beak. Aesth Plast Surg 20:421-427, 1996.

Bradley JP, Kawamoto HK, Taub P. Correction of warfarin-induced nasal hypoplasia. Plast Reconstr Surg 111:1680-1687, 2003.

Bravo FG, Schwarze HP. Closed-open rhinoplasty with extended lip dissection: a new concept and classification of rhinoplasty. Plast Reconstr Surg 122:944-950, 2008.

Burgess LP, Everton DM, Quilligan JJ, et al. Complications of the external (combination) rhinoplasty approach. Arch Otolaryngol Head Neck Surg 112:1064-1068, 1986.

Byrd S, Andochick S, Copit S, et al. Septal extension grafts: a method of controlling tip projection shape. Plast Reconstr Surg 100:999-1010, 1997.

Byrd S, Salomon J. Primary correction of the unilateral cleft nasal deformity. Plast Reconstr Surg 106:1276-1286, 2000.

Chait LA. The "C" costal cartilage graft in reconstruction of the unilateral cleft lip nose. Br J Plast Surg 34:169-172, 1981.

Chang Y, Chen Y, Noordhoff MS. One-stage salvage of fractured nasal prosthesis with immediate calvarial bone grafting. Aesth Plast Surg 12:235-237, 1988.

Cho BC. Correction of unilateral cleft lip nasal deformity in preschool and school-aged children with refined reverse-u incision and v-y plasty: long-term follow-up results. Plast Reconstr Surg 119:267-275, 2007.

Clark MP, Greenfield B, Hunt N, et al. Function of the nasal muscles in normal subjects assessed by dynamic MRI and EMG: its relevance to rhinoplasty surgery. Plast Reconstr Surg 101:1945-1955, 1998.

Cochran S, Landecker A. Prevention and management of rhinoplasty complications. Plast Reconstr Surg 122:60e-67e, 2008.

Cole RR, Myer CM III, Bratcher GO. Congenital absence of the nose: a case report. Int J Pediatr Otorhinolaryngol 17:171-177, 1989.

Collawn SS, Fix RJ, Moore JR, et al. Nasal cartilage grafts: more than a decade of experience. Plast Reconstr Surg 100:1547-1552, 1997.

Collis NM, Litherland J, Enion D, et al. Magnetic resonance imaging and explanation investigation of long-term silicone gel implant integrity. Plast Reconstr Surg 120:1401-1406, 2007.

Colton JJ, Beekhuis GJ. Use of Mersilene mesh in nasal augmentation. Facial Plast Surg 8:149-156, 1992.

Conrad K, Gillman G. A 6-year experience with the use of expanded polytetrafluoroethylene in rhinoplasty. Plast Reconstr Surg 101:1675-1683, 1998.

Conrad K, Torgerson C, Gillman G. Applications of Gore-Tex implants in rhinoplasty reexamined after 17 years. Arch Facial Plast Surg 10:224-231, 2008.

Conrad K, Yoskovitch A. The use of fibrin glue in the correction of pollybeak deformity: a preliminary report. Arch Facial Plast Surg 5:522-527, 2003.

Constantian MB. Differing characteristics in 100 consecutive secondary rhinoplasty patients following closed versus open surgical approaches. Plast Reconstr Surg 109:2097, 2002.

Constantian MB. Secondary rhinoplasty. In Goldwyn RM, Cohen MN, eds. The Unfavorable Result in Plastic Surgery. Philadelphia: Lippincott Williams & Wilkins, 2001, p 943.

Cook TA, Wang TD, Brownrigg PJ, et al. Significant premaxillary augmentation. Arch Otolaryngol Head Neck Surg 116:1197-1201, 1990.

Crysdale WS, Walker PJ. External septorhinoplasty in children: patient selection and surgical technique. J Otolaryngol 23:28, 1994.

Cussons PD, Murison MSC, Fernandez AEL, et al. A panel based assessment of early versus no nasal correction of the cleft lip nose. Br J Plast Surg 46:7-12, 1993.

Daniel RK. A 6-year experience with the use of expanded polytetrafluoroethylene in rhinoplasty. Plast Reconstr Surg 101:1684, 1998.

Daniel RK. Rhinoplasty: septal saddle nose deformity and composite reconstruction. Plast Reconstr Surg 119:1029-1043, 2007.

Daniel RK. Rhinoplasty: a simplified, three-stitch, open tip suture technique. Part I: primary rhinoplasty. Plast Reconstr Surg 103:1491-1502, 1999.

Daniel RK. Rhinoplasty: a simplified, three-stitch, open tip suture technique. Part II: secondary rhinoplasty. Plast Reconstr Surg 103:1503-1512, 1999.

Daniel RK. Secondary rhinoplasty following open rhinoplasty. Plast Reconstr Surg 96:1539, 1995.

Davis PK. Cleft lip nose tip deformity: a tutorial dissertation. Br J Plast Surg 36:200-203, 1983.

Davis PK, Jones SM. The complications of silastic implants: experience with 137 consecutive cases. Br J Plast Surg 24:405, 1971.

Deva AK, Merten S, Chang L. Silicone in nasal augmentation rhinoplasty: a decade of clinical experience. Plast Reconstr Surg 102:1230-1237, 1998.

Drake-Lee AB, Bickerton RC, Milford C. Wegener's granulomatosis and nasal deformity. Br J Clin Pract 42:348-350, 1988.

Duffy FJ, Rossi RM, Pribaz JJ. Reconstruction of Wegener's nasal deformity using bilateral facial artery musculomucosal flaps. Plast Reconstr Surg 101:1330, 1998.

Durante BJ, Porubsky ES. Reducing columella scarring in open septorhinoplasty. Laryngoscope 96:810, 1986.

Egyedi P, Müller H. Correction of the kinked nostril rim. J Max Fac Surg 14:289-290, 1986.

Elsahy NI. Prevention of parrot's beak deformity after reduction rhinoplasty. Acta Chir Plast 19:63-69, 1977.

Erlich MA, Pathiscar A. Nasal dorsal augmentation with silicone implants. Facial Plast Surg 19:325, 2003.

Fanous N, Samaha M, Yosikovitch A. Dacron implants in rhinoplasty: a review of 136 cases of tip and dorsum implants. Arch Facial Plast Surg 4:149, 2002.

Fisher DM, Mann RJ. A model for the cleft lip nasal deformity. Plast Reconstr Surg 101:1448, 1998.

Flemming I. Rhinoplasty in children. Otolaryngol Clin North Am 10:33-40, 1977.

Fodor PB. Aesthetic rhinoplasty in early adolescence. Aesth Plast Surg 12:207-216, 1988.

Fodor PB, Lemperie G, Biewener A. External skin excision in the sebaceous nose and supratip deformity. Plast Reconstr Surg 91:1180, 1993.

Fortunato G, Marini E, Valdinucci F, et al. Long-term results of hydroxyapatite-fibrin glue implantation in plastic and reconstructive craniofacial surgery. J Craniomaxillofac Surg 25:124-135, 1997.

Fujimori R, Haritz Y. Elongation of the nostril and columella using an island flap. Br J Plast Surg 35:171-176, 1982.

Furlow LT. Flaps for cleft lip and palate surgery. Clin Plast Surg 17:633-644, 1990.

Giunta SX. Premaxillary augmentation in Asian rhinoplasty. Facial Plast Surg Clin North Am 4:93-102, 1996.

Godin MS, Waldman SR, Johnson CM Jr. Nasal augmentation using Gore-Tex: a 10-year experience. Arch Facial Plast Surg 1:118-121, 1999.

Godin MS, Waldman SR, Johnson CM Jr. The use of expanded polytetrafluoroethylene (Gore-Tex) in rhinoplasty. Arch Otolaryngol Head Neck Surg 121:1131-1136, 1995.

Goodman WS, Charbonneau PA. External approach to rhinoplasty. Laryngoscope 84:2195, 1974.

Goodman WS, Zorn MLT. The unilateral cleft lip nose. J Otolaryngol 11:198-203, 1982.

Gorney M. Centripetal rotation-advancement for bilateral cleft lip nasal deformities. Ann Acad Med Singapore 12:331-336, 1983.

Goto M. Augmentation rhinoplasty by the sandbag method that uses a dermal bag containing hydroxyapatite granules. Japan J Plast Reconstr Surg 35:645-649, 1992.

Gruber RP. Open rhinoplasty. Clin Plast Surg 15:95, 1988.

Gruber RP. Primary open rhinoplasty. In Gruber RP, Peck GC, eds. Rhinoplasty: State of the Art. St Louis: Mosby, 1992, pp 61-87.

Gryskiewicz JM. Visible scars from percutaneous osteotomies. Plast Reconstr Surg 116:1771-1775, 2005.

Gryskiewicz JM. Waste not, want not: the use of AlloDerm in secondary rhinoplasty. Plast Reconstr Surg 116:1999-2004, 2005.

Gryskiewicz JM, Rohrich RJ, Reagan BJ. The use of AlloDerm for the correction of nasal contour deformities. Plast Reconstr Surg 107:561, 2001.

Gubisch W, Reichert H, Widmaier W. Six years' experience with free septum replantation in cleft nasal correction. J Craniomaxillofac Surg 17:31-33, 1989.

Guerrerosantos J, Trabanino C, Guerrerosantos F. Multifragmented cartilage wrapped with fascia in augmentation rhinoplasty. Plast Reconstr Surg 117:804-812, 2006.

Gunter JP. The merits of the open approach in rhinoplasty. Plast Reconstr Surg 99:863-867, 1997.

Gunter JP. Secondary rhinoplasty: the open approach. In Daniel RK, ed. Aesthetic Plastic Surgery: Rhinoplasty. Boston: Little Brown, 1993.

Gunter JP, Clark CP, Friedman RM. Internal stabilization of autogenous rib cartilage grafts in rhinoplasty: a barrier to cartilage warping. Plast Reconstr Surg 100:161-169, 1997.

Gunter JP, Cochran CS. Management of intraoperative fractures of the nasal septal "L-strut": percutaneous Kirschner wire fixation. Plast Reconstr Surg 117:395-402, 2006.

Gunter JP, Rohrich R. External approach for secondary rhinoplasty. Plast Reconstr Surg 80:161-173, 1987.

Guyuron B, Afrooz PN. Correction of cocaine-related nasal defects. Plast Reconstr Surg 121:1015, 2008.

Guyuron B, DeLuca L, Lash R. Supratip deformity: a closer look. Plast Reconstr Surg 105:1140-1151, 2000.

Ham KS, Chung SC, Lee SH. Complications of oriental augmentation rhinoplasty. Ann Acad Med Singapore 12:460-462, 1983.

Hansono MM, Kridel RWH, Pastorek NJ, et al. Correction of the soft tissue pollybeak using triamcinolone injection. Arch Facial Plast Surg 4:26-30, 2002.

Harashina T. Asymmetric incision for open rhinoplasty in cleft lip nasal deformity. Plast Reconstr Surg 105:805, 2000.

Herbst A. Extrusion of an expanded polytetrafluoroethylene implant after rhinoplasty. Plast Reconstr Surg 104:295-296, 1999.

Hernandez-Zendejas G. The history of augmentation rhinoplasty: implant and design. Plast Reconstr Surg 103:1802-1803, 1999.

Hiraga Y. Complications of augmentation rhinoplasty in the Japanese. Ann Plast Surg 4:495, 1980.

Hobar PC. Cleft lip II: secondary deformities. Sel Read Plast Surg 7:22, 1994.

Holmstrom H, Luzi F. Open rhinoplasty without transcolumellar incision. Plast Reconstr Surg 97:321-326, 1996.

Ishida J, Ishida LC, Ishida LH, et al. Treatment of the nasal hump with preservation of the cartilaginous framework. Plast Reconstr Surg 103:1729-1733, 1999.

Jackson IT. AlloDerm used in rhinoplasty. Plast Reconstr Surg 108:1828, 2001.

Jackson IT, Yavuzer R. AlloDerm for dorsal nasal irregularities. Plast Reconstr Surg 107:553-558, 2001.

Johnson CM, Toriumi DM. Open Structure Rhinoplasty. Philadelphia: Saunders, 1990.

Jugo SB. Total septal reconstruction through decortication (external) approach in children. Arch Otolaryngol Head Neck Surg 113:173, 1987.

Jung DH, Kim BR, Choi JY, et al. Gross and pathologic analysis of long-term silicone implants inserted into the human body for augmentation rhinoplasty: 221 revision cases. Plast Reconstr Surg 120:1997, 2007.

Juraha LZG. Experience with alternative material for nasal augmentation. Aesth Plast Surg 16:133-140, 1992.

Koh KS, Eom JS. Asymmetric incision for open rhinoplasty in cleft lip nasal deformity. Plast Reconstr Surg 103:1835-1838, 1999.

Koh KS, Kim EK. Management of unilateral cleft lip nose deformity, with retracted ala of the noncleft side. Plast Reconstr Surg 118:723, 2006.

Kornblut AD, Wolff SM, DeFries HP, et al. Wegener's granulomatosis. Laryngoscope 90:1453, 1980.

Krzysztof C, Torgerson CS, Gillman GS. Applications of Gore-Tex implants in rhinoplasty reexamined after 17 years. Arch Facial Plast Surg 10:224-231, 2008.

Krzysztof C, Yoshovitch A. The use of fibrin glue in the correction of pollybeak deformity: a preliminary report. Arch Facial Plast Surg 5:522-527, 2003.

Lam SM, Kim YK. Augmentation rhinoplasty of the Asian nose with the bird silicone implant. Ann Plast Surg 51:249, 2003.

Lee Y, Han S. Use of a temporoparietal fascia-covered silastic implant in nose reconstruction after foreign body removal. Plast Reconstr Surg 104:500-505, 1999.

Lefkovitz G. Nasal reconstruction with irradiated homograft costal cartilage. Plast Reconstr Surg 113:1291-1292, 2004.

Lewis JD. Depressed nasal fractures: a comparison of the prosthetic values of paraffin, bone, cartilage and celluloid, with report of cases corrected with celluloid implants by the author's method. Ann Otol Rhinol Laryngol 32:321, 1923.

Liou EJ, Subramanian M, Chen PKT. Progressive changes of columella length and nasal growth after nasoalveolar molding in bilateral cleft patients: a three year follow-up study. Plast Reconstr Surg 119:642, 2007.

Lipshutz HA. A clinical evaluation of subdermal and subcutaneous silicone implants. Plast Reconstr Surg 37:249, 1966.

Liu ES, Kridel RWH. Postrhinoplasty nasal cysts and the use of petroleum-based ointments and nasal packing. Plast Reconstr Surg 112:282-287, 2003.

Lo L, Kane AA, Chen Y. Simultaneous reconstruction of the secondary bilateral cleft lip and nasal deformity: Abbé flap revisited. Plast Reconstr Surg 112:1219-1227, 2003.

Lohuis PJ, Watts SJ, Vuyk HD. Augmentation of the nasal dorsum using Gore-Tex: intermediate results of a retrospective analysis of experience in 66 patients. Clin Otolaryngol Allied Sci 26:214, 2001.

Losee JE, Kirschner RE, Whitaker LA, et al. Congenital nasal anomalies: a classification scheme. Plast Reconstr Surg 113:676, 2004.

Losken A, Burstein FD, Williams JK. Congenital nasal pyriform aperture stenosis: diagnosis and treatment. Plast Reconstr Surg 109:1506, 2002.

Lovice DB, Mingrone MD, Toriumi DM. Grafts and implants in rhinoplasty and nasal reconstruction. Otolaryngol North Am 32:113, 1999.

Maas CS, Gnepp DR, Bumpous J. Expanded polytetrafluoroethylene (Gore-Tex soft-tissue patch) in facial augmentation. Arch Otolaryngol Head Neck Surg 119:1008, 1993.

Matsuya T, Lida S, Kogo M. Secondary rhinoplasty using flying-bird and vestibular tornado incisions for unilateral cleft lip patients. Plast Reconstr Surg 112:390-395, 2003.

McCurdy JA Jr. The Asian nose: augmentation rhinoplasty with L-shaped silicone implants. Facial Plast Surg 18:245, 2002.

Mendelsohn M, Dunlop G. Gore-Tex augmentation grafting in rhinoplasty: is it safe? J Otolaryngol 27:337-341, 1998.

Menick F. Anatomic reconstruction of the nasal tip cartilages in secondary and reconstructive rhinoplasty. Plast Reconstr Surg 104:2187-2198, 1999.

Millard DR, Mejia FA. Reconstruction of the nose damaged by cocaine. Plast Reconstr Surg 107:419-424, 2001.

Morehead JM, Holt GR. Soft-tissue response to synthetic biomaterials. Otolaryngol Clin North Am 27:195, 1994.

Nagasaot MJ, Yasuda S, Ogata H, et al. An anatomical study of the three dimensional structure of the nasal septum in patients with alveolar clefts and alveolar-palatal clefts. Plast Reconstr Surg 121:2074, 2008.

Neel HB III. Implants of Gore-Tex. Arch Otolaryngol 109:427, 1983.

Niechajev I. Porous polyethylene implants for nasal reconstruction: clinical and histologic studies. Aesth Plast Surg 23:395, 1999.

Ortiz-Monasterio F, Olmedo A. Corrective rhinoplasty before puberty: a long-term follow-up. Plast Reconstr Surg 68:381, 1981.

Owsley TG, Taylor CO. The use of Gore-Tex for nasal augmentation: a retrospective analysis of 106 patients. Plast Reconstr Surg 94:241-242, 1994.

Padovan IF. External approach in rhinoplasty (de-cortication). In Conley J, Dickinson JT, eds. Plastic and Reconstructive Surgery of the Face and Neck. Stuttgart: Thieme Verlag, 1972, pp 143-146.

Padovan IF, Jugo SR. Complications of external rhinoplasty. Ear Nose Throat J 70:454, 1991.

Pak MW, Chan ESY, van Hasselt CA. Late complications of nasal augmentation using silicone implants. J Laryngol Otol 112:1074-1077, 1998.

Paulus GW, Bormioli P, Steinhäuser EW. Vertical transection of the alar cartilages in unilateral cleft noses. Int J Oral Maxillofac Surg 15:225-232, 1986.

Peled ZM, Warren AG, Johnson P, et al. The use of alloplastic materials in rhinoplasty surgery: a meta-analysis. Plast Reconstr Surg 121:85e-92e, 2008.

Pigott RW. Alar leapfrog. Clin Plast Surg 12:643, 1985.

Queen TA, Palmer FR III. Gore-Tex for nasal augmentation: a recent series and a review of the literature. Ann Otol Rhinol Laryngol 104:850, 1995.

Raghavan U, Jones NS. The complications of giant titanium implants in nasal reconstruction. J Plast Reconstr Aesth Surg 59:74, 2006.

Raspall G, González-Lagunas J. Management of the nasal tip by open rhinoplasty. J Craniomaxillofac Surg 24:145, 1996.

Raszewski R, Guyuron B, Lash RH, et al. A severe fibrotic reaction after cosmetic liquid silicone injection. J Craniomaxillofac Surg, 18:225-228, 1990.

Reese BR, Koltai PJ, Parnes SM, et al. The external rhinoplasty approach for rhinologic surgery. Ear Nose Throat J 71:408, 1972.

Regnault P. Nasal augmentation in the problem nose. Aesth Plast Surg 11:1-5, 1987.

Rethi A. Raccourcissement du nez trop long. Rev Chir Plast 2:85, 1934.

Roe JO. The correction of angular deformities of the nose by a subcutaneous operation. Med Rec 40:57, 1891.

Roe JO. The deformity termed "pug nose" and its correction, by a simple operation. Med Rec 31:621, 1887.

Romo T III, Choe KS, Sclafani AP. Cleft lip nasal reconstruction using porous high-density polyethylene. Arch Facial Plast Surg 5:175-179, 2003.

Romo T III, Rizk SS, Suh GD. Mucous cyst formation after rhinoplasty. Arch Facial Plast Surg 1:208-211, 1999.

Romo T III, Sclafani AP, Sabini P. Use of porous high-density polyethylene in revision rhinoplasty and in the platyrrhine nose. Aesthetic Plast Surg 22:211, 1998.

Rothstein SG, Jacobs JB. The use of Gore-Tex implants in nasal augmentation operations. Entechnology Sept:40-45, 1989.

Sachs ME. Enbucrilate as cartilage adhesive in augmentation rhinoplasty. Arch Otolaryngol 111:389-393, 1985.

Sachs ME. Tissue clay. Arch Otolaryngol 113:289-291, 1987.

Salyer KE. Primary correction of the nasal deformity associated with cleft lip. In Cohen M, ed. Mastery of Plastic and Reconstructive Surgery. New York: Little Brown, 1994, pp 581-594.

Schubert W, Gear AJ, Lee C, et al. Incorporation of titanium mesh in orbital and midface reconstruction. Plast Reconstr Surg 110:1022-1030, 2002.

Sclafani AP, Thomas JR, Cox AJ, et al. Clinical and histologic response of subcutaneous expanded polytetrafluoroethylene (Gore-Tex) and porous high-density polyethylene (Medpor) implants to acute and early infection. Arch Otolaryngol Head Neck Surg 123:328, 1997.

Shapley H. Beyond the Observatory. New York: Charles Scribner, 1967.

Shaw RB, Kahn DM. Aging of the mid-face bony elements: a three dimensional computed tomographic study. Plast Reconstr Surg 119:675, 2007.

Sheen JH. Achieving more nasal tip projection by use of small autogenous vomer or septal cartilage grafts: a preliminary report. Plast Reconstr Surg 56:35-40, 1975.

Sheen JH. Closed versus open rhinoplasty: and the debate goes on. Plast Reconstr Surg 99:859-862, 1997.

Sheen JH. A new look at supratip deformity. Ann Plast Surg 3:498, 1979.

Sheen JH. Secondary rhinoplasty. Plast Reconstr Surg 56:137, 1975.

Sheen JH. Secondary rhinoplasty surgery. In Millard DR Jr. ed. Symposium on Corrective Rhinoplasty. St. Louis: CV Mosby, 1976.

Shiba A, Hatoko M, Okazaki T, et al. A case of human adjuvant disease after augmentation rhinoplasty. Aesth Plast Surg 23:175-178, 1999.

Shirakabe Y, Shirakabe T, Kishimoto T. The classification of complications after augmentation rhinoplasty. Aesth Plast Surg 9:185-192, 1985.

Shirakabe Y, Suzuki Y, Lam SM. A systematic approach to rhinoplasty of the Japanese nose: a thirty-year experience. Aesthetic Plast Surg 27:221-231, 2003.

Slupchynskyj O, Gieniusz M. Rhinoplasty in African American patients. Arch Facial Plast Surg 10:232-236, 2008.

Sood VP. Septoplasty in children. Indian J Otolaryngol 37:87, 1985.

Stal S, Hollier L. Correction of secondary deformities of the cleft lip nose. Plast Reconstr Surg 109:1386-1393, 2002.

Stoll W. A 5 year experience with open septorhinoplasty. Larygorhinootolgie 70:171, 1991.

Stoll W. Complications following implantation or transplantation in rhinoplasty. Facial Plast Surg 13:45-50, 1997.

Strauch B, Erhard HA, Baum T. Use of irradiated cartilage in rhinoplasty of the non-Caucasian nose. Aesthet Surg J 24:324-330, 2004.

Strauch B, Wallach SG. Reconstruction with irradiated homograft costal cartilage. Plast Reconstr Surg 111:2405-2411, 2003.

Stucker FJ. Autoalloplast. Arch Otolaryngol 108:130, 1982.

Stucker FJ. Nasal augmentation using Gore-Tex: a 10 year experience. Arch Facial Plast Surg 1:122, 1999.

Stucker FJ, Bryarly RC, Shockley WW. Management of nasal trauma in children. Arch Otolaryngol 110:190-192, 1984.

Taylor P, Kaakedjian G. Preliminary studies on the use of nail as a material for reconstructive or cosmetic surgery. Plast Reconstr Surg 101:1276-1279, 2005.

Tebbetts JB. Open rhinoplasty: more than an incisional approach. In Daniel RK, ed. Aesthetic Plastic Surgery: Rhinoplasty. Boston: Little Brown, 1993.

Tebbetts JB. Shaping and positioning the nasal tip without structural disruption: a new, systematic approach. Plast Reconstr Surg 94:61, 1994.

Teichgraeber JF, Riley WB, Russo RC. External rhinoplasty: indications for use. Br J Plast Surg 45:47, 1992.

Tessier P. Anatomical classification of facial, craniofacial, and latero-facial clefts. J Maxillofac Surg 4:69, 1976.

Tham C, Lai YL, Weng CJ, et al. Silicone augmentation rhinoplasty in an oriental population. Ann Plast Surg 54:1, 2005.

Tobin HA. Extruded nasal implant. Otolaryngol Head Neck Surg 109:552-553, 1993.

Toriumi DM, Mueller RA, Grosch T, et al. Vascular anatomy of the nose and the external rhinoplasty approach. Arch Otolaryngol Head Neck Surg 122:24, 1996.

Triglia J, Cannoni M, Pech A. Septorhinoplasty in children: benefit of the external approach. J Otolaryngol 190:274-278, 1990.

Trybus M. The harpoon-shaped nasal implant. Ear Nose Throat J 68:878-881, 1989.

Tucker K. A new look at supratip deformity. Plast Reconstr Surg 66:655, 1980.

Turegun M, Sengezer M, Guler M. Reconstruction of saddle nose deformities using porous polyethylene implants. Aesthetic Plast Surg 22:38, 1998.

Uhm K, Hwang SH, Choi BG. Cleft lip nose correction with onlay calvarial bone graft and suture suspension in oriental patients. Plast Reconstr Surg 105:499-503, 2000.

Uysal A, Ozbek S, Ozcan M. Comparison of the biological activities of high-density porous polyethylene implants and oxidized regenerated cellulose-wrapped diced cartilage grafts. Plast Reconstr Surg 112:540-546, 2003.

Van Beek A, Hatfield A, Schnepf E. Cleft rhinoplasty. Plast Reconstr Surg 114:57e-69e, 2004.

Velidedeoğlu H, Demir Z, Sahin Ǔ, et al. Block and Surgicel-wrapped diced solvent-preserved costal cartilage homograft application for nasal augmentation. Plast Reconstr Surg 115:2081, 2005.

Vilar-Sancho B. An old story: an ivory nasal implant. Aesth Plast Surg 11:157, 1987.

Vuyk HD, Adamson PA. Biomaterials in rhinoplasty. Clin Otolaryngol Allied Sci 23:209, 1998.

Vuyk HD, Kalter PO. Open septorhinoplasty: experiences in 200 patients. Rhinology 31:175, 1993.

Waldman SR. Gore-Tex for augmentation of the nasal dorsum: a preliminary report. Ann Plast Surg 26:520, 1991.

Walker PJ, Crysdale WS, Farkas LG. External septorhinoplasty in children. Arch Otolaryngol Head Neck Surg 119:984-988, 1993.

Wang TD, Madorsky SJ. Secondary rhinoplasty in nasal deformity associated with the unilateral cleft lip. Arch Facial Plast Surg 1:40-45, 1999.

Webster RC, Hamdan US, Gaunt JM, et al. Rhinoplastic revisions with injectable silicone. Arch Otolaryngol Head Neck Surg 112:269-276, 1986.

Wolfe SA. A pastiche for the cleft lip nose. Plast Reconstr Surg 114:1-9, 2004.

Wong GB, Burvin R, Mulliken JB. Resorbable internal splint: an adjunct to primary correction of unilateral cleft lip-nasal deformity. Plast Reconstr Surg 110:385, 2002.

Wright WK, Kridel RWH. External septorhinoplasty: a tool for teaching and for improved results. Laryngoscope 91:945, 1981.

Yanaga H, Yanaga K, Imai K, et al. Clinical application of cultured autologous human auricular chondrocytes with autologous serum for craniofacial or nasal augmentation and repair. Plast Reconstr Surg 117:2019-2030, 2006.

Yaremchuk MJ. Facial skeletal reconstruction using porous polyethylene implants. Plast Reconstr Surg 111:1818-1827, 2003.

Zeng Y, Wu W, Yu H, et al. Silicone implant in augmentation rhinoplasty. Ann Plast Surg 49:495, 2002.

Zhanqiang L. Carving Gore-Tex reinforced sheets for augmentation rhinoplasty in Chinese patients. Plast Reconstr Surg 117:326-328, 2006.

CHAPTER 20

Unhappy Patients and Those With Body Dysmorphic Disorder

A doctor does not treat typhoid fever, but treats the man with typhoid fever, and it is the man with his peculiarities—his body idiosyncrasies— that we have to consider.

SIR WILLIAM OSLER,
speaking of treating Walt Whitman

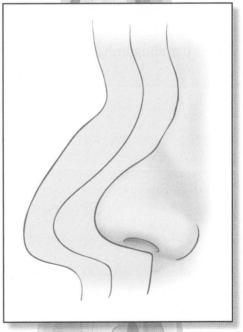

*T*his chapter is about unhappy patients, most of whom were mine—if not initially, at least eventually.

I have lectured and given courses on this topic for many years, but I have never written about it for several reasons: (1) I did not believe I knew enough, (2) I had not yet begun to put the problem together, and (3) a paper about unhappy patients that has no illustrations loses some of its teaching focus for surgeons.

Even after 30 years in practice, I do not yet feel qualified to make a diagnosis of *body dysmorphic disorder* (BDD). I am not a psychiatrist and would not qualify as an expert witness on this subject. Two of the 10 patients in this chapter were diagnosed with BDD by a psychiatrist. I do not know whether any of the others had BDD, and I do not allege that they did. There may be some surgeons who believe these patients did have BDD; there may be some who think these patients had another psychiatric disorder; or some may even take the patients' side and agree that they were justified in their unhappiness.

It is not my intent to criticize these patients for their responses to my work but rather to recount their histories, surgical procedures, and reactions so that readers might learn from them and develop their own perspectives and philosophies for handling unhappy patients.

The Problem for Surgeons

My personal introduction to BDD and unhappy surgical patients was very direct. I operated on three such persons in short succession without being aware of the possibility of BDD beforehand. A little background will put the histories of these three patients into better context. The *Diagnostic and Statistical Manual of Mental Disorders, 4th edition* (DSM-IV-TR) lists three criteria that must be met to establish a diagnosis of BDD:

1. There must be a preoccupation with an imagined defect in appearance; if a slight physical anomaly is present, the patient's concern must be markedly excessive.
2. The preoccupation must cause clinically significant distress or impairment in social, occupational, or other important areas of functioning.
3. The preoccupation must not be better accounted for by another mental disorder.

Unfortunately, psychiatrists see a different population of patients than surgeons do—that is, they see persons who (for the most part) have an established or suspected diagnosis *and who have agreed to be treated* (this latter characteristic is particularly critical, as we shall see).

Furthermore, as clear as the DSM-IV-TR criteria may seem, they are not easily applied to many rhinoplasty patients. Who decides what constitutes a deformity and therefore whether it is imagined—the surgeon, the patient, or the psychiatrist? Who defines aesthetic standards? For example, if a deformity is subtle but real, should the desire to have it corrected be an indication of BDD?

Also, who decides what is "significant distress"? If the patient has had six rhinoplasties, resulting in an increasingly deformed nose and an impaired airway, thereby creating a patient who is frustrated by failure and angry about wasted time and money, how much distress is too much? Plastic surgeons need a different context and a different set of management principles for treating such patients. In plastic surgery practices, the DSM-IV-TR criteria become less absolute.

Finally, what makes patients satisfied or dissatisfied with their surgical results, or even with their own lives? What inner forces influence patients to want further revisions, or alternatively, to decide that enough is enough? Why are some patients happy when they ought not to be, whereas others are unhappy when they should be happy? How is it possible for a surgeon to know what life events have occurred? What unknown changes color the lives of our patients, for better or worse, before we change their appearances?

The unhappiness that my three initial unhappy patients experienced and the inevitable turbulence it caused throughout their postoperative courses and in my practice sent me straight to the literature. At that time (1996), the syndrome known as BDD was being recognized with increasing frequency. But the mental health literature, although moderately extensive, had only limited value for the plastic surgeon, who treats a broader, less definable demographic. These patients often include fastidious and perfectionistic secondary rhinoplasty patients, who may have added anger, frustration, and anxiety to the mix. How would you characterize the rhinoplasty patient who has also undergone breast augmentation with reoperation for capsular contracture, blepharoplasty, and face lift? Is this individual fastidious, narcissistic, a cosmetic surgery addict, or a person with some variant of BDD? Does it matter whether this patient is 35 or 55 years old? These questions are not answered by the DSM-IV-TR criteria. What determines how many procedures a patient should undergo? Which patients are more normal: those who are delighted with imperfect results or those who are dissatisfied with postsurgical flaws? Does it matter?

In the past decade significant BDD research has appeared, and the percentage of secondary rhinoplasty patients in my practice has grown to almost 70%. Both have guided me toward the answers to some of these questions.

THE INITIAL TRIO

The following three patients introduced me to intensely unhappy surgical patients and to BDD; together they circumscribe many characteristics of the BDD spectrum.

Patient One

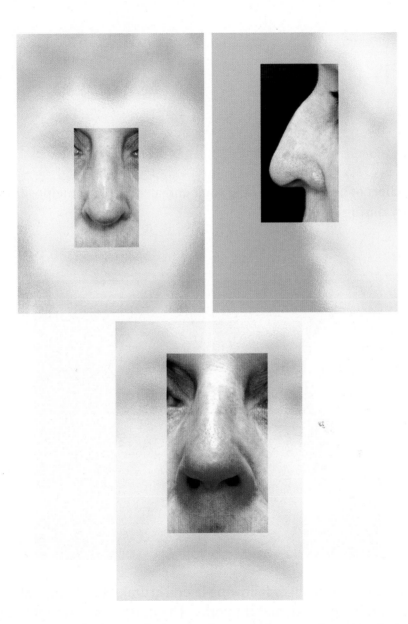

This woman was a teacher in her 60s whose goal was a functional airway and a modest dorsal hump reduction that nevertheless preserved its convexity. The patient's anatomic problems included a low radix, inadequate tip projection, a slightly narrow middle vault, and alar cartilage malposition.

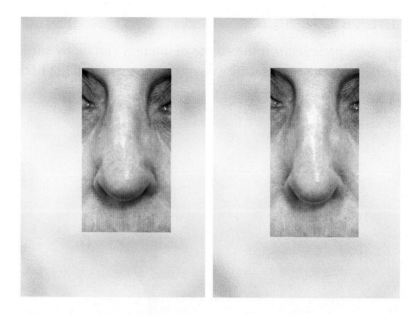

Notice the effect of her narrow middle vault and alar cartilage malposition on sidewall stability during inspiration.

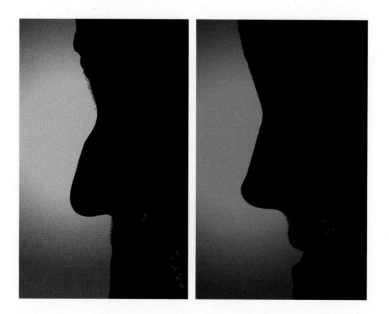

Silhouettes outline the changes following lateral crural relocation; slight dorsal reduction; and radix, spreader, and tip grafts. The dorsum was straight, the tip was above the dorsal line, and the airway was supported at both the internal and external valves. The nose looks smaller because of the rearrangement. I did not expect the patient's lax tissues to retain this shape, however. Eventually the tip would drop, thereby restoring some of the preoperative dorsal height.

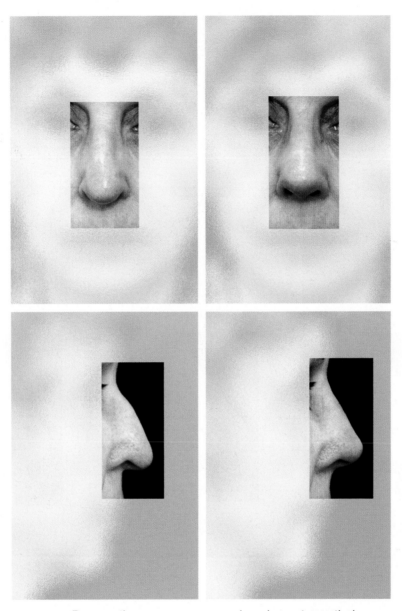

Preoperative   4 weeks postoperatively

The patient was pleased for approximately 2 weeks, at which time she called and asked to be seen. Crying and agitated, she demanded an immediate revision, because she believed that her nose had been overshortened and the tip pointed toward the ceiling. My explanation that any shortening was temporary and artifactual did not convince her. The patient resigned from her teaching position and became a recluse, remaining in her home and refusing to see friends or family. "If I return to teaching," she said, "my students will be stunned." "Everyone will ask me, 'What have you done to your nose?'" Her behavior is not uncommon among persons with BDD. In several series, 25% to 30% of patients have become housebound (see Phillips, 2005).

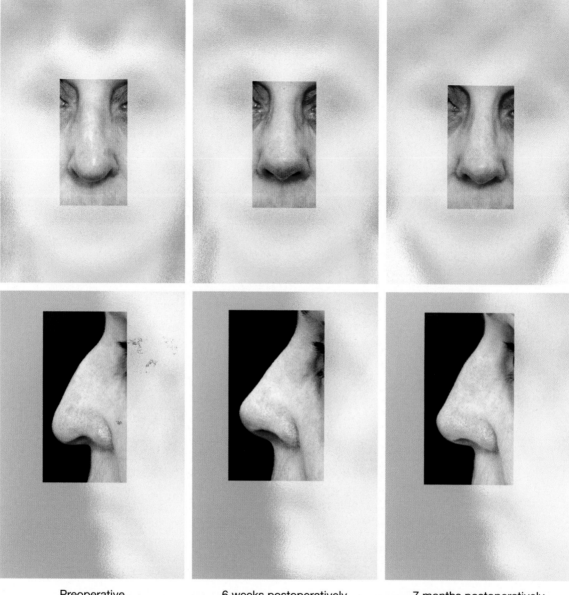

| Preoperative | 6 weeks postoperatively | 7 months postoperatively |

Note the evolving changes as the months passed—progressive narrowing and lengthening. Alar rim contours remained stable, as did middle vault stability. None of the grafts were visible, and most of the dorsal hump progressively returned, just as the patient desired.

Hoping to reassure her, I sent comparable preoperative and postoperative photographs. She returned them, covered with careful measurements, to prove what she saw instead.

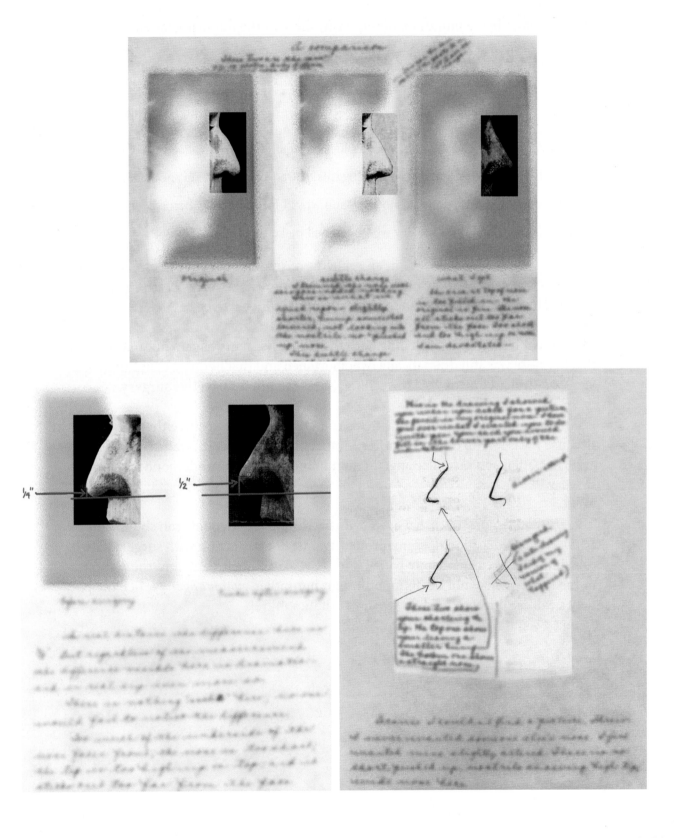

I continued to see her frequently for the first postoperative year. She repeatedly refused psychiatric counseling, which was offered as only a temporary measure until she was more emotionally equilibrated.

Shortly before her 4-month follow-up visit, she sent the following letter:

> I told you that I wanted my nose shortened by "a hair"—perhaps ⅛ inch, perhaps only 1/32 inch or 1/64 inch. . . .
>
> I never in my wildest imagination expected (nor did you ever suggest) that my nose would be this pointy, short, and turned up. This nose is a mockery of my long . . . face. It's like someone else's nose has been plucked off and put on my face. . . .
>
> I am brokenhearted and devastated [by this] sawed-off, turned-up snout. . . .
>
> How could you have done this to me—and why? I feel so terribly betrayed. . . .
>
> I am living (barely) for the day when you will make this right. . . .

At the 1-year postoperative visit, all grafts were smooth and invisible. The airway was widely patent. Airflow had increased three times over preoperative measurements. However, my reassurances were once again ineffective.

The patient had resumed teaching and was seeing her family again but maintained that her nose was still dramatically overshortened and that her nasolabial angle was almost a straight line toward the ceiling. She demanded corrective surgery.

I did not confront her with a diagnosis of BDD. I was not positive that she had it. Because I was fearful of precipitating another similar outburst, I refused to reoperate. The patient left my office angry. I do not know if she has undergone subsequent surgery.

This patient demonstrates that even primary rhinoplasty patients can show signs of BDD. Higher education does not protect against dissatisfaction with surgery. Often it is difficult to refer unhappy patients for psychiatric treatment; and the response to the surgeon may not be disappointment but rather *victim anger*. Notice the patient's words, "I feel so terribly *betrayed*" [italics mine].

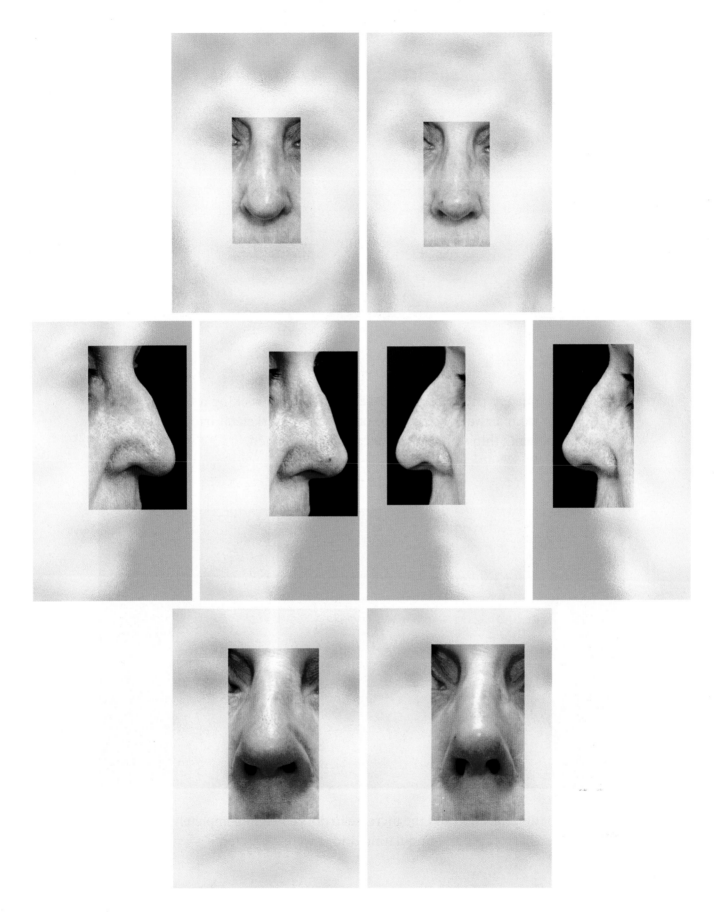

Patient Two

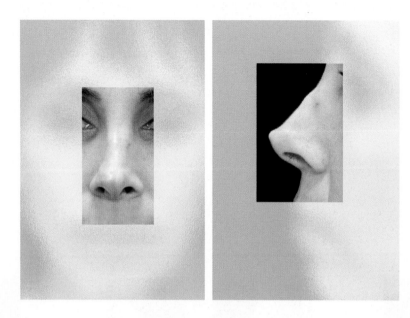

My second unhappy patient was a 44-year-old woman seeking a tertiary rhinoplasty. Aside from airway obstruction, only a series of skeletal irregularities supported the patient's thin skin. No septal cartilage remained.

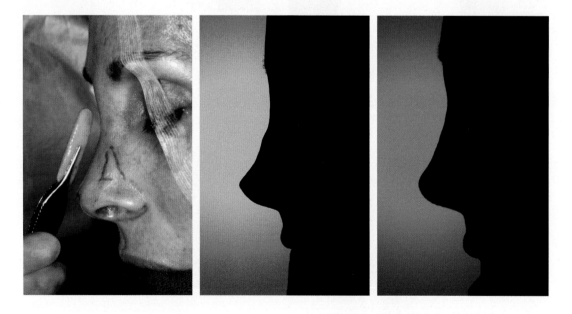

Reduction of tip projection and the increase in dorsal height completely rebalanced the nose; the sharp edges and undulating bridge were corrected.

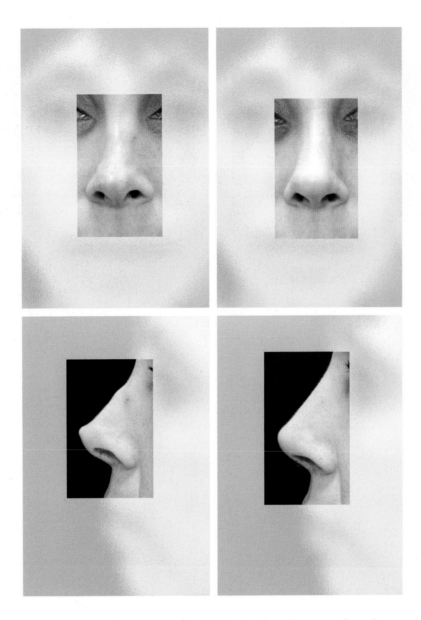

The reconstructed nose was smooth and balanced without surface distortions. Geometric mean airflow had doubled.

Initially the patient was happy with the result. Two months after surgery, however, her husband called, imploring me to revise my poor outcome. He reported that his wife had become reclusive and that my surgery had disrupted the entire family's life. I continued to see the patient at regular intervals throughout the first postoperative year. She slowly resumed her presurgery activities.

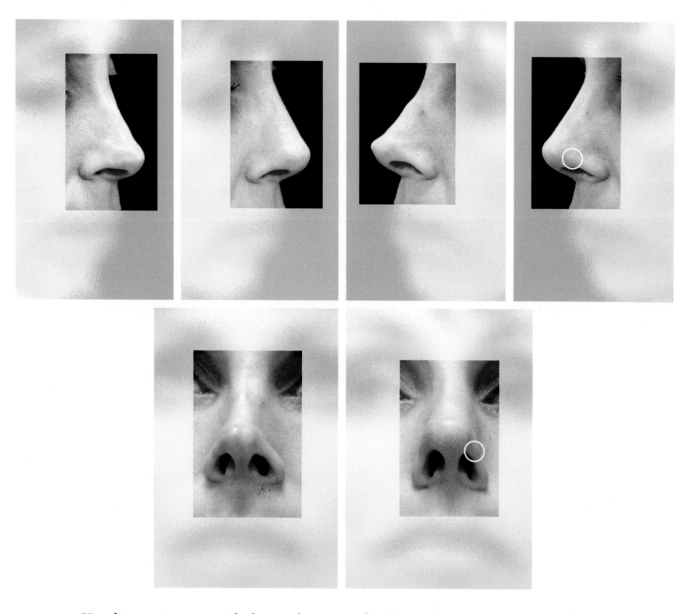

Her disappointment with the result was confined entirely to a contour irregularity of the left alar wall *(circled),* the result of a minor distortion in the underlying graft. Throughout the first year, the patient remained angry and unhappy, criticizing the result and my technique. Believing that it was my obligation to make any necessary correction, I told her the revision would be a simple adjustment of that single graft.

However, by the twelfth postoperative month, I had decided that revision was unwise. "But you told me you could fix the bump!" she exclaimed. "I can," I replied, "but I won't." I explained that the first surgery had so disequilibrated her that I did not want to risk another similar postoperative course. I meant it. I do not know if she has undergone another surgery.

Similar to the first patient, and whether or not she suffered from it, this patient demonstrates some of the hallmarks of BDD: a minor defect provokes disproportionate distress; education is no immunity against BDD; a demanding personality may mask signs that suggest BDD; and victim anger may be a clue to the disease. Finally, even the patient's husband believed that the cure was surgical and not psychiatric. My experience has been that a mental health diagnosis is unthinkable to most of these families, despite significant evidence to the contrary.

Patient Three

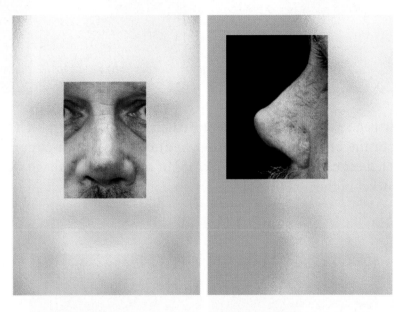

This 40-year-old autobody mechanic sought tertiary rhinoplasty to decrease the size of his lower nose and reduce tip angularity. The patient had a sophisticated grasp of nasal aesthetics, balance, and contour, an understanding that I attributed to his profession.

One previous surgery had reduced the nose, and another surgeon had added tip grafts. I explained that the size of his lower nose was partly attributable to tip cartilage distortion and excessive projection and partly to nasal length; accordingly, reducing the tip projection and increasing dorsal height would diminish the apparent size of the nasal base.

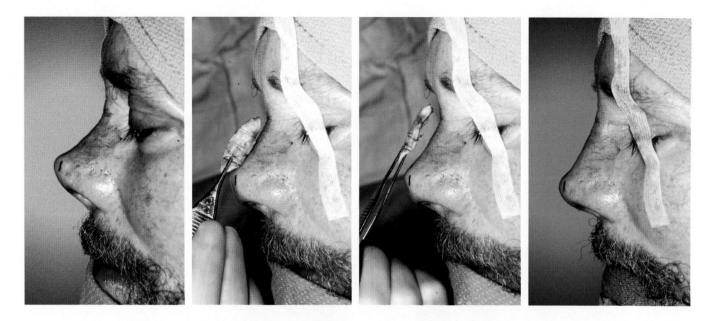

No septal cartilage was available, so I removed his previous tip grafts. Then, taking cartilage from the one remaining (untouched) ear, I placed a circumferentially wrapped, rolled ear cartilage graft. The scraps of remaining cartilage were fed into a separate pocket in the tip.

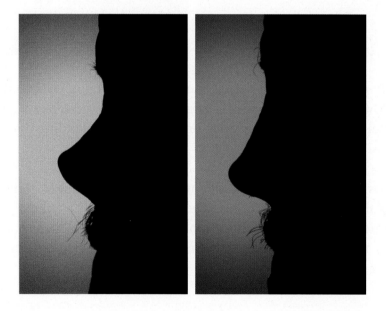

This is nasal shortening in reverse: as the dorsum goes higher, the nasal base rotates caudally because of increased anterior pressure on the dorsal skin. Caudally placed tip grafts only help to force the skin further downward so that there is a relative and absolute increase in nasal length.

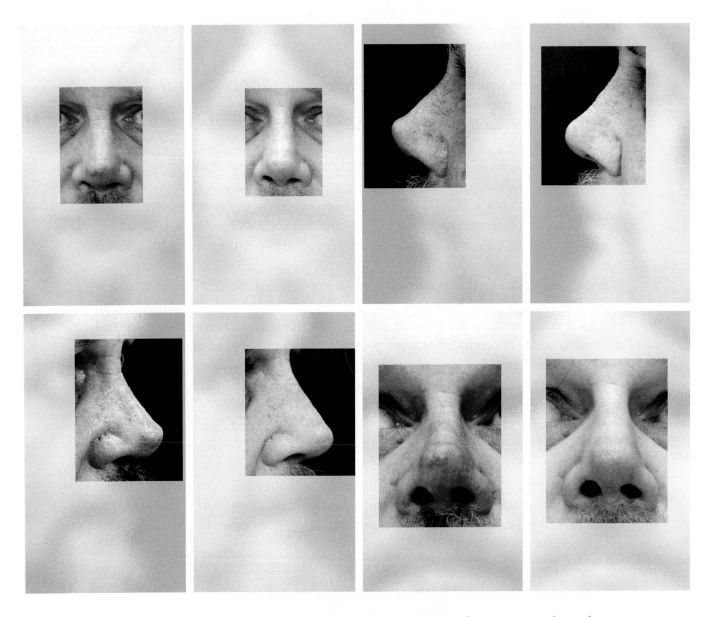

Unlike the previous two patients, this man was not happy for even 2 weeks. When I removed his splint, he looked in the mirror and said, "You have destroyed my face." During that visit and subsequent ones, I was unable to reassure him, even with comparative photographs and a lengthy review of our preoperative plan. He closed his business (36% of BDD patients are unemployed and unable to work; Phillips, 1996), his alcohol intake increased, and he became unable to work or leave his home.

At his 1-year visit, he returned to my office with his son and ex-wife, armed with desperate appeals for a surgical solution. My attempt to refer him for psychiatric treatment was unsuccessful.

Eventually, the patient tried to use a razor to reduce the dorsal height, but he succeeded only in lacerating himself. After treatment in the emergency room, he was admitted to the psychiatric unit and later referred to a psychiatrist with special expertise in BDD. The patient continued to request more surgery, but I did not reoperate.

This episode demonstrates the more extreme variant of BDD. The common characteristics, in my experience, are as follows:

1. The entire family believes that the patient's distress reflects the need for surgery.
2. The response to postoperative emotional pain in these unhappy patients may be addiction.
3. Some patients with BDD will inflict injury on themselves to correct their perceived deformities (45% to 71% of affected patients have suicidal ideation, and 24% to 28% attempt suicide; Veale et al, 1996; Phillips et al, 2005).

It is important to note that none of these patients fulfilled the DSM-IV-TR criteria for BDD preoperatively. None had unusual distress about their deformities. In all cases the deformities, as the patients saw and described them, seemed accurate and appropriate. All of the patients were pleasant preoperatively; all saw examples of my treatment results for similar deformities, and all agreed to my surgical plan in detail. Their presenting deformities were neither trivial nor imagined. These patients exhibited no signs of obsessive behavior or distress in daily functioning: all were active and productive in their work. For these reasons, the usual screening methods and checklists suggested for making a diagnosis of BDD would not have applied here. Nevertheless, the patients' postoperative signs of distress were indeed real, significant, and debilitating, but the treatment they presumably needed, according to these patients and their families, was entirely surgical. It is also sobering to wonder to what degree surgery can precipitate BDD in patients who are predisposed but not previously afflicted.

SUMMARY OF BODY DYSMORPHIC DISORDER CHARACTERISTICS IN THE LITERATURE

BDD is not a new disorder. It is the term currently used for a disease that was previously called *dysmorphophobia* in Eastern European, German, and Russian psychiatric literature. Freud described a patient he called "The Wolf Man," whose behavior included the obsessive and mirror-checking traits of the disease. Having previously treated the patient for "compulsive neurosis," Freud later commented that the patient "neglected his daily life and work because he was engrossed, to the exclusion of all else, in the state of his nose. . . . His life was centered on the little mirror in his pocket, and his fate depended on what it revealed or was about to reveal" (Hay, 1970).

Based on its similarity to obsessive-compulsive disorder (OCD), BDD has been characterized as part of that spectrum (Richter et al, 2004). However, there are ways in which BDD fits that conceptualization and ways in which it does not. The primary similarities between BDD and OCD are their responses to pharmacotherapy and cognitive behavioral therapy. However, patients with BDD are notorious for their poor insight (between 35% and 40% are delusional; Phillips, 2004). Also, the intensity with which BDD patients experience their perceived flaws is uncharacteristic of OCD.

There is evidence that BDD is a heritable disorder, which is particularly relevant to the histories of some rhinoplasty patients, as we shall see. Eight percent of patients with BDD have a family member with BDD, which is four to eight times the prevalence in the general population (Bienvenue et al, 2000). Patients with BDD appear to have abnormal perceptual and emotional information-processing capabilities and deficits in memory organization (Hanes, 1998). Interestingly, the brains of patients with BDD emphasize negative words and interfere with the processing of positive words, making these patients more hypersensitive to criticism and therefore less amenable to reassurance by the surgeon (Buhlmann et al, 2002). Similarly, patients with BDD are much more likely than control subjects or patients with OCD to interpret others' descriptive or neutral comments as criticism (Buhlmann et al, 2002). Patients with BDD are therefore much more sensitive than control subjects to teasing and are more likely to misidentify facial expressions as angry or contemptuous. Even more important, BDD patients imagine distortions in their own faces when judging computerized images (Yaryura-Tobias et al, 2002). This characteristic has encouraging implications for surgeons who may try to screen patients for BDD by using computer-imaging software.

Characteristically, BDD has its onset in childhood or adolescence, most commonly between the ages of 12 and 14 years. Although the disease usually arises in the early teen years, the diagnosis is often delayed for an average of 11 years after its onset. As many as one third of patients with BDD also have an eating disorder (Ruffolo et al, 2006). It should not be surprising to plastic surgeons that the disease is as common in men as in women, because male rhinoplasty patients are so widely believed to be troublesome.

Particularly troublesome for surgeons is the delusional variant seen in some patients with BDD. At least 35% to 40% of patients have no insight into their disease. Nearly all patients with BDD try to cope with their disease by adopting behaviors designed to diminish the anxiety they feel—for example, camouflaging a perceived defect with makeup, hair, or their hands; constantly comparing the area of the body they consider "defective" to that of other individuals; frequently checking the mirror; excessive grooming; and a continuous need for reassurance. The literature indicates a prevalence of 3% to 15% in surgical practices. In my own practice the prevalence is 0.5% of primary rhinoplasty patients and 4% (operated) to 12% (interviewees) of secondary patients.

There are significant comorbidities: 76% of those with BDD also have major depressive disorder; 37% have social anxiety disorder; 32% have OCD; and 25% to 35% have an eating disorder and associated substance abuse and impulse control disorder (Hadley et al, 2006).

Particularly relevant is the fact that, across all cultures, the most common area of the body for which BDD patients seek surgical treatment is the nose (45%; Phillips, 2005). Unfortunately, as my own earlier patients and subsequent cases indicate, surgery is almost always ineffective, and many patients with occult disease exhibit full-blown BDD postoperatively. Most studies show a surgical dissatisfaction rate of 80% to 90% in patients with BDD. Furthermore, not all unhappy patients go away quietly. In a 2002 survey, 40% of plastic surgeons stated that a patient with BDD had threatened them physically or with legal action (Sarwer, 2002). In one prominent New York case, a patient with BDD sued her plastic surgeon, asserting that, despite undergoing successful previous operations performed by him, she was unable to give informed consent because of the cognitive distortion produced by her disease (Leonardo, 2001). Several unhappy plastic surgery patients have murdered their physicians; however, it has not been established whether the patients' psychopathology in these cases was BDD.

THE PROBLEM FOR PLASTIC SURGEONS

In reviewing these data, the most pressing question continues to be whether to operate. How does the surgeon decide? All of us who treat cosmetic surgery patients see those who are anxious, depressed, or significantly distressed by a rather minor flaw. But there are other considerations. Secondary rhinoplasty patients who have already spent a significant amount of money and emotional energy to achieve a certain result, who may have had one undesirable outcome after another, who may have exhausted family support (after all, how many operations can you have on your nose?), and who may be, justifiably or unjustifiably, angry at the previous surgeon or surgeons, do not all have BDD. Many can be helped by a proper diagnosis and skillful, compassionate surgery. As important as the psychiatric literature is, all plastic surgeons must develop their own individual criteria for accepting or rejecting patients, and these criteria should reflect each surgeon's safe zone.

A number of surgeons have observed that one key factor may not be simply the size of the defect but rather *the patient's response to it* (Gorney, 2006). Therapists using cognitive-behavioral therapy to treat patients with BDD note the black-and-white, all-or-nothing thought patterns of these patients. The challenge for therapists, and for surgeons, is not necessarily to change the patient's belief but rather its *significance*. For better or worse, it is the patient's reality that really counts.

HOW THE SIGNS AND SYMPTOMS OF BODY DYSMORPHIC DISORDER HAVE MANIFESTED THEMSELVES IN MY RHINOPLASTY PRACTICE

Most of the characteristics of BDD that are identified in the psychiatric literature are found in the following case studies.

Patient Four

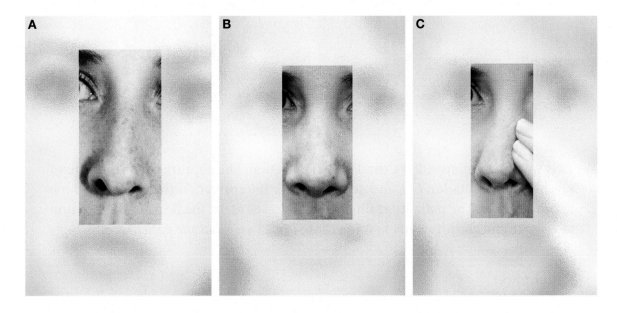

The first photograph shown here was taken before this patient had any surgery *(A)*. The second image is from when I saw her after she had undergone several rhinoplasties *(B)*. Her nose was symmetrical, the contour was smooth, and the airway was wide open. But the patient complained that her nose was crooked. The crookedness was so significant, she said, that others constantly noticed it; even her fiancé had left her because of the asymmetry. When I asked her to demonstrate the correction that she would like, she pushed her nose to the side *(C)*.

Patient Five

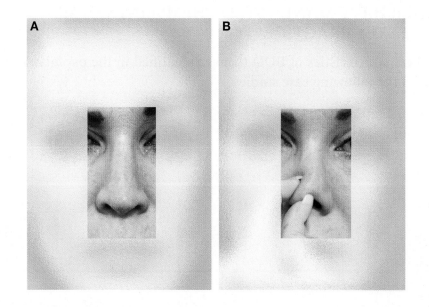

This woman demonstrated a similar dissatisfaction. She appears as she did when I saw her in consultation *(A)*, and demonstrating the correction that she wanted me to produce *(B)*. The patients' realities in these cases are at the heart of the decision to operate and constitute my first criterion: *I must see what the patient sees.*

Patient Six

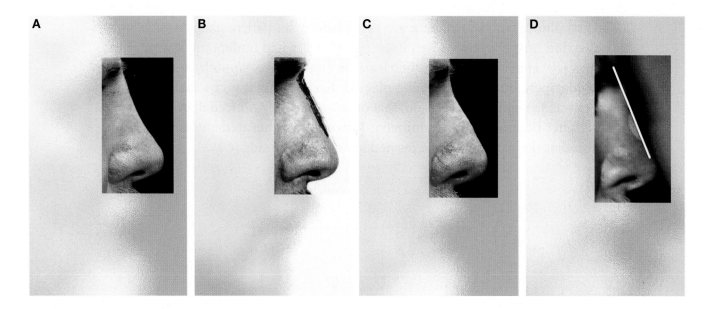

This patient had undergone 10 previous rhinoplasties. I was going to be surgeon number eight. He was agreeable and calm when he saw me, and he appeared as he did in photo *A*; he requested a change that he had drawn on a photo *(B)*. Believing that the request was reasonable and that I could achieve it, I reduced and re-created a new dorsum with rib cartilage *(C)*. However, as he had done when he first saw me, the patient wore a small adhesive bandage to hide the deformity *(D)*—no longer the original deformity, but rather the one he believed I had produced. The sense of deformity can be a lifelong affliction.

Patient Seven

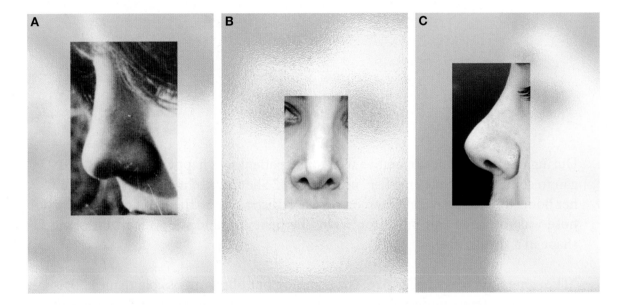

Photo *A* shows the patient's nose before several rhinoplasties (*B* and *C*). She presented with a supratip deformity, despite having undergone a homograft dorsal implant, and requested restoration of her original appearance. Because no septal cartilage was available, I augmented the dorsum, tip, and lateral walls with rib cartilage.

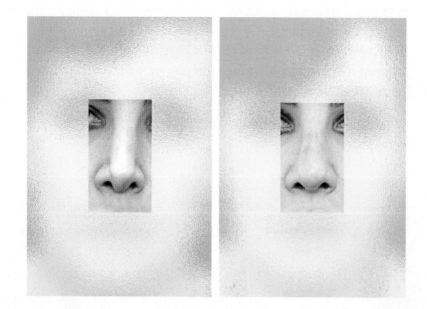

During the first few postoperative weeks, the patient was happy. But soon she began to contact me requesting her "next surgery." She traveled a great distance from her home to see me several times, on occasion distraught to the point of tears. The nose was too large and much too wide, she believed, and she wanted the same shape in a smaller size.

"The same nose in a smaller size" is a common but often impossible request. Particularly in patients undergoing secondary or tertiary rhinoplasty, where the soft tissues have already contracted maximally, the skin sleeve is a fixed rather than a variable parameter. Thus a straight nose in only one size is possible. Less augmentation would leave a residual supratip deformity, and more augmentation would simply make the nose larger and risk graft visibility.

To convince the patient that we had achieved her goals of autogenous reconstruction, correction of the supratip deformity, and a restoration that resembled her presurgical appearance, I sent her a series of comparative photographs.

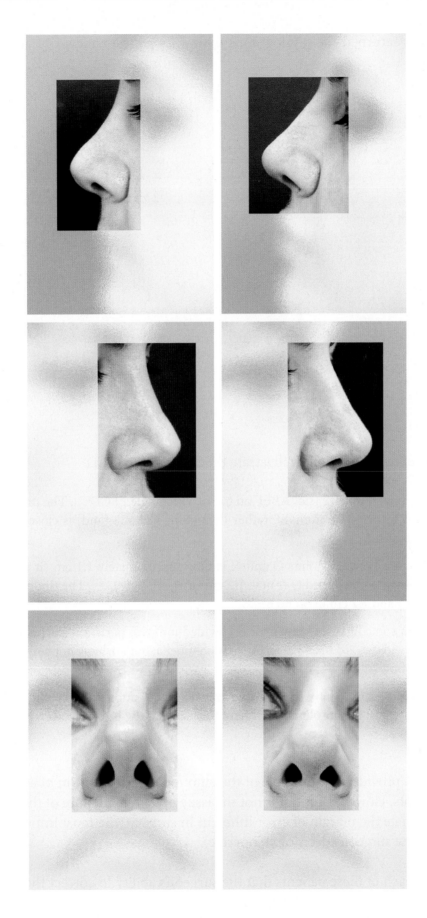

The patient returned the photographs with a four-page analysis of all aesthetic problems.

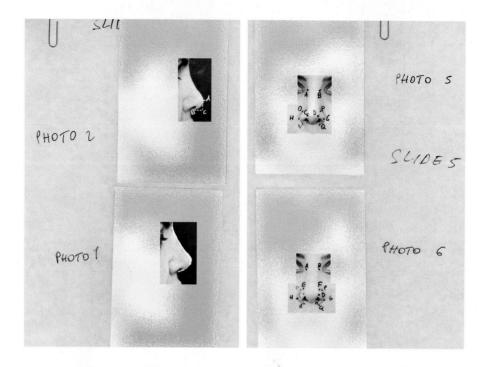

The short excerpts that follow illustrate the crossover to OCD.

> Now, we have a trapeze [sic] ABEF on top of a rectangle EFCD . . . The most protruding point seems to lie along EF rather than along CD. . . . [and] is closer to an ideal vertical tangent. . . .
>
> The distance between points O and N is now approximately 1.1 cm (it was 1.0 cm), and between points P and Q is now 1.2 cm (it was 1.1 cm). . . . The tip lobule is 1 cm in photo 5 and 1.2 cm in photo 6. . . .
>
> In fact, in some light the nose appears divided into two parts; the part above EF and the part below. . . . I'd like to keep the new columella, but it is now not compatible with the tip lobule. . . .
>
> The nostrils seem to have stretched horizontally. . . . I am ready to come and see you personally. . . . I am absolutely confident that you are the best person to help me with my nose. . . .

This patient provides one example of the emotional perfectionism of some dissatisfied patients. However, insight is not the issue here. It is a failure of the patient to fully appreciate the margin of error inherent in surgery (the most important of all criteria in the surgeon's decision to operate).

Notice for each of these patients that the surgeon's ability to correct the deformity does not guarantee a satisfied patient.

The Link to Relational Trauma

Patients with BDD are obviously troubled, but where does the problem begin? This question, I believe, has received too little attention in the literature. My current answer reflects observations of the effects of trauma in dysfunctional families and the experiences of some of my patients.* Relational trauma and its lifelong aftershocks circumscribe many features relevant to our discussion of patients with BDD and the spectrum of affective and behavioral dysfunction in which BDD is only a single point.

Trauma, Core Issues, Addictions, and Relational Problems

Nurturing parents raise their children to understand five concepts *(core issues)* that form the basis for mature adult behavior: (1) their vulnerabilities, (2) their strengths and weaknesses, (3) their dependency, and (4) the importance of moderation. *But most of all, nurturing parents teach their children that* (5) *they are valuable*—that they are neither less than nor better than others but are precious simply because they are alive. Their value does not need to be earned.

When dysfunction in a family causes relational trauma or abuse of any kind, the core issues develop differently. The child may learn distorted self-esteem, develop poor boundaries, have an imperfect sense of reality, and struggle with self-reliance or living in moderation.

We all know patients who display the extremes of these types of dysfunctional upbringing. At one end of the spectrum are arrogant, resentful, self-important patients who are rude to office and hospital personnel and want to dictate the operative procedure. At the other end are passive, hypersensitive, indecisive, dependent patients whose neediness places special burdens on both surgeon and staff.

Although dysfunctional behavior appears along a spectrum, the extremes are easiest to identify as the *love (or relational) addict* and the *love (or relational) avoidant*. Love addicts, in particular, have a special capacity to create fantasies that significantly complicate the surgeon-patient relationship and may contribute to the unhappiness and emotional intensity felt by patients with BDD.

---

*My ideas have been heavily influenced by the model elaborated by Pia Mellody, to whom I am grateful for her interest and comments on my thesis.

Relational Addiction

Both love addicts and love avoidants are subsets of individuals known as *codependents,* a term that itself is more broadly used to indicate immaturity caused by childhood trauma. Codependents suffer from five primary, or core, symptoms:

1. Difficulty experiencing an appropriate level of self-esteem
2. Difficulty protecting themselves by setting proper boundaries
3. Difficulty defining their reality; in other words, knowing who they are
4. Difficulty with self-care
5. Difficulty living in moderation

As a result, codependents interpret the behaviors of others inaccurately, which in turn impairs their relationships. However, the primary problem of codependents is their relationship with themselves. As a result, secondary symptoms develop that directly interfere with a healthy surgeon-patient relationship. These include the following:

1. Negative control. Codependents either try to control others or allow others to control them.
2. Resentment as a form of self-protection. From this resentment develops victim anger, as already seen in patients one, two, and five. This resentment may generate not only anger but also desire for revenge.
3. Impaired spirituality. Codependents improperly view others with godlike powers through hate, fear, or worship or may attempt to be another's higher power.
4. Addictions and mental or physical illness.
5. Difficulty with intimacy (healthy, close relationships).

As a subcategory of codependency, love (or relational) addicts share three common traits that directly affect their ability to establish and maintain a healthy surgeon-patient relationship:

1. Love addicts assign a disproportionate amount of time and attention to the person to whom they are addicted, often obsessively.
2. Love addicts have unrealistic expectations for unconditional positive approval from the person to whom they are addicted.
3. Love addicts are unable to value or care for themselves in that relationship.

It is not difficult to imagine what problems these personal characteristics can create in marriages or other intimate relationships, but imagine also what problems they can create when the love addict is a patient.

Love addicts commonly rate their surgeons as superior to (or more powerful than) themselves. In fact, patients who assign more power to a surgeon than he or she truly possesses will always expect a more flawless surgical result than is ever possible. Beyond the surgical result, love addicts can expect the other party (the surgeon, in this situation) to rescue them from their own unhappiness, protect them from pain, and nurture them—exactly what they never received from their parents. Thus the surgeon becomes the savior, and the object of an addiction that is no different from an addiction to alcohol, gambling, drugs, sex, or work. However, the surgeon, who has now become the love addict's drug, can never fulfill these impossible expectations, and so the patient experiences repeated disappointments. When the patient experiences enough pain, he or she may move to another surgeon, begin the cycle again, and only suffer subsequent disappointments.

The toxicity of the patient's disappointment fuels victim anger, complaints to medical boards, or retaliation against what the patient believes is a deliberate failure to nurture and rescue, which is what the patient expected.

The Physician Component

In the midst of this bewildering morality play, the surgeon plays a primary role. Trained and disciplined as we are, our behavior only fuels the flames. Matching the patient's sense of low self-esteem is the surgeon's (perceived or real) high self-esteem. Matching the patient's boundaryless vulnerability is the surgeon's apparent unflagging strength and invulnerability. Matching the patient's physical (nasal) and psychological sense of imperfection is the surgeon's apparently needless and wantless perfection.

And So the Play Begins

We have our protagonist. The patient, wounded through improper parenting into a painful reality of shame and inadequacy (or superiority), the specter of which has followed the patient into adulthood camouflaged, copes with greater or lesser success through years of adaptation. Just as the child adapted to survive in a dysfunctional family unit, he or she has adapted to survive in life. The variations of this compensatory behavior are as limitless as the human personality. Examples of these behaviors include the successful executive who nevertheless swamps the surgeon's office with fussy, worried telephone calls about each step of the preoperative and postoperative care; or the charming, voluble, cooperative, and grateful woman who has no questions about the surgical procedure but who nevertheless remains dismally dissatisfied with every one of her numerous previous cosmetic operations. My first clue to adaptations of the wounded child is usually a sense of discomforting incongruence—that is, the demeanor of worried indecision does not match that of the successful executive; neither does the unhappiness with previous results match the charming, unquestioning persona of the patient in front of me. I try not to brush aside bewilderment in these circumstances.

A patient drawn to surgery to increase his or her sense of self-worth seeks a surgeon-patient relationship that simulates the unconditional, positive regard that the patient wanted from his or her parents as a child but may not have received. The attention, the careful instructions, and the solicitousness of the staff, which appears to be merely competent care to a conscientious surgeon, may look like the behavior of loving parents to a patient who has seemed to adapt but, in reality, has no idea of his or her self-worth. The entire experience is intensified by expectations of improvement after surgery. Similar to Sleeping Beauty waking to new happiness with her prince, the love-addicted patient expects to wake up from anesthesia to a transformed life.

As noted earlier, love addicts can neglect self-care when they enter into an addictive relationship. As surgeons we see these manifestations in a different setting, such as when an apparently self-sufficient, competent patient deteriorates after surgery and becomes passive, excessively needy, and childlike. For example, I treated one tertiary rhinoplasty patient whose preoperative complaints were well circumscribed and achievable but who, after surgery, had difficulty expressing herself in moderation and difficulty containing her anger.

Patient Eight

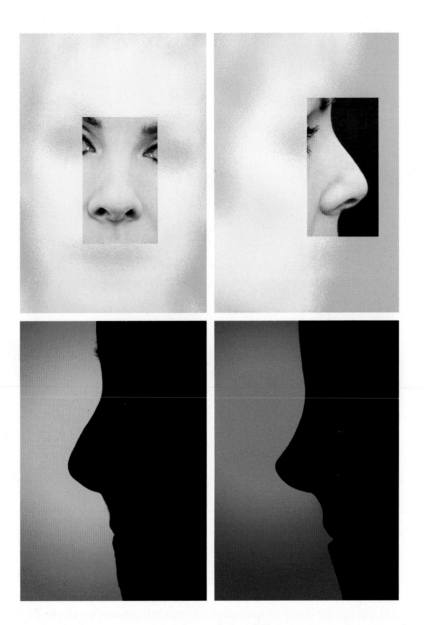

This primary rhinoplasty patient requested the following conservative changes: reduce the hump, but do not create a pinched tip, retroussé, or tip angularity. Silhouettes dramatize the rearrangement.

The patient's sister came with her when the dressings were removed and remarked, with apparent annoyance, "*I told her* she should never have gone through this."

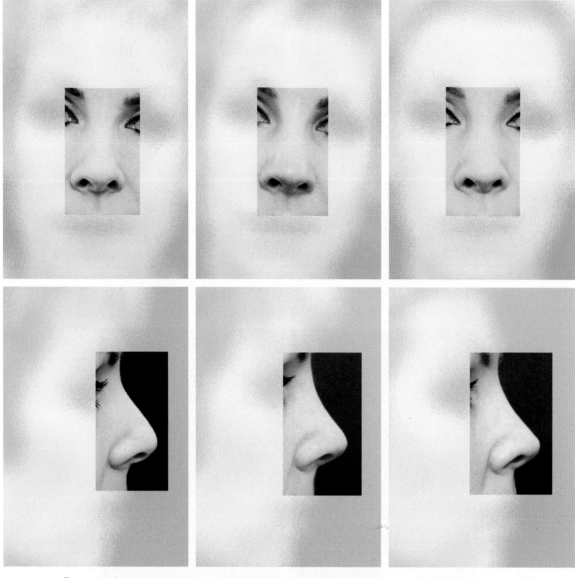

| Preoperative | 1 month postoperatively | 18 months postoperatively |

Notice, as you compare the preoperative, 1-month postoperative, and 18-month postoperative photographs, that things change only as they should. The nose progressively narrows, but the middle vault remains stable. Frontal symmetry and balance have improved. In the lateral views, the nose appears smaller where it was reduced, but (despite tip grafting that has brought the tip above the septal angle) the lower nose does not appear larger because it is offset by the radix graft. As the edema resolves, contours improve but remain stable.

The patient was almost immediately unhappy. It was futile to reassure her that the swelling would be transient. She was inconsolable.

She wrote a letter pleading for revision. Although my staff and I had spent many hours trying to reassure her, her response was not disappointment but rather victim anger. The following are excerpts from our correspondence (italics are mine):

> I have a few more questions [based on what I have read on the Internet]. . . . I am wondering if [the osteotomy] was made sufficiently thin enough? If this wasn't made thin enough, then it seems I could wait forever and still not have the look I was hoping to achieve. . . . If this is the case, then the mental distress of having to wait another 6 months for more surgery and then having to go through another year of swelling is almost more than I can bear. . . .

> *I know that you don't consider me an attractive person. My sister told me that at this point my looks are ruined—that my nose is way too wide and I am missing a certain more feminine look I had before. You may not agree, but I have not heard one positive comment from anyone: friends, family, co-workers, or even casual acquaintances. . . .*

> It is now the start of the seventh month with no change. . . . Doctors on the Internet say that their patients do not swell and are happy right away. . . . I just expected to feel more attractive, not less so. . . .

> Why did you use a spreader graft in my nose when, according to the attached articles, it is not generally recommended for nasal refinement?

> *I feel, at this point, that it is cruel to continue making me walk around looking like this.* Why do people on the *Extreme Makeover* shows have noses that look so good and are hardly swollen after 6 weeks to 4 months when their noses were worse than mine to begin with?

> *I have lost hope, 18 months after surgery, that my nose is going to turn into something I can live with. Nothing has changed—it is larger than ever. I cannot tolerate any more remarks such as: "why is your nose so large after you had rhinoplasty?" "why did you have it made so wide?" "when are you going to do something about it?" "how can you walk around like that?" "I would be so disappointed if I were you," etc. . . .*

> It is the extreme width from the front view that is very disturbing to me. . . . I am relying on you for compassion and help. . . .

> *I just wanted to thank you for effectively ruining my life. Each plastic surgeon I have seen has admitted that my nose is too wide but that I should go back to you because you are such a "professional" and would be able to fix it, and you certainly would not want an unhappy patient. Well, as we know, you don't care if I am unhappy or not. . . .*

You have made my nose wider and bigger than any woman I know. I feel, literally, like a freak. I am having a hard time even leaving the house each morning. Now, let's see— what kind of drug would help that problem? How many years of counseling will help with having an oversized nose that I actually paid for?

A better profile doesn't make up for having what my brother-in-law calls a "clown" nose. Why you have turned against me and abandoned me when I am in need of help, I just cannot understand. If you don't believe the comments I am hearing, I can get sworn affidavits. *I think you are just stubbornly refusing to acknowledge that this look has not worked out for me. . . .*

Throughout these excerpts, notice the patient appears to be mind reading ("I know that you don't consider me an attractive person"), an unusual remark to make to one's surgeon. Recall the patient's victim anger ("I feel, at this point, that it is cruel to continue making me walk around looking like this"), alternating with desperation, and her inability to nurture herself ("I have lost hope at this point").

Finally, notice that the patient believes that the relationship is deteriorating (because I will not agree to schedule another surgery), the patient's seductive pleas ("I *know,* with your expertise, that something can be done about it. . . . I am relying on you for compassion and help"). At last, the patients' victim anger resurfaces ("I just wanted to thank you for effectively ruining my life. . . . You don't care if I am happy or not. . . . I feel, literally, like a freak"), and she states her real distress ("Why you have turned against me and abandoned me when I am in need of help, I just cannot understand").

I did not manage this case expertly. I was responding in a logical manner, answering questions about spreader grafts, and explaining osteotomies when I might have been more successful if I had addressed her pain and fear. Unfortunately, the patient's solution is more surgery (as we have seen in each of the preceding patients). This is one of the characteristics that distinguishes surgical patients from psychiatric patients. In the latter, a diagnosis of BDD has already been made and the patient has accepted it.

I speculate that many patients with love-addicted personalities see their surgeons as nine-foot-tall, bulletproof saviors who will "rescue" them from their inadequacies and, through the miracle of surgical intervention, will fix what is wrong in these patients' lives. When this does not occur, these patients become angry. As in patient one, the reaction is not disappointment but rather victim anger: "How could you have done this to me, and why? . . . I feel so terribly betrayed."

Evidence From a Patient's Story

Patient Nine

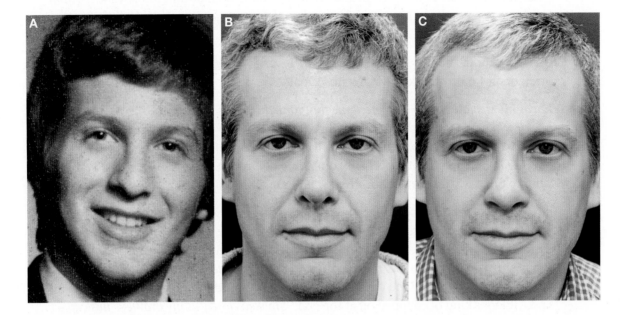

The history of this patient from 2001 was my first clue to the link between relational trauma and BDD. The above photographs show the patient's preoperative appearance *(A)*, his appearance when he first consulted me, requesting a reduction of nostril visibility *(B)*, and 4 years postoperatively after conchal skin/cartilage composite grafts *(C)*.

At the beginning of his interview, the patient explained that he had previously been diagnosed as having BDD. He had been treated and believed he had recovered. I sought confirmation from his therapist, who concurred.

After his surgery, through which he was an excellent patient, I asked, "If I write you a letter with a series of questions, will you describe for me what it was like being inside BDD?" He agreed, and the following is his fascinating letter, printed in its entirety. The sections with the greatest relevance to the etiologic factors of BDD are in italics.

Here are some thoughts that I hope touch on some of the questions you asked me to answer about my experiences with BDD.

Before the First Surgery: Summer of 1978

I was an extremely shy, self-conscious, and unconfident child and adolescent. I could barely get two words out in history class without becoming tongue-tied, blushing, and my voice becoming quivery.

I felt OK about the way I looked. *I wished I wasn't so thin and scrawny,* but I didn't dwell on it. I didn't think about my nose at all.

It was my stepfather who convinced me that something was wrong with the way I looked. Looking back on it, he spent a lot of time and creativity trying to convince me that my nose looked weird. I suppose he didn't feel too good about himself—he was a 50-year-old parking lot attendant with, probably not coincidentally, a large "Greek" nose that had a bump on it. My mother, my brothers, and I are all 100% Jewish.

It took years for him to convince me that something was wrong with my nose. *He said to me, "Your nose droops. I'm going to call you 'droopy nose' from now on," doing his best imitation of a 7-year-old.* I looked in the mirror, turning my head from side to side, but everything looked OK to me. *I was mostly angry just for the very idea that my stepfather was trying to upset me.* One day, he pointed out my brother's nose to me. "Look," he said. "It looks kind of chopped off at the end." *I looked closely at my brother's nose apart from his face for probably the first time in my life.* My stepfather was right; my brother's nose looked different from what most people think a nose should look. I'd never noticed it before.

The harassment from my stepfather continued through the years. "Your nose goes down straight like this," he said, while tracing his finger through the air, "and then . . . it droops. I don't know; it looks funny." My stepfather also described my nose as if it were in the process of getting worse. "It's starting to droop. It's turning into a [family name] nose." My biological father was mentally ill, so I found this frightening. *Finally, the summer before my senior year in high school, I submitted two photographs taken by my stepfather with the express purpose of showing me what was wrong with my nose. My stepfather struggled to find the perfect angle to capture the flaw of my nose. And I let him do it.*

That year, which was kind of a lonely one for me, I got dumped by my first girlfriend, among other things, and I would take out the photographs whenever I felt in a down mood. I noticed my nose looked a little flat at the end, but that it was at 90 degrees in profile (which I felt was good). With a pen, I drew in my own tip graft to make my nose look like an average nose. One day, I got angry and scribbled through the tip of my nose angrily. It's clear in retrospect that *my generalized self-hatred had transferred to my nose.* I remember the following "conversation" with my stepfather:

ME: Other people have noses like mine.
HIM: No they don't.

The battle was over. I believed my stepfather.

I started looking at my nose in the mirror with a second mirror so I could scrutinize my nose in profile. *I'd work myself into a state of agitation at how my nose "drooped."* After 10 minutes or so, I would stop. I don't believe I thought about my nose too much when I was out in public, but the little I did, I found to be painful. "Why not change the thing I hated about myself?" I thought. *I thought by changing my nose, I would stop thinking about it for even a second, and free my mind from this obstacle.* My stepfather and mother were against surgery, but I was convinced there was something wrong with my nose. I didn't give too much detailed instruction to [the doctor]. "I don't like the way it droops. I just want a slight change. Don't make me look like a pig." I had seen two of my classmates' "nose jobs" and didn't like their unnatural look. I thought that if I told [the doctor] to be conservative, he would be and everything would be OK. *I had grown up with the TV shows* Medical Center *and* Marcus Welby, MD, *and in those shows doctors were gods and never made mistakes.*

After Primary Surgery: 1978-1982

I didn't like the way I looked after surgery, but I wasn't horrified. I hoped that I had broken even—that my nose had looked weird before the surgery, and now it looked weird still, but at least I had actively tried to change something I didn't like about myself. My stepfather's reaction: "It still looks weird." My brother's reaction: "It still looks Jewish."

I had a goal in mind when I went to college: to become a doctor myself. I focused on that goal as much as I could and tried to forget about my nose. On my first day at the University of Massachusetts, I bumped into a high school acquaintance who lived in my dorm: "I hate nose jobs," she said, apropos of nothing—other than seeing my nose, that is. I was an erratic student: some days I'd study all day, and the next day I'd skip all my classes. I had around a 3.5 GPA after 2 years, and I worried all the time about my future, to the point of waking up with my heart pounding. *Occasionally I would use two mirrors to look at myself in profile, vacillating back and forth about whether my nose looked OK.* I don't remember looking at it too closely from the front.

In the summer of 1980, my brother committed suicide. I blamed myself for not being more involved in my brother's life and concentrating on my pre-med obsession instead. *I felt I didn't cry enough, I felt numb. I hated myself so much, and considered myself an uncaring person.* I lost my ambition to be a doctor, reasoning that if I couldn't help or care about my brother, how could I care about strangers. I switched majors from premed to psychology, then English. *As my life lost meaning, I started to get obsessed with my nose for the first time. I felt sure that it looked operated on and strange, and I started to avoid socializing. I asked all my friends, old and new, about whether they had noticed anything weird looking about my nose.* No one said they did. I had very nice friends as roommates, and they kept me from being totally isolated. *Unfortunately, I can't remember how long it took to grow into an obsession. I think it was a fairly short period of time. I remember wanting to drown myself when I went on an outing to the beach with my friends; that's how bad I felt about how I looked.* I felt my nose looked shapeless, short, and snubby in profile, but I don't remember thinking much about how my nostrils looked from the front.

Hope came when a psychologist I was seeing suggested that I go to a medical library to find out more about my nose. I saw an article by one surgeon about something called a "supratip deformity." I felt very happy that there was a name and a solution for my problem. I had a feeling that this surgeon was a maverick, a man who cared about quality in what I had started to feel was a pretty sloppy and careless profession. *He was my only hope, so perhaps I built him up in my mind.* But he was so busy in those days that I think it took me 6 months just to get an appointment and another 3 to have the surgery. *I stayed pretty isolated before surgery,* and I was still very self-conscious about my nose, but I think I might have taken a class or two and was somewhat relaxed and hopeful before surgery. I signed up for a summer class at UCLA so that I could hang around Los Angeles for awhile after surgery.

Surgery: 1982

It was quite an experience going to another city for the surgery. I stayed at a house for out-of-town patients, and got to know a few people who were in the same boat as I was, and I didn't feel so isolated. I have fond memories of the woman who owned the house; among her kindnesses, she served us fresh-squeezed orange juice, even after we had had our surgeries and couldn't appreciate it. I remember catching a glimpse of myself after the bandages were removed and noticing a lot of nostril show for the first time. I quelled that thought and walked around UCLA fairly happy, even with my glasses taped to my forehead, because I knew that my profile looked better. *I had gone to the best doctor in the world:* What else could I do? It was time to forget about my nose.

I pretty much did. I struggled to finish college and find a new purpose in life now that my dream of being a doctor was over. Every day I would wake up and think about my brother, and what an asshole I was. I tried desperately to feel some grief and a connection to him. *I went to a psychiatrist with the goal of learning how to cry about my brother, and to feel less like an evil person who had somehow caused him to kill himself.* I somewhat succeeded in my goal of grieving the loss of my brother. I cried a lot, but it was difficult for me. Every time I cried, I thought I was breaking through to a more real and passionate and compassionate life.

I read a book by Noam Chomsky called *Turning the Tide* and became wildly political. This book changed my whole view of the world. The book was about the U.S. government supporting the brutal Salvadoran government, and the counterrevolutionaries in Nicaragua. *I had a found a new obsession, a purpose to life.* I would stop moaning about things I should have done for my brother, but couldn't do anything about now, and become a Central America activist. I imagined my brother as a Nicaraguan or Salvadoran peasant whom I would save. I worked really hard trying to do that for a few years, from 1986 to 1988. *My guilt about my brother was transferred to these political issues.* I don't remember looking at my nose at all, or thinking much about it.

1988-1992

My inheritance from my father ran out. The Central America issue was fading from the news. With no money, I moved back to my parents' house. *I felt like a complete failure.* With my new political beliefs, I didn't want to work in the corporate world. I felt a sense of dissatisfaction with the political world, a lack of a sense of accomplishment or of developing my skills. Could I really hand out fliers for the rest of my life? I signed up for computer science classes at the University of Massachusetts in Boston. I had no car and practically no friends in my old hometown. *I tried to concentrate on my classes, but I felt a sense of guilt about abandoning the Central America issue. I had become very sensitive to the fact that there was a huge amount of suffering in the world and I was doing very little to help alleviate it. I wasn't doing well in my computer science classes. In this maelstrom of negative feeling, my nose obsession grew to its greatest level ever.* It began in January 1992, perhaps related to a medical experiment I had signed up for: $1200 to be a guinea pig for a blood pressure medication. Somewhere between January and June of 1992, *I developed a full-blown obsession with how my nostrils looked from the front. My nose looked "suspended" up above where it should be. I tried to pull my nose down. I pushed my nostril sills up. My nostrils looked very round, noticeable, and unnatural to me,* which they hadn't before, except right after surgery, and I had quickly forgotten about it. *I wrote to my surgeon, hiding my great distress.* By this time I was looking at my nose for hours at a time, arguing with myself. "If it's so obvious to me, why isn't it obvious to everyone else? Why didn't I think or notice it much in the last 10 years when it looks so obvious now?" *I would walk around the house looking at my nose in various lighting, trying to see when the nostril problem was most noticeable.* The surgeon wrote back to me and said "further improvement was possible," but I had no money. I begged my brother Michael and my parents for money, but they wouldn't give it to me. I was currently working for $7.50 an hour, and *I had a sense of hopelessness* about raising the money. Looking back on it, I don't know why. Why couldn't I have gotten a second or even a third job if I was so desperate for "further improvement"? *I felt totally helpless, and I went the mental health route instead.*

1992-1996: A Trip Through the Mental Hell-th System

Various medications were tried, mixed with others, and abandoned. My nose obsession continued. *I grew suicidal because I couldn't stop thinking about how deformed my nose looked to me and, I imagined, to others. Some medications made me sick, some made me confused. My life was out of control as I looked for a magic pill. I was in and out of hospitals.* In 1996 I remember being so confused that I spent a whole night trying to figure out how to put on my t-shirt. I failed. I went into a 10-day coma from what afterward doctors said was serotonin poisoning. I was released from the hospital a month later. *I was in the blackest mood of my life, and I stayed in bed sleeping as much as possible. I went back into the hospital.* I got electroshock therapy and was released in, I think, October 1996. *I went to a group home to live, because my mother couldn't stand the stress anymore. I spent my days in treatment chatting with other nuts. At first the ECT made me so confused I didn't know who I was or what my problems were. A lot of the negative energy was removed from my nose. I started to think that my problem was not my nose, but that I was 36 years old and didn't know how to support myself finan-cially, and that I'd never had a girlfriend, and that I would be in this awful situation for the rest of my life unless I worked to change it.* I forgot about the poor people of El Salvador, Nicaragua, and everywhere. I thought, *"My life sucks almost as bad as theirs does, I had better do something about helping myself before I can help them."* I got a job delivering newspapers early in the morning. Then I got a job as a substitute teacher. I sold my brother's vintage guitar for $2000 and moved out of the group home and into a nice apartment near the ocean. I got my first real girlfriend at age 37. I got certified as a teacher and got my first real job as a math teacher at 38. I still didn't like my nose: the nostrils, the idea that I even got that first nose job in the first place, *but instead of carrying the obsession with myself all day, the last thing I said to myself as I left the mir-ror was, "That's not your real problem."* And I was able to forget about it as I went about my business.

In 2000, I got married. In 2001 my marriage wasn't going well, and my stepfather died. My work as a teacher at an alternative school was a strain, because I was still shy and not a strict-enough disciplinarian. I went to Portugal with my wife and felt guilty be-cause the whole time I was thinking about how I was going to tell her I wanted a sep-aration. *My wife spoke Portuguese and we were staying with her brother there, and I was totally dependent on her. In this context I developed nose consciousness for the first time since being released from the hospital in 1996.* I got in contact with my surgeon again, and then you.

Now, let me read your questions again to make sure I touched on them in my "nose biography":

Q: Are there stages to developing BDD?

A: In my experience, there are different levels of BDD, but the onset is fairly abrupt.
Level 0: Lack of nose consciousness.
Level 1: Nose consciousness in private moments; dissatisfaction, mostly forgotten in public.
Level 2: On the brink. Carrying nose consciousness around while in public, fight-ing it off with varying degrees of success, struggling, wasting time in front of the mirror.
Level 3: Over the edge. Full-blown obsession, spending several hours in front of the mirror, difficulty thinking of anything else.

Q: Were all my perceptions distorted, or just my body image, or just my nose?

A: Just my nose.

Q: Did I view my surgeon's surgery differently [when BDD developed]? Was it no longer successful in my eyes?

A: Since I didn't notice my nostril visibility before the surgery, I wondered whether in fixing my supratip deformity, my surgeon inadvertently created the nostril visi-bility problem. I knew my surgeon was regarded as the best rhinoplasty surgeon in the world, so I figured the nostrils were probably a preexisting problem that I had not noticed before. I wondered why my surgeon did not fix the nostril problem at the same time as the supratip problem. At the same time that I developed BDD with regard to my nostrils, I was grateful that my surgeon had done such a nice job on my profile. At the same time, I wished that my nose was longer, but I knew that shortening of my nose had occurred in the first operation, and my surgeon was probably unable to do anything to correct that. As far as my profile went, even with BDD, I thought my surgeon did a great job with what he had to work with, but I figured that the material just wasn't there.

Q: How did my friends and associates view this period? Did anyone understand?

A: My friends were very supportive for long periods, although many gave up on me because I was sick for a very long time. Overall, I think my friends were probably more understanding than I would have expected them to be.

Q: How easy was it to find a psychiatrist who understood this problem?

A: I didn't really find anyone who I felt helped me, but I don't think there is really any way to help someone with BDD, other than hit-or-miss methods. ECT helped me, I guess, but I worry that I may have sustained brain damage in the process, because I am definitely more forgetful than I was in the past, but it may be because of age.

Q: [What are the] clues for a surgeon to make the diagnosis of BDD?

A: Honest patients will tell you if they have BDD, or if they don't know about BDD. If they answer questions posed to them honestly about how much they think about their appearance and if they believe their obsession is negatively affecting their lives, the surgeon will be able to determine whether or not these persons have BDD.

I can see reading over what I wrote, that I wrote mostly about my life, to give a context in which BDD developed. *Not surprisingly, when my life is not going well, I have a tendency to develop BDD.* I may take another shot at this, with a greater focus on the questions you specifically asked, but I am afraid if I don't send what I have written so far, you won't get anything. I hope what I have written is of some use to you, and perhaps other doctors and patients, in understanding BDD.

If I needed evidence that some patients with BDD come from dysfunctional families, this was it. His letter told a compelling story of systematic child abuse by his stepfather. He describes the early attention the stepfather brought to his nose, his initial resistance to the stepfather's beliefs, and his ultimate growing obsession with his perceived nasal deformity once the stepfather's view prevailed.

This patient had an epiphany, completed his education, created a family, and became a school teacher. Many patients are not that fortunate and spend years pursuing a dizzying array of operations that are never successful.

Narcissism in the Classical Sense: A Factor in Body Dysmorphic Disorder

Surgeons have a tendency to label patients with BDD, and many other difficult patients, as narcissistic. The DSM-IV-TR defines *narcissistic personality disorder* as a preoccupation with an exaggerated sense of self-importance, brilliance, or beauty. But who was Narcissus? Ovid's *Metamorphoses* notes that Narcissus was the son of the nymph Liriope. Anxious to know if her son would live to see a ripe old age, she consulted the seer Tiresias. The prophet answered, "If he never knows himself."

Seeing his reflection in a pool of water, Narcissus was engulfed by the beauty of his own image. "He fell in love with an image without reality, and he mistook for reality what was only an image. Narcissus was held spellbound by himself and lay there motionless . . . gazing into his own eyes . . . the beauty of his face, the rosy glow on his snow-white skin, and he admired all that he saw. . . . Foolishly he longed for himself. . . . So Narcissus, pining with love, wasted away and was gradually consumed by the fire of love buried within him. . . . Narcissus laid his weary head upon the green grass as death closed the eyes that wondered at the beauty of the sight that held them."

Narcissus, filled with "such chill pride," was unable to establish an authentic relationship, and instead became captivated and eventually destroyed by the illusory beauty of his own reflection. In *I Don't Want to Talk About It*, therapist Terrence Real agrees with the Renaissance philosopher, Marsilio Ficinio, that Narcissus suffered not from an overabundance of self-love but rather from a deficiency of it.

The myth of Narcissus is a parable about the absence of self-esteem. Rather than an internal sense of preciousness and value instilled by his parents, Narcissus formed his sense of himself entirely from the external: his beautiful appearance. In this way, he is no different from the man who only believes that he has self-worth when he earns more money than I do, or drives a bigger car, or performs more rhinoplasties. Like anyone addicted to reflected glory, Narcissus cannot break free, even at the cost of his own life. As such, Narcissus is not self-obsessed; rather he is image-obsessed.

Put some of your unhappy patients in this context. I believe that many of the patients who seek one cosmetic procedure after another or one rhinoplasty touchup after another, who are never quite happy but never quite able to articulate why, are searching for a sense of self-worth that surgery cannot provide. The operation is irrelevant. These patients see themselves as imperfect and worthless because their noses are not perfect. They unconsciously believe that once the surgical correction is made, an internal sense of self-worth will appear. This, it seems to me, is narcissism in the classical sense, and it explains not only why the surgery is not helpful but why entire families concur that the problem is surgical and not psychological. It is not uncommon for families to share the same mistaken beliefs about self-esteem, because parenting values continue from generation to generation unless someone breaks the pattern. Traditional socialization teaches young women that self-worth depends on appearance, whereas it teaches young men that self-worth depends on performance. In each case the filter is external, and so something internal is always missing.

Patient Ten

This young woman underwent rhinoplasty when she was a college student; at that time I had been in practice for only 2 years.

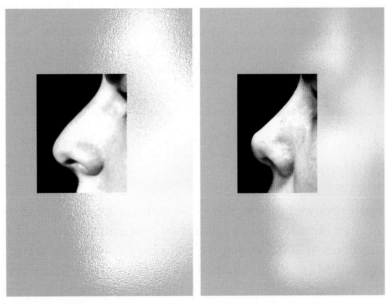

Preoperative   10 years postoperatively

A very bright young woman, she went on to practice law and then abandoned it to help her husband in his business. She suffered chronically from clinical depression that did not respond to a change in careers.

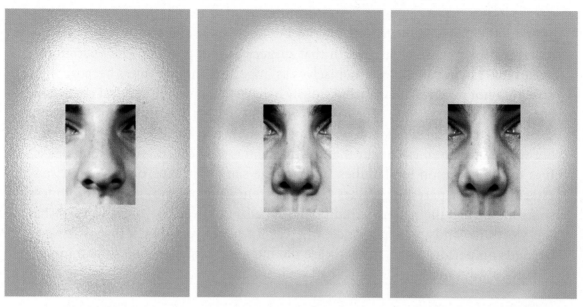

Preoperative   7 years postoperatively   10 years after the initial surgery

Periodically she would call to ask about revisions, an idea that I always discouraged despite the fact that she had received advice about "easy touch-ups" from other surgeons. Some 20 years after her rhinoplasty, she committed suicide. Nothing external in this woman's life apparently created a sufficient sense of self-worth. I have listened to the histories of many unhappy patients and others treated for BDD; virtually every one used the words, "I was never quite good enough," or "I always felt that there was something wrong with me." "I must have surgery," one patient confided, "because inside I am fundamentally flawed."

The Incidence of Body Dysmorphic Disorder in Private Practice

Some years ago I reviewed the records of 50 consecutive primary rhinoplasty patients and 75 consecutive secondary rhinoplasty patients whom I had seen in consultation, in addition to 200 consecutive secondary patients on whom I had performed rhinoplasty. My staff and I looked for the following primary and secondary personality traits as we saw them: normal, depressed, demanding, perfectionistic, undiagnosed but real surgical problem, functional problem, minimal defect, and, finally, no insight. This last trait is notoriously characteristic of patients with BDD.

Primary and Secondary Personality Characteristics of 200 Consecutive Operated Secondary Rhinoplasty Patients

Personality Trait	Number	Percent*
Primary Characteristics		
Unremarkable	81	41
Undiagnosed surgical pathology	51	26
Perfectionistic	25	13
Functional airway pathology	18	9
Depressed	9	5
Demanding	8	4
Minimal defect	8	4
No insight	0	0
Secondary Characteristics		
Functional airway pathology	103	52
Depressed	48	24
Demanding	30	15
Perfectionistic	27	14
Undiagnosed surgical pathology	21	11
Minimal defect	15	8
No insight	7	4
Unremarkable	2	1

*Percentages may exceed 100 because numbers were rounded off.

Personality Characteristics of 325 Rhinoplasty Patients

Personality Trait	50 Primary Rhinoplasty Patients Seen in Consultation (%)	75 Secondary Rhinoplasty Patients Seen in Consultation (%)	200 Secondary Rhinoplasty Patients (%)
Unremarkable	50	7	41
Undiagnosed surgical pathology	16	36	26
Perfectionistic	10	19	13
Functional airway pathology	14	7	9
Depressed	0	4	5
Demanding	8	11	4
Minimal defect	0	5	4
No insight	2	12	4

We rated our patients according to their most prominent primary and secondary personality characteristics. For example, if a patient had a functional problem but was also depressed, each characteristic was listed according to its dominance.

When both primary and secondary traits were pooled, 61% of secondary rhinoplasty patients had functional problems that justified their unhappiness, and 37% had an undiagnosed pathologic condition that was treatable and directly related to their chief complaints.

However, 29% of these patients were depressed, 27% were perfectionistic, 19% were demanding, and 4% had apparent BDD that I did not perceive before surgery.

As expected, secondary rhinoplasty patients as a whole were more demanding and perfectionistic and had more minimal defects than primary rhinoplasty patients. They also had more undiagnosed deformities (but fewer functional problems, surprisingly). Although 12% of secondary rhinoplasty patients seen in consultation had no insight into their BDD, most were eliminated before surgery. Four percent of the operated secondary rhinoplasty patients later showed signs of BDD. Finally, even the primary rhinoplasty patients are not a "safe" group: 2% had no insight and therefore saw something I did not.

So what was my rationale for operating on that 4%? Examining their records, in each case I made a diagnosis of perfectionism, depression, or a functional problem that I believed justified the surgery. In focusing on the surgical deformity, I overlooked the BDD.

A Survey of 1000 Consecutive Rhinoplasty Patients

Some patients may have BDD, but equally troublesome are those who are disruptive and consume unusual amounts of staff and surgeon time. How common are they?

To determine this, I reviewed the records of 1000 consecutive rhinoplasty patients: 78% women and 22% men, 35% primary and 65% secondary rhinoplasty patients, which was my consistent demographic over the years. Patients were rated for their impact on the practice (that is, the level of disruption they caused) and on their insight.

Of 1000 patients, 9.1% were taxing, disruptive, narcissistic, or needy, and 2.5% had no insight into their behavior; thus 11.6% were deemed difficult patients.

Within the 11.6% who were labeled difficult, men were disproportionately represented: among the disruptive or needy patients, 30% were men, and of those with BDD, 40% were men. However, men represented only 22% of the total population. Other surgeons have made the same observation (Gorney, 2006).

As was identified in the survey, even primary rhinoplasty patients can be disruptive or have BDD. Of all the disruptive or needy patients, 6.5% were primary rhinoplasty patients; of all the patients with no insight (or BDD), 5% were primary rhinoplasty patients.

According to these data, therefore, if you perform only primary rhinoplasty, your chances of having a patient with BDD are 0.5%. If you also perform secondary rhinoplasty and your practice composition and diagnostic skills resemble mine, your chances are 4.5% of encountering a patient with BDD. However, 11.6% of your rhinoplasty patients will require extra time from you and your staff.

Putting It All Together

My current thesis is this: The degree of difficulty that patients demonstrate to surgeons and staff is partly related to their narcissism in the true sense of the word. Their self-worth is not internal but rather dependent on appearance. The conversion to BDD, in many cases, is related to childhood trauma. There is recent corroborating evidence to support my theory (Didie et al, 2006). The particularly troublesome subset of these difficult patients is the love addicts, as defined by Pia Mellody (1992): those unfortunate persons whose childhood experiences have engendered poorly functioning adults who cannot value themselves; who have poorer protective capacities (boundaries); who have distorted senses of reality ("My nose is abnormal; therefore I am worthless"); who have difficulty with self-care (particularly during the postoperative course) as well as with living and behaving moderately. In surgical situations, love addicts see the surgeon as a rescuer and therefore place unrealistic expectations not only on the surgeon but also on the effect that rhinoplasty will have on their lives. Preoperatively and postoperatively, these patients may experience an emotional high. As one patient told me, "I am never as happy as when I am recovering from cosmetic surgery." However, when the "rescue" does not occur, the fantasy transforms into victim anger and fear of abandonment, not just by the patient but by the plastic surgeon as well. The patient may plan how to entice the surgeon to operate again and reestablish the relationship, leave and find another surgeon, begin a secondary addiction (just as one of these patients did to alcohol), or think of ways to retaliate, through the medical boards, the Internet, destruction of personal property, or even bodily harm. Many of these patients demonstrate and recount significant relational trauma and self-esteem issues that lead them to multiple surgeries, endless revisions, unhappiness with the result, anger against the surgeon, a sense of betrayal, and sometimes a desire to "get even"—hence the importance of recognizing language and behavior that connote victim anger.

Who, Then, Are the Surgical Candidates?

Determining who are candidates for surgery is, of course, the critical question. Although screening surveys have proved useful in some dermatologic practices, I have not had the same experience in my practice. Even those developed by experts are too easily discovered by the patients: for my own practice, the questions are too transparent, and many patients will not admit that their distress level is as high as it feels, because they are seeking surgery, not psychiatric treatment, and therefore will not risk disqualifying themselves. However, there is a bigger issue: a decision to operate cannot rest simply on the size of the deformity—that is, if the deformity is large, surgery is always indicated, but if it is "slight" (in DSM-IV-TR language), surgery is not indicated.

Not every patient unhappy with prior surgery has BDD and, conversely, some patients who may have BDD seem reasonable, even charming, but are still not candidates for surgery. Therefore I believe it is most useful to use criteria that extend beyond the patients' level of distress and even the magnitude of their deformities. Any decision to operate must reflect both the surgical problem and the rapport between patient and surgeon.

Independent of the magnitude of the deformity or the emotions that may be felt by the patient or the surgeon are the answers to the following five questions:
1. *Can I see the deformity?* This question eliminates delusional patients, or patients whose problem shows only in "certain lights and certain mirrors in my house" and may be a clue to the patient for whom the nose has become a physical manifestation of an internal imperfection.
2. *Can I fix it?* This criterion will vary from surgeon to surgeon and must be based on operative experience and ease in correcting specific problems.
3. *Can I manage the patient?* A patient who is unacceptably nervous, impossible to examine, or unwilling to comply with preoperative and postoperative instructions is a poor candidate, even if all other conditions are met.

4. *If there is a complication, will the patient remain controlled and cooperate with treatment?* No patient enjoys a complication, but there are those who, although disappointed, quietly understand and will await the proper time for revision. There are others who become hysterical, angry, disruptive, or accusatory and want an immediate correction. Most surgeons can sense with accuracy which patients fall into which groups. I know from experience that the personal stress of operating on the latter group and anticipating the outcome if something goes wrong is agonizing. More than that, patients whose emotions are poorly controlled are in no position to withstand the additional trauma of surgery.

5. *Does the patient accept the margin of error inherent in surgery?* In dealing with patients with BDD, perfectionists, or those biased by a previous negative surgical experience, this is the most important criterion. Some patients (and even some surgeons) have unrealistic views concerning the degree to which any surgeon can control wound healing; the quality and availability of building materials, the patient's immune competence, or myriad other factors, currently known and unknown, that influence surgical outcomes.

    Even more important, a patient's willingness to accept the imperfection that is inherent in surgery is a willingness to accept the imperfection that is inherent in being human. Finally, acceptance of postoperative imperfection indicates recognition that surgeons themselves are not perfect.

This last recognition flies in the face of one of the strongest beliefs held by love addicts: that there is, somewhere out there, a savior who can correct what is wrong in the patient's life and create self-esteem. Failure to accept the fifth criterion is an absolute contraindication to elective aesthetic surgery, in my opinion.

Unless I can answer "yes" to each of these questions, I will not operate.

Conclusion

BDD is a troublesome disease. Because patients and their families are generally unaware of the disordered thought processes associated with it, BDD is extremely difficult to treat once surgery has been performed. BDD is common enough that every plastic surgeon will encounter it. My experience has generated the hypothesis that BDD is the result of narcissism, compounded in many instances by childhood trauma or abuse, which correlates with the increased incidence in other family members. Does the degree of childhood trauma correlate with the severity of symptoms of BDD? At present, I do not know. But I do believe that you cannot have BDD if you have self-esteem.

However, BDD is only one end of the spectrum. There are other difficult patients who are still not surgical candidates, even though they do not meet the criteria for BDD. Ultimately the decision to operate is a personal one between the patient and the surgeon. It depends on the ability of the surgeon to make the diagnosis, his or her comfort with its correction, and the personality characteristics *of the individual patient and surgeon.*

To that end, there is no substitute for taking the time needed during the initial patient interview, because rhinoplasty is brain surgery.

BIBLIOGRAPHY

Allen F, Pincus HA, First MB (Chair, Vice-Chair, Editor). Diagnostic and Statistical Manual of Mental Disorders (DSM-IV-TR), 4th ed. (text revision). Washington, DC: American Psychiatric Association, July 2000.

Andreasen NC. Dysmorphophobia: symptom or disease? Am J Psychiatry 134:673-676, 1977.

Bernstein DP, Fink L. Childhood Trauma Questionnaire: A Retrospective Self-Report (CTQ). San Antonio: Harcourt Assessment, 1998.

Bernstein DP, Fink L, Handelsman L, et al. Initial reliability and validity of a new retrospective measure of child abuse and neglect. Am J Psychiatry 151:1132-1136, 1994.

Bienvenu OJ, Samuels JF, Riddle MA, et al. The relationship of obsessive-compulsive disorder to possible spectrum disorders: results from a family study. Biol Psychiatry 48:287-293, 2000.

Book HE. Psychiatric assessment for rhinoplasty. Arch Otolaryngol 94:51-55, 1971.

Borah G. Psychological complications in 281 plastic surgery practices. Plast Reconstr Surg 104:1241-1246, 1999.

Brown J, Cohen P, Johnson JG, et al. Childhood abuse and neglect: specificity of effects on adolescent and young adult depression and suicidality. J Am Acad Child Adolesc Psychiatry 38:1490-1496, 1999.

Brunswick RM. A supplement to Freud's "History of an Infantile Neurosis." Int J Psychoanal 9:439-476, 1928.

Buhlmann U, Wilhelm S, McNally RJ, et al. Interpretive biases for ambiguous information in body dysmorphic disorder. CNS Spectr 7:435-443, 2002.

Byram V, Wagner HL, Waller G. Sexual abuse and body image distortion. Child Abuse Neglect 19:507-510, 1995.

Carter LS. Katharine Phillips '87: shedding light on BDD. Dartmouth Med, Spring 2001, pp 60-64.

Castello JR. Body dysmorphic disorder and aesthetic surgery: case report. Aesthetic Plast Surg 22:329-331, 1998.

Clarkson P, Stafford-Clark D. Role of the plastic surgeon and psychiatrist in the surgery of appearance. Br J Med 2:1768-1771, 1960.

Cole RP, Shakespeare V, Shakespeare P, et al. Measuring outcome in low-priority plastic surgery patients using Quality of Life indices. Br J Plast Surg 47:117-121, 1994.

Constantian MB. Closed rhinoplasty: current techniques, theory, and applications. In Mathes SJ, Hentz VR, eds. Plastic Surgery, vol 2, 2nd ed. Philadelphia: Elsevier, 2006, p 565.

Constantian MB. Relationship between patient and surgeon. In Goldwyn RM, Cohen MN, eds. The Unfavorable Result in Plastic Surgery, 3rd ed. Lippincott Williams & Wilkins, 2001, p 940.

Crerand CE, Franklin ME, Sarwer DB. Body dysmorphic disorder and cosmetic surgery. Plast Reconstr Surg 118:167e-180e, 2006.

Crisp AH. Dysmorphophobia and the search for cosmetic surgery. Br Med J 282:1099-1100, 1981.

Davis J, Petretic-Jackson PA, Ting L. Intimacy dysfunction and trauma symptomatology: long-term correlates of different types of child abuse. J Trauma Stress 14:63-79, 2001.

Deckersbach T, Savage CR, Phillips KA, et al. Characteristics of memory dysfunction in body dysmorphic disorder. J Int Neuropsychol Soc 6:673-681, 2000.

Didie ER, Tortolani CC, Pope CG, et al. Childhood abuse and neglect in body dysmorphic disorder. Child Abuse Negl 30:1105-1115, 2006.

Dinis PB. Psychosocial consequences of nasal aesthetic and functional surgery: a controlled prospective study in an ENT setting. Rhinology 36:32-36, 1998.

Doheny K. Cosmetic surgeries don't always end in a smile. Los Angeles Times, August 21, 1998.

Drapeau M, Peny JC. Childhood trauma and adult interpersonal functioning: a study using the core conflictual relationship theme method. Child Abuse Negl 28:1049-1066, 2004.

Dufresne RG. A screening questionnaire for body dysmorphic disorder in a cosmetic dermatologic surgery practice. Dermatol Surg 27:457-462, 2001.

Edgerton MT. Plastic surgery and psychotherapy in the treatment of 100 psychologically disturbed patients. Plast Reconstr Surg 88:594-608, 1991.

Evans E, Hawton K, Rodham K. Suicidal phenomena and abuse in adolescents: a review of epidemiological studies. Child Abuse Negl 29:45-58, 2005.

Ficino M. Commentary on Plato's symposium on love (translated by Jayne S). Dallas TX, Spring, 1985.

Gipson M, Connoly FH. The incidence of schizophrenia and sincere psychological disorders in patients 10 years after cosmetic rhinoplasty. Br J Plast Surg 28:155-159, 1975.

Glasgold AI. Psychological effects of rhinoplasty. J Med Soc N J 81:187-189, 1984.

Goin JM, Goin MK. Changing the Body: Psychological Effects of Plastic Surgery. Baltimore: Williams & Wilkins, 1981.

Goin MK. Psychological understanding and management of rhinoplasty patients. Clin Plast Surg 4:3-7, 1977.

Goldwyn RM. Beyond Appearance: Reflections of a Plastic Surgeon. New York: Dodd, Mead, 1986.

Goldwyn RM. The dissatisfied patient. In Goldwyn RM, Cohen MN. The Unfavorable Result in Plastic Surgery, 3rd ed. Philadelphia: Lippincott, 2001, pp 8-13.

Goldwyn RM. The Patient and the Plastic Surgeon, 2nd ed. Boston: Little Brown, 1991.

Goldwyn RM. Why we fail. In Goldwyn RM, Cohen MN, eds. The Unfavorable Result in Plastic Surgery, 3rd ed. Philadelphia: Lippincott, 2001, pp 3-7.

Gorney M. Professional and Legal Considerations in Cosmetic Surgery. In Sarwer DB, Pruzinsky T, Cash TF, et al, eds. Psychological Aspects of Reconstructive and Cosmetic Plastic Surgery. Philadelphia: Lippincott, 2006, pp 315-327.

Groves JE. Taking care of the hateful patient. N Engl J Med 298:883-887, 1978.

Guggenheim FG. Body dysmorphic disorder. In Sadock BJ, Sadock VA, eds. Kaplan and Sadock's Comprehensive Textbook of Psychiatry, vol 1, 7th ed. Philadelphia: Lippincott Williams & Wilkins, 2000, pp 1527-1531.

Guyuron B. Patient satisfaction following rhinoplasty. Aesthetic Plast Surg 20:153-157, 1996.

Hadley SJ, Kim S, Priday L, et al. Pharmacologic treatment of body dysmorphic disorder. Prim Psychiatry 13:61-69, 2006.

Hanes KR. Neuropsychological performance in body dysmorphic disorder. J Int Neuropsychol Soc 4:167-171, 1998.

Haraldsson PO. Psychosocial impact of cosmetic rhinoplasty. Aesthetic Plast Surg 23:170-174, 1999.

Harris D. The benefits and hazards of cosmetic surgery. Br J Hosp Med 41:543-545, 1989.

Hauptfuhrer F. Face to face with a nose? Asks Desmond Morris—look closely, it may be telling you something. People 25:57-61, 1986.

Hay GG. Psychiatric aspects of cosmetic nasal operations. Br J Psychiat 116:85-97, 1970.

Haybashi K, Miyachi H, Nakakita N, et al. Importance of a psychiatric approach in cosmetic surgery. Aesthet Surg J 27:398-401, 2007.

Hinderer UT. Dr. Vazquez Anon's last lesson. Aesthetic Plast Surg 2:375-382, 1978.

Hodgkinson DJ. Identifying the body-dysmorphic patient in aesthetic surgery. Aesthetic Plast Surg 29:503-509, 2005.

Hollander E. Body dysmorphic disorder. Psychiatr Ann 223:359-364, 1993.

Hollander E, Allen A. Beauty is in the eye of the beholder: new insights in imagined ugliness. Prim Psychiatry 13:37-38, 2006.

Honigman RJ. A review of psychological outcomes for patients seeking cosmetic surgery. Plast Reconstr Surg 113:1229-1237, 2004.

Ishigooka J, Iwao M, Suzuki M, et al. Demographic features of patients seeking cosmetic surgery. Psychiatry Clin Neurosci 52:283-287, 1998.

Jakubietz M, Jakubietz RJ, Klose DF, et al. Body dysmorphic disorder: diagnosis and approach. Plast Reconstr Surg 119:1924-1930, 2007.

Josephson SC. Obsessive-compulsive disorder, body dysmorphic disorder and hypochondriasis: three variations on a theme. CNS Spectr 1:24-31, 1996.

Kaplan HI. Somatoform disorders. In Kaplan HI, Sadock BJ, eds. Comprehensive Textbook of Psychiatry/VI, 6th ed. Baltimore: Williams & Wilkins, 1995, p 1268.

Kearney-Cooke A, Striegel-Moore RH. Treatment of childhood sexual abuse in anorexia nervosa and bulimia nervosa: a feminist psychodynamic approach. Int J Eat Disord 15:305-319, 1994.

Klassen A, Jenkinson C, Fitzpatrick R, et al. Patients' health-related quality of life before and after aesthetic surgery. Br J Plast Surg 433-438, 1996.

Knorr NJ. Feminine loss of identify in rhinoplasty. Arch Otolaryngol 96:11-15, 1972.

Kurtz RM. Sex differences and variations in body attitudes. J Consult Clin Psychol 33:625-629, 1969.

Last U, Moses S, Mahler D. Mental health correlates of valid perception of nasal deformity in female applicants for aesthetic rhinoplasty. Aesthetic Plast Surg 7:77-80, 1983.

Leonardo J. New York's highest court dismisses BDD case. Plast Surg News July:1-9, 2001.

Macgregor FC. Facial disfigurement: problems and management of social interaction and implications for mental health. Aesthetic Plast Surg 14:249-257, 1990.

Mancini C, Van-Ameringen M, Macmillan H. Relationship of childhood sexual and physical abuse to anxiety disorders. J Nerv Ment Dis 183:309-314, 1995.

Marcus P. Psychological aspects of cosmetic rhinoplasty. Br J Plast Surg 37:313-318, 1984.

Marcus P. Some preliminary psychological observations on narcissism, the cosmetic rhinoplasty patient and the plastic surgeon. Aust N Z J Surg 54:543-547, 1984.

McElroy SL, Phillips KA, Keck PE Jr, et al. Body dysmorphic disorder: does it have a psychotic subtype? J Clin Psychiatry 54:389-395, 1993.

Mellody P, Freundlich LS. The Intimacy Factor: The Ground Rules for Overcoming the Obstacles to Truth, Respect, and Lasting Love. New York: HarperCollins, 2003.

Mellody P, Miller AW, Miller JK. Facing Love Addiction: Giving Yourself the Power to Change the Way You Love. New York: HarperCollins, 1992.

Moses S. After aesthetic rhinoplasty: new looks and psychological outlooks on postsurgical satisfaction. Aesthetic Plast Surg 8:213-217, 1984.

Muhlbauer W, Wood DL, Home C. The Thersites complex in plastic surgical patients. Plast Reconstr Surg 107:319-326, 2001.

Newell R. Attitude change and behaviour therapy in body dysmorphic disorder: two case reports. Behav Cogn Psychother 22:163-169, 1994.

Ovid's Metamorphosis II: Echo and Narcissus (translated by Hendricks RA). In Hendricks Rhoda A. Classical Gods and Heroes: Myths as Told by the Ancient Authors. New York: William Morrow, 1974, p 339.

Phillips KA. Body dysmorphic disorder: diagnosis and treatment of imagined ugliness. J Clin Psychiatry 57(Suppl 8):61-65, 1996.

Phillips KA. Body dysmorphic disorder: the distress of imagined ugliness. Am J Psychiatry 148:1138-1149, 1991.

Phillips KA. Body dysmorphic disorder. In Oldham JM, Riba MB, eds. Review of Psychiatry Series, No 20. Somatoform and Factitious Disorders. Arlington, VA: American Psychiatric Publishing, 2001.

Phillips KA. The Broken Mirror—Understanding and Treating Body Dysmorphic Disorder. New York: Oxford University Press, 2005.

Phillips KA. Letter to the editor. Am J Psychiatry 149:577-578, 1992.

Phillips KA. Letter to the editor. Am J Psychiatry 149:719, 1992.

Phillips KA. Psychosis in body dysmorphic disorder. J Psychiatr Res 38:63-72, 2004.

Phillips KA, Coles M, Menard W, et al. Suicidal ideation and attempts in body dysmorphic disorder. J Clin Psychiatry 66:717-725, 2005.

Phillips KA, Diaz SF. Gender differences in body dysmorphic disorder. J Nerv Ment Dis 185:570-577, 1997.

Phillips KA, Dufresne RG. Body dysmorphic disorder: a guide for dermatologists and cosmetic surgeons. Am J Clin Dermatol 4:235-243, 2000.

Phillips KA, Grant J, Siniscalchi J, et al. Surgical and nonpsychiatric medical treatment of patients with body dysmorphic disorder. Psychosomatics 42:504-510, 2001.

Phillips KA, Kim JM, Hudson JI. Body image disturbance in body dysmorphic disorder and eating disorders—obsessions or delusions? Psychiatr Clin North Am 18:317-334, 1995.

Phillips KA, McElroy SL. Insight, overvalued ideation and delusional thinking in body dysmorphic disorder: theoretical and treatment implications. J Nerv Ment Dis 181:699-702, 1993.

Phillips KA, McElroy SL, Keck PE Jr, et al. Body dysmorphic disorder: 30 cases of imagined ugliness. Am J Psychiatry 150:302-308, 1993.

Phillips KA, McElroy SL, Keck PE Jr, et al. A comparison of delusional and nondelusional body dysmorphic disorder in 100 cases. Psychopharmacol Bull 30:179-186, 1994.

Powley KR. Brochure for Neysa Jane Body Dysmorphic Disorder Fund.

Real T. I Don't Want to Talk About It: Overcoming the Secret Legacy of Male Depression. New York: Scribner, 1997, p 43.

Richter MA, Tharmalingam S, Burroughs E, et al. A preliminary genetic investigation of the relationship between body dysmorphic disorder and OCD. Neuropsychopharmacology 29(Suppl 1):S200, 2004.

Robin AA. Reshaping the psyche: the concurrent improvement in appearance and mental state after rhinoplasty. Br J Plast Surg 152:539-543, 1988.

Rosen JC. Development of the body dysmorphic disorder examination. Behav Res Ther 34:755-766, 1996.

Roth RS, Lowery JC, Davis J, et al. Psychological factors predict patient satisfaction with postmastectomy reconstruction. Plast Reconstr Surg 119:2008-2015; discussion 2016-2017, 2007.

Ruffolo JS, Philips KA, Menard W, et al. Comorbidity of body dysmorphic disorder and eating disorders: severity of psychopathology and body image disturbance. Int J Eat Disord 39:11-19, 2006.

Ruhlmann U, McNally RJ, Wilhelm S, et al. Selective processing of emotional information in body dysmorphic disorder. J Anxiety Disord 16:289-298, 2002.

Sarwer DB. Awareness and identification of body dysmorphic disorder by aesthetic surgeons: results of a survey of American Society of Aesthetic Plastic Surgery members. Aesthet Surg J 22:531-535, 2002.

Sarwer DB. Body image dissatisfaction and body dysmorphic disorder in 100 cosmetic surgery patients. Plast Reconstr Surg 101:1644-1649, 1998.

Sarwer DB. Female college students and cosmetic surgery: an investigation of experiences, attitudes and body image. Plast Reconstr Surg 115:931, 2004.

Sarwer DB. Mental health histories & psychiatric medication usage among persons who sought cosmetic surgery. Plast Reconstr Surg 114:1927-1935, 2004.

Savage CR, Deckersbach T, Wilhelm S, et al. Strategic processing and episodic memory impairment in obsessive compulsive disorder. Neuropsychology 14:141-151, 2000.

Silverman AB, Reinherz HZ, Giaconia RM. The long-term sequelae of child and adolescent abuse: a longitudinal community study. Child Abuse Negl 20:709-723, 1996.

Slator R. Are rhinoplasty patients potentially mad? Br J Plast Surg 45:307-310, 1992.

Slator R. Rhinoplasty patients revisited. Br J Plast Surg 46:327-331, 1993.

Slaughter JR, Sun AM. In pursuit of perfection: a primary care physician's guide to body dysmorphic disorder. Am Fam Physician 60:1738-1742, 1999.

Smith TW. The selection of patients for rhinoplasty. Arch Otolaryngol 94:56-58, 1971.

Stewart EJ. Assessment of patient's benefit from rhinoplasty. Rhinology 34:57-59, 1996.

Stroomer JWG. The effects of computer simulated facial plastic surgery on social perception by others. Clin Otolaryngol 23:141-147, 1998.

Terino E. Psychology of the aesthetic patient: the value of personality profile testing. Facial Plast Surg Clin North Am 16:165-171, 2008.

Thomas CS. Appearance, body image and distress in facial dysmorphophobia. Acta Psychiatr Scand 92:231-236, 1995.

Thomas JR. Analysis of patient response to preoperative computerized video imaging. Arch Otolaryngol Head Neck Surg 115:793-796, 1989.

Tobin HA. The less-than-satisfactory rhinoplasty: comparison of patient and surgeon satisfaction. Otolaryngol Head Neck Surg 94:86-95, 1986.

Veale D. Outcome of cosmetic surgery and "DIY" surgery in patients with body dysmorphic disorder. Psychiatr Bull 24:218-221, 2000.

Veale D, Boocock A, Gournay K, et al. Body dysmorphic disorder: a survey of fifty cases. Br J Psychiatry 169:196-201, 1996.

Vilar-Sancho B. Present and future of rhinoplasty: an editorial. Aesthetic Plast Surg 9:181-184, 1985.

Waller G, Hamilton K, Rose N, et al. Sexual abuse and body image distortion in the eating disorders. Br J Psychiatry 32:350-352, 1993.

Wenninger K, Heiman J. Relating body image to psychological and sexual functioning in child sexual abuse survivors. J Trauma Stress 11:543-562, 1998.

Wright MR. How to recognize and control the problem patient. J Dermatol Surg Oncol 10:389-395, 1984.

Wright MR. The male aesthetic patient. Arch Otolaryngol Head Neck Surg 113:724-727, 1987.

Wright MR. Management of patient dissatisfaction with results of cosmetic procedures. Arch Otolaryngol 106:466-471, 1980.

Yaryura-Tobias JA, Neziroglu F, Torres-Gallegos M. Neuroanatomical correlates and somatosensorial disturbances in body dysmorphic disorder. CNS Spectr 7:432-434, 2002.

CREDITS

Unless otherwise indicated, page numbers listed include all photographs.

Legend: *T,* top; *B,* bottom; *C,* center; *L,* left; *R,* right

Figures pp. 6, 8 (R), *1443, 1444* (L), *1444* (R)
Constantian MB. Toward refinement in rhinoplasty. Plast Reconstr Surg 74:19-32, 1984.

Figure p. 8 (L)
Hartt F. Donatello, Prophet of Modern Vision. New York: Harry N. Abrams, 1972. (Original photograph by David Finn.)

Figures pp. 13, 33 (T), *34* (BL), *595* (L), *598* (T), *900* (L), *900* (C), *904* (L), *904* (R), *905* (B), *906* (B), *911, 914* (BCR), *915* (T), *995* (BL), *995* (BCL), *1352* (BCR)
Tables pp. 900, 901, 902
Constantian MB. The boxy nasal tip, the ball tip, and alar cartilage malposition: variations on a theme, a study in 200 consecutive primary and secondary rhinoplasty patients. Plast Reconstr Surg 116:268-281, 2005.

Figures pp. 19 (TR), *690* (L), *690* (C), *691* (TL), *691* (TR), *691* (B)
Constantian MB. A model for planning rhinoplasty. Plast Reconstr Surg 79:472-481, 1987.

Figures pp. 25 (TL), *280* (CR), *917* (T), *917* (BL), *919, 921* (TR), *924* (T), *924* (BR), *926* (TL), *926* (BL), *926* (BCL), *937* (TL), *937* (BL), *940* (BL), *1282* (L), *1282* (R), *1284* (T), *1285* (T), *1351* (T)
Constantian MB. The two essential elements for planning tip surgery in primary and secondary rhinoplasty. Plast Reconstr Surg 114:1571-1581, 2004.

Figures pp. 26 (T), *40* (BL), *40* (BCL), *61, 62* (T), *62* (BL), *62* (BR), *64* (TL), *65* (TC), *80, 82* (BL), *93* (TR), *93* (B), *97* (T), *97* (C), *97* (BL), *98* (T), *98* (BL), *122* (TR), *123* (BR), *143* (T), *144* (CR), *144* (R), *151* (CR), *151* (R), *156* (TL), *156* (TR), *163* (T), *190* (L), *190* (R), *209* (T), *212* (TL), *220* (TC), *224* (BL), *224* (BR), *228* (R), *232* (TL), *233* (TL), *234* (C), *237* (T), *238* (BL), *238* (BCR), *313* (T), *439* (BR), *745* (T), *745* (BR), *753* (T), *759* (T), *971* (BR), *978* (TL), *978* (BR), *1286* (TCR), *1286* (TR), *1287* (BCR), *1291* (BCR), *1322* (R), *1324* (T), *1345* (TL), *1386* (BL), *1389* (TL), *1389* (TCL)
Constantian MB. Closed rhinoplasty: current techniques, theory, and applications. In Mathes SJ, Hentz VR, eds. Plastic Surgery, 2nd ed. Philadelphia: Saunders, 2006.

Figures pp. 38 (TCR), *38* (TR), *660* (TL), *660* (BL), *662, 1251* (BL), *1251* (BCL)
Constantian MB, Clardy RB. The relative importance of septal and nasal valvular surgery in correcting airway obstruction in primary and secondary rhinoplasty. Plast Reconstr Surg 98:38-54, 1996.

Figure p. 44 (L)
Constantian MB. An alternate strategy for reducing the large nasal base. Plast Reconstr Surg 83:41-52, 1989.

Figures pp. 51 (B), *74* (B), *91* (TL), *700* (TR), *700* (BR), *703* (T), *703* (BL), *703* (BCL)
Constantian MB. The middorsal notch: an intraoperative guide to overresection in secondary rhinoplasty. Plast Reconstr Surg 91:477-484, 1993.

Figures pp. 99, 102 (L), *103* (T), *103* (B), *151* (L), *151* (CL), *154, 155* (T), *156* (BR), *1124* (TL), *1124* (B), *1127, 1165* (BL), *1166* (R), *1171* (L), *1171* (R), *1176* (T), *1176* (BCR), *1176* (BR), *1292* (R), *1300* (C), *1300* (R), *1302, 1303* (TL), *1303* (TCL), *1312, 1314* (TL), *1314* (BL), *1315* (TL), *1315* (BC), *1322* (L), *1322* (C), *1323, 1329* (T), *1332* (TL), *1332* (BL), *1333* (TL)

> Constantian MB. Indications and use of composite grafts in 100 consecutive secondary and tertiary rhinoplasty patients: introduction of the axial orientation. Plast Reconstr Surg 110:1116-1133, 2002.

Figure p. 136 *(adapted)*

> Doty RL, Frye R. Influence of nasal obstruction on smell function. Otolaryngol Clin North Am 22:397-411, 1989; and Howard BK, Rohrich RJ. Understanding the nasal airway: principles and practice. Plast Reconstr Surg 109:1128-1146, 2002.

Figures pp. 168 (T), *169* (CL), *170, 215* (BL), *654* (L), *657* (TL), *657* (BL), *1306* (R), *1307, 1311* (B)

> Constantian MB. The incompetent external nasal valve: pathophysiology and treatment in primary and secondary rhinoplasty. Plast Reconstr Surg 93:919-931, 1994.

Figures pp. 195 (T), *198* (T), *200* (L), *200* (C), *201* (C), *201* (R), *205* (TR), *226, 744* (TL), *836* (CR), *845* (TL), *845* (TCL), *856* (L), *858* (B), *976* (L), *977* (T), *1047* (L), *1048* (TL), *1048* (TCL), *1048* (BCR), *1048* (BR), *1132* (TL), *1132* (TCL)

> Constantian MB. Four common anatomic variants that predispose to unfavorable rhinoplasty results: a study based upon 150 consecutive secondary rhinoplasties. Plast Reconstr Surg 105:316-331, 2000.

Figures pp. 313 (B), *850* (TL), *850* (TC), *934* (CR), *935* (BCR), *935* (BR), *1389* (BCR)

> Constantian MB. Elaboration of an alternative, segmental, cartilage-sparing tip graft technique: experience in 405 cases. Plast Reconstr Surg 103:237-253, 1999.

Figures pp. 330 (L), *331* (L), *332* (TL), *332* (TC), *332* (BC), *333* (TL), *333* (B), *334* (TL), *334* (TC), *336* (TL), *1065* (BL), *1065* (BCL), *1244* (L), *1247* (BL), *1247* (BCL)

> Constantian MB. Rhinoplasty in the graft-depleted patient. Oper Tech Plast Reconstr Surg 2:67-81, 1995.

Figures pp. 376 (L), *378* (BC), *378* (BR), *379* (T), *1026, 1029* (T), *1029* (BL), *1029* (BCL)

> Constantian MB. Distant effects of dorsal and tip grafting in rhinoplasty. Plast Reconstr Surg 90:405-418, 1992.

Figures pp. 441 (L), *442, 446* (TL), *446* (BC), *447* (TL), *448* (BL), *1309* (TL)

> Constantian MB. Functional effects of alar cartilage malposition. Ann Plast Surg 30:487-499, 1993.

Figures pp. 576 (L), *576* (CR), *576* (R), *577* (TL), *577* (TCL), *577* (B), *743* (TR), *861* (T), *863* (T)

> Constantian MB. Experience with a three-point method for planning rhinoplasty. Ann Plast Surg 30:1-12, 1993.

Figures pp. 836 (L), *845* (BCR), *1286* (TL), *1386* (BR), *1389* (TCR)

> Constantian MB. Closed rhinoplasty. In Goldwyn RM, Cohen MN, eds. The Unfavorable Result in Plastic Surgery: Avoidance and Treatment. Philadelphia: Lippincott, 2001.

Figures pp. 865 (T), *968* (TL), *971* (T), *971* (BL), *971* (BCL)

> Constantian MB. Differing characteristics in 100 consecutive secondary rhinoplasty patients following closed versus open surgical approaches. Plast Reconstr Surg 109:2097-2111, 2002.

Figures pp. 987 (TR), *987* (BCL), *987* (BR), *988* (R)

> Postoperative photographs courtesy John R. McGill, MD.

Figures pp. 997 (L), *998* (TL), *998* (B)

> Constantian MB. An algorithm for correcting the asymmetrical nose. Plast Reconstr Surg 83:801-811, 1989.

Figures pp. 1102, 1107 (BL), *1317* (R), *1372* (L), *1372* (C), *1373* (TL), *1373* (BL)

> Constantian MB. An alar base flap to correct nostril and vestibular stenosis and alar base malposition in rhinoplasty. Plast Reconstr Surg 101:1666-1674, 1998.

Figures pp. 1112 (BCR), *1112* (BR), *1278* (L), *1278* (C), *1281* (T), *1281* (BCR)

> Constantian MB. The septal angle: a cardinal point in rhinoplasty. Plast Reconstr Surg 85:187-195, 1990.

INDEX